Rehabilitation
NURSING
Procedures
MANUAL

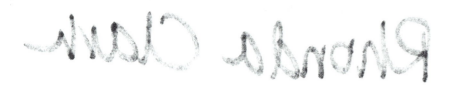

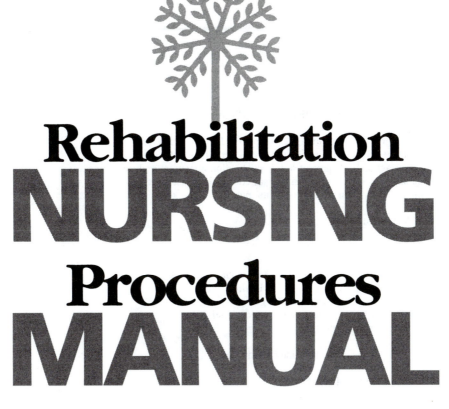

Rehabilitation NURSING Procedures MANUAL

Second Edition

Editors

Therese T. Alexander, MSN, CRRN
Educator, Center for Clinical Excellence
Rehabilitation Institute of Chicago
Chicago, Illinois

Roberta J. Hiduke, MS, RN
Nursing Education Program Coordinator
Rehabilitation Institute of Chicago
Chicago, Illinois

Kathleen A. Stevens, MS, CRRN
Director, Center for Clinical Excellence
Rehabilitation Institute of Chicago
Chicago, Illinois

McGraw-Hill
Health Professions Division

New York • St. Louis • San Francisco • Auckland • Bogotá • Caracas • Lisbon • London • Madrid
Mexico City • Milan • Montreal • New Delhi • San Juan • Singapore • Sydney • Tokyo • Toronto

McGraw-Hill

*A Division of The **McGraw·Hill** Companies*

REHABILITATION NURSING PROCEDURES MANUAL, 2/e

1234567890 MALMAL 99

ISBN 0-07-048266-7

This book was set in Times Roman by V & M Graphics, Inc.
The editors were Stephen Zollo and Steven Melvin;
the production supervisor was Catherine Saggese.
Edward Smith Design, Inc., was text and cover designer.
Geraldine Beckford prepared the index.

Malloy Lithographers, Inc., was the printer and binder.

This book is printed on acid-free paper.

Library of Congress Cataloging-in-Publication Data

Rehabilitation nursing procedures manual / editors, Therese T.
    Alexander, Roberta J. Hiduke, and Kathleen A. Stevens.—2nd ed.
        p.   cm.
    Includes bibliographical references and index.
    ISBN 0-07-048266-7
    1. Rehabilitation nursing—Handbooks, manuals, etc.
I. Alexander, Therese T. II. Hiduke, Roberta J. III. Stevens,
Kathleen A.
    [DNLM: 1. Rehabilitation Nursing. WY 150.5 R3451 1999]
RT120.R4R42   1999
610.73—dc 21
DNLM/DLC
for Library of Congress   99-10684

CONTENTS

CONTRIBUTORS

General Editors

Therese T. Alexander, MSN, CRRN
Educator, Center for Clinical Excellence
Rehabilitation Institute of Chicago
Chicago, Illinois

Roberta J. Hiduke, MS, RN
Nursing Education Program Coordinator
Rehabilitation Institute of Chicago
Chicago, Illinois

Kathleen A. Stevens, MS, CRRN
Director, Center for Clinical Excellence
Rehabilitation Institute of Chicago
Chicago, Illinois

Chapter Authors

Therese T. Alexander, MSN, CRRN [1, 2, 7]
Educator, Center for Clinical Excellence
Rehabilitation Institute of Chicago
Chicago, Illinois

Kathleen H. Culler, MS, OTR/L [7]
Educator, Center for Clinical Excellence
Rehabilitation Institute of Chicago
Chicago, Illinois

Mary E. Dillon Grant, MS, RN [9]
Outpatient Clinical Nurse
Rehabilitation Institute of Chicago
Chicago, Illinois

Eileen T. French, BSN, CRRN [3, 4]
Formerly, Nursing Supervisor
Rehabilitation Institute of Chicago
Chicago, Illinois

Charles Gutfeld, BSN, MBA, MPH [3]
Nursing Supervisor, Outpatient
Rehabilitation Institute of Chicago
Chicago, Illinois

Numbers in brackets refer to chapters written or cowritten by the contributors.

Diane Hartwig, MS, RN, CS-ACNP, CRRN [5]
Nurse Practitioner
Rehabilitation Institute of Chicago
Chicago, Illinois

Roberta J. Hiduke, MS, RN [9]
Nursing Education Program Coordinator
Rehabilitation Institute of Chicago
Chicago, Illinois

Judy Hill, MS, OTR/L [7]
Clinical Administrative Director
Rehabilitation Institute of Chicago
Chicago, Illinois

Jordess Isaac, BSN, RN [2]
Nursing Supervisor
Rehabilitation Institute of Chicago
Chicago, Illinois

Sandra Keller, MSN, CRRN [1]
Nursing Supervisor
Rehabilitation Institute of Chicago
Chicago, Illinois

Karen M. LeFevour, BSN, RN, CRRN [1]
Nursing Supervior
Rehabilitation Institute of Chicago
Chicago, Illinois

Kathy M. Martinez, PT [2]
Clinical Educator
Center for Clinical Excellence
Rehabilitation Institute of Chicago
Chicago, Illinois

Arlynne Ostlund, MA, RN, CRRN [3]
Nursing Supervisor
Rehabilitation Institute of Chicago
Chicago, Illinois

Adrienne Sarnecki, RN, MSN, CRRN [8]
Administrative/Clinical Director of Subacute/Acute
    Orthopedic Programs and Pharmacy Department
Rehabilitation Institute of Chicago
Chicago, Illinois

Kathleen A. Stevens, MS, CRRN [6]
Director, Center for Clinical Excellence
Rehabilitation Institute of Chicago
Chicago, Illinois

Randy Temple, RN, CRRN [4]
Infection Control Nurse
Rehabilitation Institute of Chicago
Chicago, Illinois

Laura Leigh, MBA, MSN, RN, CRRN

GENERAL DESCRIPTION AND OBJECTIVES

Rehabilitation nursing is defined as "the diagnosis and treatment of human responses of individuals and groups to actual or potential health problems relative to altered functional ability and lifestyle" (ARN, 1994). This procedure manual is built on the foundation and definition of rehabilitation nursing practice.

The purpose of any procedural manual is to provide a foundation for the delivery of safe, effective care. The procedures defined in Rehabilitation Nursing Procedures Manual have been carefully developed by expert rehabilitation nurses. They are based on the standards of care that are used by the Rehabilitation Institute of Chicago. The primary objective of the book is to provide the learner with guidelines for practice of common rehabilitation procedures. These specific procedures should be reviewed and adapted as necessary before approval for use in a particular practice setting.

These procedures are commonly used for persons with disabilities including spinal cord injury, stroke, brain injury, multiple sclerosis, cerebral palsy, orthopedic dysfunctions, and musculoskeletal problems. It is also intended to assist in providing care for persons with alterations in function such as mobility, dysphagia, incontinence, and respiratory problems.

INTENDED AUDIENCE

The intended audience for this manual is primarily rehabilitation nurses. However, this manual can also be very helpful for any member of the interdisciplinary team including physical therapists, occupational therapists, speech-language pathologists, and unlicensed assistive personnel. The principles of these procedures are based on collaborative, interdisciplinary practice. Many of the procedures can be adapted for home use by patients and families.

LEVELS OF CARE IN REHABILITATION

Rehabilitation nursing is a relatively new area of specialty nursing. The dimensions of our practice have grown immensely over the past 10 years. Rehabilitation nursing has now evolved into a continuum of services provided through multiple levels of care. It is practiced in the inpatient acute, inpatient subacute, long-term care or skilled nursing, day rehabilitation, outpatient, home care, and assisted or transitional living venues of care. This procedure manual can be used by nurses practicing in any of these levels of care where they will be responsible for prescribing, delegating, and coordinating rehabilitation nursing care.

FORMAT

The procedures are organized in nine chapters that cover nutrition, mobility, bowel and bladder elimination, skin care, respiratory care, safety management, self-care, community re-entry, and patient-family teaching.

Each procedure within the chapter will follow the same format, which will include:

Name of the procedure
Purpose
Staff responsible
Equipment
General considerations
Procedure step-by-step
Documentation
Patient/Family Teaching
References

LEVEL OF STAFF TO PERFORM

We have not indicated level of staff to perform the procedures. It is clear that some procedures or components of procedures can be performed by unlicensed assistive personnel. However, it is the decision of each institution based on their state's Nurse Practice Act to establish standards regarding appropriate personnel to perform specific tasks and procedures.

DOCUMENTATION

Documentation of specific procedures must be done per your institution's policies. Many institutions/organizations are moving toward charting by exception. Manual forms, flow charts, and care plans have been traditional means for nursing documentation. Information technology has furthered our practice by documentation on-line and at point of care, moving us toward a paperless medical record. Outcomes measurement should be included in documentation of specific procedures. Because tools vary from institution to institution, we have not included this specifically with each procedure.

LIABILITY

Although the authors hope that the use of the procedures included in this book will benefit all populations served, we must expressly disclaim liability for any injury resulting from the improper or negligent use of the procedures. Further, references to and opinions expressed regarding the efficacy of any product or piece of equipment are based on the subjective experience of the staff of the Rehabilitation Institute of Chicago and not on statistical data. Such references and opinions do not constitute an endorsement of any product or equipment.

Every effort has been made to base procedures on the most current research in nursing and related fields. In the absence of research results, procedures are developed on the basis of clinician experience.

CONCLUSION

For more than 40 years, the Rehabilitation Institute of Chicago has been a trusted source of rehabilitation care, education, and advocacy for people with disabilities. The Rehabilitation Institute of Chicago has also been a major force in education and training and provides formal education to thousands of students annually. We have also produced many training manuals for clinicians providing care for people with disabilities. We hope in offering the Rehabilitation Nursing Procedures Manual that we have provided you with a much-needed resource.

ACKNOWLEDGEMENTS

This Rehabilitation Nursing Procedures Manual has been developed by many individuals within the Nursing Division of the Rehabilitation Institute of Chicago. Each chapter editor spent numerous hours researching their topic to be sure we are providing current state-of-the-art information related to each procedure. They all are to be commended for taking on this monumental task, in addition to their daily responsibilities, and doing it with enthusiasm. These nurses have a passion for educating other nurses and providing them with information that will ensure good nursing care and practice for all persons with disabilities.

I especially want to thank Kathleen Stevens, Therese Alexander, and Roberta Hiduke for their leadership and direction in this project. They developed the vision for all of us and led endless meetings where nurses collaborated together in chapter writing.

I must also acknowledge all writers from the first edition of Rehabilitation Nursing Procedures Manual. They provided the foundation upon which we built this manual. They were the pioneers in rehabilitation nursing and the role models that helped formulate our current nursing practice. These individuals include Nancye B. Holt, Carolyn E. Carlson, Winona P. Griggs, and Rosemarie B. King. We are carrying their torch forward in rehabilitation nursing into the next millennium.

Finally, I wish to thank three key administrative leaders at the Rehabilitation Institute of Chicago: Dr. Henry B. Betts, our former CEO & President, whose leadership and vision has opened the world for persons with disabilities; Dr. Elliot J. Roth, our Medical Director and Sr. Vice President of Clinical Affairs, who challenges nursing to constantly analyze our practice and scientifically search for opportunities to improve the quality of care we deliver to our patients; and lastly, Dr. Wayne M. Lerner, our CEO & President, who has supported all of us in the development of this book.

Laura Leigh, MBA, MSN, RN, CRRN
Vice President, Patient Care Services &
Chief Nurse Executive

BASIC GUIDELINES FOR INFECTION CONTROL

Randy Temple, RN, CRRN

The performance of any hands-on procedure has the subtext of providing an opportunity for the trade or transmission of host flora between the provider and recipient of care. The opportunity does not equal the inevitability however. There are several basic principles and guidelines the healthcare provider can follow that will aid to minimize the risk of disease transmission. Key among them is proper handwashing. Handwashing has been shown time and again to be the single most effective means of interrupting the transmission of potential pathogens between persons. Hands should be washed prior to performing any procedure and upon completing any direct care procedure and between clients.

In addition to handwashing there are other guidelines that need to be closely observed to minimize risks to the provider and recipient of care during the performance of the direct care procedure. These guidelines, and any subsequent policies and procedures arising from them, should be applied consistently to all direct care situations within the limitations imposed by patient and provider safety, patient clinical status, product availability, and environment of service provision.

Personal protective equipment (PPE)—gloves, gowns or aprons, masks, and protective eyewear (goggles or eyeshields)—is a necessary and federally mandated adjunct to proper handwashing for specific types of direct care procedures. PPE should be used with consistent guidelines as well for the provision of direct care.

Hands should be washed, using soap and running water or an effective waterless sanitizer

- Before and after all direct patient care
- After any activity or procedure requiring contact with excreta or secreta of the patient *or* self
- After any activity requiring handling an item or equipment that has been soiled with excreta or secreta of any person

All fluids and wastes produced by the human body have the ability to serve as a source of potentially infective organisms. The only fluids produced by the human body that one can reasonably assume safe are sweat and tears. Activities or procedures requiring contact with the excreta or secreta of the human body—urine, feces, sputum, vomitus, saliva, as well as blood, blood products, wound drainage, and intracorporeal fluids, collectively referred to as body fluids—require the use of appropriate PPE. Gloves should be appropriate for the procedure performed. Latex gloves are appropriate for many chemical and organic exposures. Certain chemical exposures may require gloves of alternate composition. Gowns or aprons should be minimally moisture-resistant to limit the potential for fluid strike through. Masks should be of adequate size to cover both the mouth and nostrils. Eyeshields or goggles should be of a design that will protect both direct and lateral sprays or splashes. Reusable equipment is acceptable if properly decontaminated between uses. Disposable equipment may be preferred for routine nonsurgical activities.

Gloves should be worn for

- Any activity that may involve direct contact with body fluids
- Any activity involving handling equipment or objects that may be contaminated with body fluid
- Hands-on contact with a patient by any person with an exudative dermatitis or open lesion on their own hands

Moisture-resistant or moisture-impervious aprons or gowns should be worn for

- Any activity that may involve contamination of the provider's clothing or body fluids either directly through splashing or spraying or indirectly by contact with a contaminated object
- Any activity that may involve contamination of the provider's clothing by excessive soilage or contamination of the environment during the provision of care

Protective masks and eyewear should be worn for

- Any activity that may result in the spray or splashing of body fluids towards the provider's face
- Any activity that may result in the aerosolization of body fluids

Used equipment should be disposed of in accordance with all applicable local ordinances regarding the disposal of potentially infectious medical waste. The requirements for labeling and bagging may vary with site of service. "Red bagging" may not be required in the home setting for items that may require segregation from the general waste stream in the institutional setting. Double bagging is generally no longer mandated although it may still be required by facility policy.

Needles and other sharps should be discarded in puncture-resistant or puncture-proof containers unbroken. Needles should never be bent after use on a person in an attempt to prevent re-use. Needles used for injection attached to a disposable syringe should be discarded while still attached to the syringe. An attempt should not be made to remove them.

Rehabilitation
NURSING
Procedures
MANUAL

CHAPTER 1

Procedures to Establish, Maintain, and Improve Oral and Enteric Intake

Introduction

Proper nutrition and hydration are important components of the care of the patient in rehabilitation. There are special nutritional and fluid considerations to assist in increasing the patient's strength and energy, to sustain life, and promote quality of life. A complete assessment by the rehabilitation team is important to prevent complications that can occur due to alteration of nutrition or oral intake such as weight loss, dehydration, or skin breakdown.

Dysphagia is a common occurrence in patients with disabilities that can alter nutrition or oral intake. Early identification of dysphagia is essential to development of a treatment plan, reduce complications, promote well being, and alleviate patient and family anxiety. Dysphagia assessment and treatment must be done by individuals, regardless of discipline, with specialized training in that area. A patient suspected of aspiration should have a video fluoroscopic swallow study (sometimes called a modified barium swallow or cookie swallow test) performed. Video fluoroscopy is the only reliable way to detect aspiration, and its findings will help determine the treatment plan. Silent aspiration, when the patient aspirates without coughing or choking, may occur and if suspected should be vigorously investigated and treated.

Many patients because of dysphagia or altered mental status are unable to tolerate oral feedings. Enteral feedings may be required. The nursing management of a variety of feeding tubes should include general care, insertion, dressing care, stabilization, administration of feedings and medication, and troubleshooting of possible problems.

Utilization of resources by the rehabilitation nurse is imperative to provide the best possible care. The nutritionist is a valuable resource for determining adequate nutritional needs and diet. The speech language pathologist is an expert in dysphagia management and feeding techniques. The occupational therapist is a valuable resource for provision of adaptive equipment and techniques used for feeding.

The rehabilitation nurse has an important role in communicating with the interdisciplinary team regarding the patient's overall nutritional status and its impact on achieving optimal health. All team members must collaborate on ways to implement the treatment plan and achieve desired outcomes. The patient is the most important team member and determines if the individualized nutritional plan and goals can be met.

Nutritional and Fluid Considerations for Rehab Patients

PURPOSE

To identify nutritional and fluid special considerations for various rehab populations; perform a simple nutritional assessment

STAFF RESPONSIBLE

EQUIPMENT

No equipment necessary

GENERAL CONSIDERATIONS

1. Nutrients are considered to include: protein, carbohydrates, fat, calories, vitamins, minerals, fluids, and electrolytes.

2. Factors that interfere with adequate intake of nutrients include diseases or disabilities that alter appetite, smell, taste, access to food, attentiveness, dexterity, mastication, swallowing, digestion, absorption, transport, storage, metabolic demand, and excretion.

3. Neurologic injury/illness alters the metabolic rate and places patients at risk for protein and caloric deficits. Decreased oral intake with simultaneous increased nutritional requirements result in inadequate protein, and decreased carbohydrates and fat for energy. Protein is necessary for building and sustaining tissue, maintaining energy, and maintaining various physiologic processes, including hormone, enzyme, and antibody activity and tissue repair synthesis.

4. Traumatic spinal cord injury (SCI), brain injury (BI), and burns produce acute hypermetabolic states, which trigger a catabolic response where endogenous proteins are broken down. Potential complications resulting from catabolism are:
   - Protein and/or caloric malnutrition
   - Increased susceptibility to infection
   - Respiratory distress
   - Poor wound healing
   - Slowed recovery

5. With trauma, glycogen stores in the liver and muscle cells are temporarily converted to glucose for energy (glycogenolysis), and because of the high energy demands, proteins, rather than stored fats, are used as energy sources, so further protein depletion occurs. Trauma and/or sepsis can also cause high nitrogen excretion from breakdown of muscle and lean body mass. The muscle flaccidity associated with acute SCI enhances nitrogen and calcium losses even more than immobilization.

6. Nitrogen, necessary for tissue synthesis, comes from dietary protein. Food protein is essential because once eaten, it is digested and converted into amino acids in the alimentary tract. These amino acids are absorbed and transported to cells where they are converted to substances such as collagen and myosin.

7. Effects of traumatic brain injury (TBI) on nutrition can include damage to the hypothalamus, which can produce hyperphagia (loss of satiety, desire to eat and/or drink constantly—especially sweets—and hoarding of food or eating nonedible items) and frontal lobe damage, which can create problems with initiation.

8. Elderly stroke patients might have malnourishment and vitamin deficiencies on admission. Nutritional status of those with right arm paresis is worse than those with left arm paresis.

9. Effects of respiratory disease on nutrition can include depression, anorexia, side effects of medication, fatigue, and difficulty eating during dyspneic episodes and are often associated with less-than-adequate intake of nutrients; caloric needs are increased due to increased work of breathing, increased dead space ventilation, inefficient gas exchange, and increased oxygen consumption; and excessive carbohydrate intake (>500 g/day) results in increased oxygen consumption and CO_2 production and retention, compounding already existing respiratory insufficiency. Adequate nutrition is essential to optimal respiratory function.

10. In pediatrics, one must consider alterations in growth, body composition, energy requirements, and feeding difficulties. A dietary assessment should include both what and how much the child eats. The family's perception of the child's nutritional status is a critical factor in selecting a therapeutic approach, which may include food supplements, nighttime nasogastric feedings, nasojejunal feed-

ings if esophageal reflux is a problem, and feeding via gastrostomy. Oral food intake and activities involved in chewing, sucking, and swallowing help to develop the oropharyngeal musculature needed for speech. Children receiving long-term anticonvulsant therapy are at high risk for vitamin D and folate deficiencies, altered calcium metabolism, and pathologic fractures.

PATIENT AND FAMILY EDUCATION

1. Teach patient and family about adequate nutritional and fluid intake.
2. Use dietary teaching materials available from the dietitian.

Procedure

Brief Nutritional Assessment

 Steps

 Additional Information

1. Review patient's chart/referral material and interview patient for needed information:

   - Nutritional intake: Amount and type, calorie count, intake/output, food preferences and/or cultural patterns, food intolerances, appetite
   - Height, premorbid weight
   - Activity level (voluntary and involuntary)
   - Ability to swallow
   - Medication

   Consider the patient's recent pattern (last 3 days) and past patterns as well as future patterns.

2. Measure patient's height and current weight

   Use a tape measure to measure height and an accurate scale for weight. If unable to measure height due to deformity in children, measure ulnar length, fibula length, arm-span or arm, thigh, and calf circumference.

3. Observe patient's activity level

   Compare patient's current activity level to activity levels for able-bodied individuals.

4. Inspect hair and skin

   Observe the skin for itching, rash, lesions, color, pigmentation, hydration, texture and thickness, turgor and elasticity, vascularity, erythema, and edema. Observe hair for dryness, brittleness, or fragility; quantity, quality, and distribution of hair; pattern of hair loss; if it comes out easily.

5. Test ability to smell, taste, and swallow

   To test smell: occlude one nostril while testing the other—use several familiar odors, such as tobacco, coffee, perfume (not alcohol!). To test taste: test anterior two-thirds of tongue (CN VII) and posterior one-third of tongue (CN IX)—use several familiar items, such as fruit, sugar, pepper. To test swallowing, ask patient to dry swallow, observing for laryngeal elevation. Some patients can swallow saliva but silently aspirate on it; if this is suspected, consult with speech-language pathologist (SLP).

6. Observe dentition

   Use a light source to inspect the teeth. Normally, an adult has 32 teeth, 8 on each side of each jaw. Look for obvious caries and any teeth that are missing, broken, stained, or displaced. Ask patient if (s)he uses dentures or partials and where they are.

7. Measure body temperature

8. Observe patient's affect

Is patient yes/no reliable? Is (s)he cooperative? Is (s)he attentive?

9. Estimate ideal body weight

Estimate ideal weight according to a height and weight formula, skin fold thickness, past healthy weight, or whatever technique your dietitian/institution uses. One way to calculate ideal body weight (IBW):

Female: For 5' = 100 lb, then add 5 lb for each inch over 5'

Male: For 5' = 106 lb, then add 6 lb for each inch over 5'

10. Determine caloric needs

To determine caloric needs, multiple IBW by the activity factor to obtain an estimate of kcal/day. The activity factors are: "13" if sedentary; "15" if moderately active; "20" if very active.

11. Review laboratory values

Review laboratory values, such as hemoglobin and hematocrit (looks at iron and O_2 binding capabilities), total protein (reflects current serum protein levels), albumin (often more accurate than total protein), triglycerides and cholesterol levels (saturated fatty acids), and total lymphocyte count (WBC × 1000 − % lymphocytes, indicates the amount of protein and how well the immune system is functioning).

12. Consider malnutrition

To determine if severe malnutrition exists, calculate the percent of body weight lost. If >2% in 1 week, >5% in 1 month, >7.5% in 3 months, or >10% in 6 months, then the person is considered malnourished.

 ## DOCUMENTATION

1. Assessment data and treatment plan.

REFERENCES

Buelow, J.M. and Jamieson, D. (1990) "Potential for Altered Nutritional Status in the Stroke Patient" *Rehabilitation Nursing* 15(5):260–263.

Cherney, L.R. (1994) *Clinical Management of Dysphagia in Adults and Children*, 2d ed. Gaithersburg, MD: Aspen Publishers, Inc.

Cherney, L.R. and Souder, T.S. (1996) "Evaluating Swallowing Disorders: The Speech-Language Pathologist's Perspective" *Topics in Stroke Rehabilitation* 3(3):14–26.

Ford, R.D. (Ed.) (1985) *Health Assessment Handbook*. Springhouse, PA: Springhouse Corp.

Haynes, M.K.M. (1992) "Nutrition in the Severely Head-Injured Patient" *Clinical Rehabilitation* 6:153–158.

Logemann, J. (1983) *Evaluation and Treatment of Swallowing Disorders*. Boston: College-Hill Press, Inc.

Martin-Harris, B. and Cherney, L.R. (1996) "Treating Swallowing Disorders following Stroke" *Topics in Stroke Rehabilitation* 3(3):27–40.

McCourt, A.E. (Ed.) (1993) *The Specialty Practice of Rehabilitation Nursing: A Core Curriculum*, 3d ed. Skokie, IL: Rehabilitation Nursing Foundation.

McHale, J.M., Phipps, M.A., Horvath, K., and Schmelz, J. (1998) "Expert Nursing Knowledge in the Care of Patients at Risk of Impaired Swallowing" *Image: Journal of Nursing Scholarship* 30(2):137–141.

Mullen, M. (1995) "Dietitians and Nurses: Building Partnerships for Tomorrow's Health Care Market" *Food & Nutrition News* 67(3):19–20.

Newmark, S.R., Sublett, D., Black, J., and Geller, R. (1981) "Nutritional assessment in a rehabilitation unit." *Archives of Physical Medicine and Rehabilitation* 62:279–282.

Patrick, J. and Gisel, E. (1990) "Nutrition for the Feeding Impaired Child" *Journal of Neurologic Rehab* 4:115–119.

Perlman, A. (1996) "Neuroanatomy and Neurophysiology: Implications for Swallowing" *Topics in Stroke Rehabilitation* 3(3):1–13.

Dysphagia Assessment

PURPOSE

To identify persons with dysphagia

STAFF RESPONSIBLE

EQUIPMENT

1. Suction machine and equipment
2. Feeding utensils (small Teflon-coated spoon, metal spoon, and utensils)
3. Cups (30 to 200 ml)
4. Modified cups with cut-outs
5. Food or liquid for trial feeding
6. Pillows for positioning

GENERAL CONSIDERATIONS

1. Chewing and swallowing dysfunction may be seen in patients with diagnosis of:
   - Vascular-related disorders (cortical involvement, brain stem stroke)
   - Brain injury
   - Degenerative neurologic disease [parkinsonism, amyotrophic lateral sclerosis (ALS), multiple sclerosis (MS), myotonic dystrophy, oculopharyngeal muscular dystrophy, myasthenia gravis (MG), Huntington's chorea]
   - Other neurologic etiologies including poliomyelitis, Guillain-Barré syndrome, scleroderma, systemic lupus erythematosus (SLE)
   - Spinal cord injury
   - Debilitation and extreme weakness
   - Dementia or confusion
   - Burn injury
2. Suspect dysphagia if any of the following are noted:
   - Uncoordinated chewing and swallowing
   - Presence of dysarthria
   - Drooling
   - Choking
   - Coughing while or immediately after eating or drinking
   - Aspiration of food or saliva (not observable like the other signs)
   - Pocketing of food
   - Absence of gag reflex
   - Moist quality of voice
3. The major complications associated with dysphagia are choking, aspiration, dehydration, and malnutrition.

PATIENT AND FAMILY EDUCATION

1. Catalogs of patient teaching materials:
   - Pro-ed, 8700 Shoal Creek Boulevard, Austin, Texas 78757-6897
   - Imaginart, 307 Arizona Street, Bisbee, Arizona 85603.
   - Interactive Therapeutics, Inc., PO Box 1805, Stow, Ohio 44224-0805.
   - Pritchett & Hull Associates Inc. 3440 Oakcliff Road NE, STE 110d, Atlanta, Georgia 30340-3079.
   - The Speech Bin, 1965 Twenty-Fifth Avenue, Vero Beach, Florida 32960.
   - For professional education only:
     - Applied Symboliz, 800 North Wells Street, Suite 200, Chicago, Illinois 60610
     - Canyonlands Publishing, Inc., 141 South Park Avenue, Tucson, Arizona 85719.
2. Patient and family teaching to include dysphagia definition, treatment plan, special equipment and techniques, and potential outcomes.

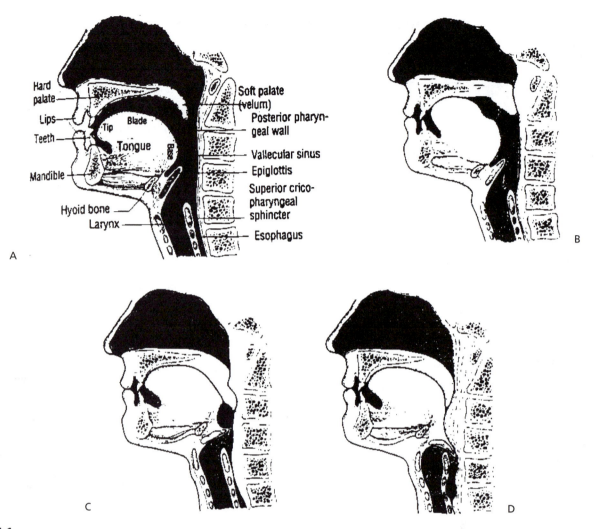

Figure 1-1

Procedure

Dysphagia Assessment

 Steps

I. Obtain data from referral material or referring agency
  1. History or etiology of swallowing dysfunction
  2. Weight loss
  3. Diagnostic testing results
  4. Type of diet
  5. Results from previous attempts to feed
     • Any problems or difficulties chewing or swallowing
        • Solids
        • Liquids
     • Fatigue
        • With repetition
        • At certain hours of the day
     • Pocketing of food particles and in what part of mouth
     • Coughing or choking
     • Nasal regurgitation
     • Wet, gurgly voice quality
     • Aspiration, history of aspiration pneumonia or other respiratory problems
  6. Current feeding method
     • Oral
     • Enteral
     • Parenteral

II. Assessment
  1. Mobility: Can the patient assume an appropriate feeding position?

- Head and trunk aligned with midline
- Good head control
- Neck slightly flexed
- Hips flexed
- Ability to sit at 90 degrees
- Assistance or assistive devices needed to maintain position
2. Respiratory: Can the patient protect his or her airway?
   - Cough reflex
   - Phonation characteristics
   - Secretions (amount and type)
   - Breath sounds
   - Tracheostomy (type)
   - Suctioning requirements
3. Cognition and behavior
   - Level of responsiveness
   - Lethargy
   - Impulsiveness
   - Memory problems

- Ability to follow simple commands
- Attention span
4. Oral sensory and motor
   - Swallow response
   - Response to stimuli
   - Mouth posture at rest
   - Oral and facial sensation
   - Voluntary movement
     - Opens and closes mouth
     - Opens and closes lips
     - Moves tongue (in and out, side to side, up and down)
5. Functional
   - Use of empty cup, straw, and spoon—can patient use them appropriately?
   - Upper extremity function
   - General coordination
III. Consult with rehab physician, SLP, and dietitian to formulate a safe feeding program.

DOCUMENTATION

Record assessment findings in medical record with treatment plan.

REFERENCES

Cherney, L.R. (1994) *Clinical Management of Dysphagia in Adults and Children*, 2d ed. Gaithersburg, MD: Aspen Publishers, Inc.

Cherney, L.R., Cantieri, C.A., and Pannell, J.J. (1986). *Clinical Evaluation of Dysphagia*. Rockville, MD: Aspen

DiIovio, C., and Price, M.E. (1990) "Swallowing: An Assessment Guide" *American Journal of Nursing* July 38–41.

Emick-Herring, B. and Wood, P. (1990) "A Team Approach to Neurologically Based Swallowing Disorders" *Rehabilitation Nursing* 15(3):126–132.

Ergun, F. and Miskovitz, P.F. (1992) "Aging and the Esophagus: Common Pathologic Conditions and Their Effect upon Swallowing in the Geriatric Population" *Dysphagia* 7:58–63.

Herrera, W., Zeligman, B.E., Gruber, J., et al. (1990) "Dysphagia in Multiple Sclerosis: Clinical and Videofluoroscopic Correlations" *Journal of Neurologic Rehab* 4:1–8.

Langmore, S.E., Terpenning, M.S., Schork, A., et al. (1998) "Predictors of Aspiration Pneumonia: How Important is Dysphagia?" *Dysphagia* 13:69–81.

Martin-Harris, B. and Cherney, L.R. (1996) "Treating Swallowing Disorders following Stroke" *Topics in Stroke Rehabilitation* 3(3): 27–40.

McCourt, A.E. (Ed.) (1993) *The Specialty Practice of Rehabilitation Nursing: A Core Curriculum*, 3d ed. Skokie, IL: Rehabilitation Nursing Foundation.

Perlman, A. (1996) "Neuroanatomy and Neurophysiology: Implications for Swallowing" *Topics in Stroke Rehabilitation* 3(3):1–13.

Price, M.E. and DiIovio, C. (1990) "Swallowing: A Practice Guide" *American Journal of Nursing* July 42–46.

Safe Feeding and Stimulation Techniques of the Patient with Dysphagia

PURPOSE

To reinforce and initiate the stages and movements of normal chewing and swallowing; to prevent the complications related to swallowing dysfunction (i.e., aspiration, choking, pocketing, dehydration, and malnutrition); to monitor and provide safety measures for the patient with swallowing dysfunction

STAFF RESPONSIBLE

EQUIPMENT

1. Ice
2. Cotton-tipped applicators or stainless-steel spoon
3. Straw
4. 1-oz medication cup
5. Laryngeal mirror (size 00)
6. 200-ml cut-out cup
7. Nonsterile gloves
8. Patient's food tray

 GENERAL CONSIDERATIONS

1. The stages of swallowing are:
   - Oral preparatory phase, in which food is manipulated in the mouth
   - Oral phase, in which lingual movement propels the bolus posteriorly
   - Pharyngeal phase, which is the swallowing response (primarily involuntary)
   - Esophageal phase, during which peristaltic waves carry food through the esophagus
2. Feeding techniques deal with the preparatory and oral stages of the swallow, which terminate when the swallow response is triggered.
3. Feeding techniques include:
   - Positioning of material (food) in the mouth
   - Manipulating food in the mouth with the tongue
   - Chewing boluses of food of various consistencies
   - Recollecting the bolus into a cohesive mass before initiation of the swallow
   - Organizing lingual peristalsis to propel the bolus posteriorly
4. Swallowing techniques deal with the stimulation of the swallowing response, improvement of pharyngeal transit time, airway protection, and improvement of the preparatory and oral stages of the swallow.
5. Food is one of the primary facilitators of oral movement because it stimulates sensations of touch, taste, and temperature as well as provide visual and olfactory input.
6. Direct feeding involves introducing food into the mouth and attempting to reinforce the appropriate behaviors during the stages of swallowing.

7. Physiotherapeutic interventions utilize exercises to improve motor controls that are prerequisites for normal swallowing. Many of these exercises are done by the speech pathologist.
8. Thermal stimulation is a method used to stimulate the swallowing response in patients whose swallowing response does not trigger or triggers late (Fig. 1-2).

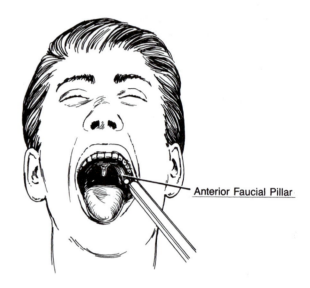

Anterior Faucial Pillar

Figure 1-2

9. It is unlikely that an actual swallow will be triggered with thermal stimulation. The purpose of the exercise is to heighten sensitivity to the swallowing response so that, when food or liquid is presented and the patient attempts a voluntary swallow, the response will be triggered.
10. The SLP evaluates the patient and makes recommendations on the use of thermal stimulation and other feeding techniques.
11. Contraindications for thermal stimulation include hypertonicity of the oral musculature and abnormal reflexes. Stimulation may accentuate these problems.
12. The techniques included in this procedure are ones that the nursing staff can utilize as appropriate. There are other techniques that only the speech pathologist should perform.
13. When dysphagia is suspected, contact the SLP for a video fluoroscopy. A thorough evaluation and guidelines for feeding techniques for each individual patient need to be developed. Incorporate these techniques into the plan of care.
14. Criteria for food selection to facilitate chewing and swallowing are as follows:
    - Semisolid foods such as purees or foods that hold some shape are often the easiest to swallow. Form provides stimulation to initiate the swallow.

- Foods with texture stimulate chewing. Chewing assists in stimulating the swallow response.
- Liquids, such as water and juices, are often difficult to swallow because they are thin and have no texture. Also, water is tasteless.
- Milk, ice cream, and milkshakes, although they have some form, are difficult to clear rapidly because they form excessive mucus in the mouth and throat.
- Ice cream, ice chips, and Jell-O, although semisolid in form, usually melt to a thin liquid by the time the patient with dysphagia finally swallows the bolus.
- Meats require a great deal of chewing and, therefore, are difficult to manage. Ground meats may crumble and be aspirated. Chicken may be the easiest to chew and holds its form as a bolus.
- Sweet, sour, and salty foods may stimulate chewing, which potentiates swallowing.
- Foods at body temperature are not stimulating enough; foods slightly warmer or colder than body temperature are better.

15. The patient with dysphagia should be well rested and as calm and undistracted as possible at the time of eating.

16. Criteria to be met before feeding include that the patient
    - Is alert and responsive
    - Has control of oral movements
    - Protects the airway
    - Holds and swallows saliva

17. Before feeding patients with dysphagia or potential chewing and swallowing problems, staff should demonstrate knowledge of and skill in performing Heimlich's maneuver. Family members may need to learn this as well. Recommended approaches are as follows:
    - Conscious patient, standing or sitting
        - Stand behind with one foot beside and the other foot behind the patient (this braces you to support the patient and positions you for performing abdominal thrusts).
        - Wrap your arms around the patient's waist.
        - Make a fist with one hand, and grab it with the other. The fist is placed with the thumb side against the patient's abdomen, slightly above the navel and below the rib cage.
        - Press your fist into the patient's abdomen with a quick, forceful, inward and upward thrust. Repeat thrusts in rapid sequence if necessary.

- Unconscious patient, lying
    - Position the patient on his or her back.
    - Kneel straddling his or her thighs.
    - With one hand directly over the other, place the heel of the bottom hand in the middle of the patient's abdomen a little above the navel (avoid pressure over or near the xiphoid or rib areas).
    - Press quickly into the abdomen with a forceful upward thrust along the midline of the body. Repeat if necessary.

18. In the home setting, ongoing instruction is provided by the nurse or SLP.

19. Evaluate upper extremity function and individual's ability to perform feeding activities with or without assistance.

PATIENT AND FAMILY EDUCATION

1. Educate the patient and caregivers as to the proper method of feeding the individual. Include potential complications, risks, and signs and symptoms indicative of the need to discontinue oral feeding.

2. Teach the Heimlich maneuver to family members responsible for feeding the patient.

3. Catalogs of patient teaching materials:
    - Pro-ed, 8700 Shoal Creek Boulevard, Austin, Texas 78757-6897
    - Imaginart, 307 Arizona Street, Bisbee, Arizona 85603.
    - Interactive Therapeutics, Inc., PO Box 1805, Stow, Ohio 44224-0805.
    - Pritchett & Hull Associates Inc. 3440 Oakcliff Road NE, STE 110d, Atlanta, Georgia 30340-3079.
    - The Speech Bin, 1965 Twenty-Fifth Avenue, Vero Beach, Florida 32960.
    - For professional education only:
        - Applied Symboliz, 800 North Wells Street, Suite 200, Chicago, Illinois 60610
        - Canyonlands Publishing, Inc., 141 South Park Avenue, Tucson, Arizona 85719.

4. Patient and family teaching to include dysphagia definition, treatment plan, special equipment and techniques, and potential outcomes.

Procedure

Safe Feeding and Stimulation Techniques of the Patient with Dysphagia

 Steps

 Additional Information

1. Initiate intake and output flow sheet, calorie count, food diary, or count number of spoonfuls of food taken at each meal. This may be partial spoonfuls (e.g., ¼-tsp amounts).

The patient with dysphagia may not be taking in enough fluids because of difficulty swallowing; this potentially jeopardizes his or her hydration status. Observation and assessment of intake and output provide information about patient's hydration status and also can indicate cardiac, endocrine, or renal problems. Additional hydration assessment includes observation of skin turgor, condition of mucous membranes, and urine specific gravity. Foods that are easiest to swallow for the patient with dysphagia may not be the most nutritious. Patients with dysphagia eat slowly and often become fatigued or cannot consume enough at each meal to maintain adequate nutritional intake. Calorie counts provide information about nutritional status. Consult dietitian for appropriate management of nutritional needs. This record keeping is essential in the home setting.

2. Weigh patient twice a week or on a routine basis.

Patient's weight will assist in determining adequacy of caloric intake.

3. Position patient in these positions for feeding:
   - In bed
     - Patient at head of bed
     - Head of bed raised 90 degrees
     - Neck slightly flexed
     - Pillows supporting position if necessary
   - In chair
     - Patient sitting at 90 degrees with trunk extended
     - Head aligned with midline
     - Neck slightly flexed
     - Feet flat
     - Table or lapboard at proper height

Appropriate positioning improves patency of pharyngeal pathway, allows epiglottal closure, and helps prevents aspiration. Flexion also encourages a swallow. Proper table or lapboard height would allow patient to rest forearms flat on surface with elbows flexed more than 90 degrees and shoulders neutral and symmetric. These positions most commonly are the best for feeding. There may be instances when this is not so, and the SLP will identify the best positions, in those special situations. If 90-degree sitting position cannot be achieved, maintain patient at no less than 60 degrees.

4. Modify feeding environment when appropriate:
   - Decrease distractions
   - Find a quiet, low-stimulus place (e.g., patient's room with curtains drawn, private room, empty part of hallway)
   - Keep patient focused on task of eating
   - Keep conversation to a minimum
   - Focus on one food item at a time

Patients who cannot attend to more than one task at a time require environmental modifications. Place only one food item in front of patient.

5. Reinforce rate and amount of feeding:
   - Give ⅓ to ½ tsp at a time, place food on intact side or side without sensory or motor loss
   - Put spoon down between portions
   - Check for empty mouth before proceeding
   - Encourage patient to take a sip of fluid at slow rate

Teach patient correct rate and amount. If swallowing problem is not severe, promote independence and encourage slower rate.

6. Food temperature should be slightly warmer or colder than body temperature.

This will heighten patient's awareness of food present in mouth and stimulate swallow response. Hot foods can burn tongue, cold foods can numb tongue, and foods at room temperature do not provide enough stimulation.

7. Feeding equipment suggestions are:
   • Use cut-out cup or small, 1-oz medication cup
   • Cut straws shorter, or do not use a straw
   • Do not have patient drink out of cartons
   • Use an iced spoon or cold stainless-steel spoon to feed patient, alternating between cold and regular temperature
   • Feed patient at same level you are, otherwise patient may have to tilt head back to look up

The use of cut-out cups or small medicine cups helps limit volume of fluid and amount of neck extension. Slight flexion makes swallowing easier. Straws are difficult to use with facial weakness and paralysis. A short straw may be used because it requires less effort and muscle strength than a long one.

8. Reinforce voluntary swallow. Say to patient:
   • "Hold the food in your mouth."
   • "Hold your breath."
   • "Think about swallowing."
   • "Swallow." Hold patient's mouth or lips closed if mouth or lip closure is not adequate.
   • "Breathe."
   • "Swallow again."

This technique works best for patients who are cognitively intact or have a tracheostomy. Keep directions short and direct for increased understanding and emphasis. Practice steps with a dry swallow or empty spoon before starting.

9. Place hand on sagging or drooping facial muscles to support them during feeding.

Mouth and lips must close to initiate and stimulate swallowing. This is the first step in swallowing. Providing support to drooping facial muscles from facial paralysis will give better control over food particles.

10. Place food in back of mouth for patients with hyperactive or hypoactive tongues.

This will inhibit hyperactive tongue and assist hypoactive tongue during oral phase of swallowing only if the swallow response is adequate and patient can protect his or her airway.

11. Do not combine solids and liquids in same mouthful.

The combination of textures and thicknesses is too confusing and will not enhance the swallowing response.

12. Assist with swallowing.
   • Apply gentle pressure or massage over larynx.
   • Stroke digastric muscle on either side or both sides.
   • Place ice at sternal notch.

These activities may help stimulate a swallow.

13. Ask patient to wipe his or her lips with napkin.

The automatic response that usually follows is a swallow. Use of napkin also provides pressure on lips and may assist with lip closure.

14. Check patient has swallowed:
   • Watch for rise of larynx to indicate that swallowing has occurred.
   • Check for clear mouth before proceeding.

Give patient enough time to swallow. Teach patient to insert a finger to check oral cavity for food. Look for signs that may indicate aspiration (wet or moist-sounding voice, shortness of breath, difficulty breathing and decreased lung sounds, cyanosis, regurgitation of food particles). Staff and family should be able to perform emergency interventions, such as suctioning or Heimlich's maneuver, as well as call for help.

15. Thermal stimulation (as directed by SLP):
   • Wash hands
   • Position patient at 80 to 90 degrees
   • Place cotton-tipped applicator and laryngeal mirror in ice for 10 s
   • Lightly brush base of anterior faucial pillar (Fig. 1-2)

This will provide more sensory stimulation than a room temperature or plastic spoon. If patient begins to gag, stop procedure. This may help elicit a swallow.

- Five to ten strokes should be done on each anterior faucial pillar
- If procedure does not produce an involuntary swallow, instruct patient to swallow voluntarily
- Stimulation will need to be repeated four or five times daily for 5 to 10 min each time for several weeks to 1 month

ADDENDUM: SPECIAL CONSIDERATIONS FOR PATIENTS WITH TRACHEOSTOMY

Follow steps 1 through 14 above. In addition:

 Step

 Additional Information

1. If patient has cuffed tracheostomy tube, cuff should be deflated during feeding.

   Suctioning should be done before deflating in case food has pocketed above cuff. If patient needs cuff inflated, then (s)he should not be fed orally.

2. Add blue food coloring to food. Show patient food and let him or her smell it before adding coloring to food.

   If patient coughs or is suctioned and substance is blue, aspiration can be determined because food has been dyed a distinct color. Glucose strips are also used on trachea secretions to determine aspiration.

 DOCUMENTATION

1. Document the stimulation techniques used.
2. Record the results and any unusual occurrences during the procedures.
3. Document the recommended changes in the procedure based on patient responses.
4. Record the result of assessments.
5. Document safety measures and effectiveness.
6. Record nutritional intake and output, calorie count, food diary, and weights.
7. Document patient and family teaching.

REFERENCES

Cherney, L.R. (1994) *Clinical Management of Dysphagia in Adults and Children*, 2d ed. Gaithersburg, MD: Aspen Publishers, Inc.

Cherney, L.R. and Souder, T. S. (1996) "Evaluating Swallowing Disorders: The Speech-Language Pathologist's Perspective" *Topics in Stroke Rehabilitation* 3(3):14–26.

Kaatzke-McDonald, M.N., Post, E. and Davis, P.J. (1996) "The Effects of Cold, Touch and Chemical Stimulation of the Anterior Faucial Pillar on Human Swallowing" *Dysphagia* 11(3):198–206.

Martin-Harris, B. and Cherney, L.R. (1996) "Treating Swallowing Disorders Following Stroke" *Topics in Stroke Rehabilitation* 3(3):27–40.

McCourt, A.E. (Ed.) (1993) *The Specialty Practice of Rehabilitation Nursing: A Core Curriculum*, 3d ed. Skokie, IL: Rehabilitation Nursing Foundation.

Perlman, A. (1996) "Neuroanatomy and Neurophysiology: Implications for Swallowing" *Topics in Stroke Rehabilitation* 3(3):1–13.

Rosenbek, J.C., Roecker, E.B., Wood, J.L. and Robbins, J. (1996) "Thermal Application Reduces the Duration of Stage Transition in Dysphagia after Stroke" *Dysphagia* 11(4):225–233.

Steele, C.M., Greenwood, C., Ens, I., et al. (1997) "Mealtime Difficulties in a Home for the Aged: Not Just Dysphagia" *Dysphagia* 12(1):43–50.

Transition from Enteral to Oral Feeding

PURPOSE

To determine the patient's readiness for oral feeding and the level of oral feeding needed for the patient with chewing and swallowing difficulties; to determine the appropriate feeding method (enteric or oral) for patients with chewing and swallowing difficulties.

GENERAL CONSIDERATIONS

1. Effective control of swallowing implies the use of the lips, cheeks, tongue, palate, larynx, and respiratory musculature (Fig. 1-1A).

2. There are no absolute guidelines to determine whether a patient should or should not be given oral feedings. However, according to Logeman (1983), a patient aspirating more than 10 percent of every bolus and taking more than 10 s to swallow a single bolus, regardless of the consistency of the food, should not be fed orally.

3. The decision to use oral or enteral feeding is based on the physician's, nurse's, and SLP's assessments of oral and pharyngeal transit time and potential for aspiration. Ideally, these can be verified by video fluoroscopy.

4. The amount of time it takes to swallow a single bolus is an important factor in nutritional management. If the patient cannot consume enough nutrition orally, enteric supplements are necessary.

5. The nursing assessment should include:
   - Soft palate reflex
   - Swallow reflex
   - Function of the cranial nerves—trigeminal (V), facial (VII), glossopharyngeal (IX), vagus (X), spinal accessory (XI), and hypoglossal (XII)
   - Labial function
   - Lingual function
   - Respiratory status—history of aspiration, requirement for suctioning, tracheostomy, and so forth
   - Level of responsiveness

6. Other factors that could inhibit oral feeding are degree of head control, general level of endurance, upper extremity function, general coordination, or specific dietary or dentition problems.

7. The managing physician makes the final decision regarding oral feeding.

8. The following may indicate that the patient is at high risk for aspiration and should remain prohibited from oral intake:
   - Reduced alertness
   - Reduced responsiveness to stimulation
   - Absent swallow
   - Absent protective cough
   - Difficulty handling secretions, for example, excessive coughing and choking, copious secretions, and a wet, gurgly voice quality
   - Significant reductions in the range and strength of oral motor and laryngeal movements

9. The length of time that it takes to progress from enteric to oral feeding is determined by the speech pathologist and the physician. This information will assist in the decision-making process about whether to place a gastrostomy tube or to utilize a nasogastric tube.

10. Nasogastric tube feeding is generally considered a temporary solution and is used with patients whose chewing and swallowing problems are thought to be short term. If swallowing rehabilitation is anticipated to be long, a gastrostomy tube would be more appropriate.

11. Enteric feedings should stabilize a patient's nutritional needs.

12. Functional severity levels for dysphagia (Cherney et al., 1996) are outlined in Table 1-1.

13. Diet types for solid food (Steffel, 1981) are outlined in Table 1-2.

14. Diet types for liquids are outlined in Table 1-3.

PATIENT AND FAMILY EDUCATION

Teach the patient and family about the transition process, their roles, and the importance of following the treatment plan.

Table 1-1 Functional Severity Levels for Dysphagia

Functional Level	Characteristics
Severe (Nonfunctional)	All nourishment from alternate feeding method Patient receives nothing by mouth Trial oral feeding, by SLP or feeding specialist with physician's order
Moderately severe (Interferes with function)	Alternate feeding method is primary source of nourishment Limited, inconsistent success with oral intake Patient requires constant supervision Some team involvement is needed, but only the SLP or feeding specialist introduces new food items or techniques
Moderate (Interferes with function)	Alternate methods may be withdrawn on a trial basis Patient is fairly reliable with a prescribed diet of specific items Constant supervision is still needed Nursing is most involved and follows the instructions of SLP or feeding specialist Introduction of new food items or techniques is supervised by SLP or feeding specialist
Mild moderate (Interferes with function)	Patient is fairly reliable with defined level of food consistency Clear liquids or solids may still cause difficulty Nursing takes primary responsibility for supervision of feeding Self-feeding instruction is initiated if upper extremity function permits
Mild (Adequate but reduced)	Patient receives regular diet with only some foods restricted because of particular difficulty with them Patient may require some special techniques or procedures to achieve successful swallowing Less close staff supervision is needed
Minimal (Adequate but reduced)	Patient receives a regular diet without any restrictions No supervision is required Occasional episodes of coughing with liquids or solids
Normal (Adequate)	Patient is independent in oral intake of all food consistencies Safe and efficient swallowing competency

Procedure

Transition from Enteral to Oral Feeding

 Steps

 Additional Information

1. Complete the dysphagia assessment

If aspiration is still a possibility, another video fluoroscopy should be performed.

2. Consult with SLP and physician about assessment findings and treatment plan

Specific treatment techniques should be identified for each individual patient.

3. Follow procedure for safe feeding of dysphagic patient

See procedure on Safe Feeding.

4. Remove tube only after adequate oral feeding (calories and fluids) has been consistently attained for 3 to 5 days

Tube use may continue indefinitely if inadequate fluids or food can not be ingested orally.

Table 1-2   Diet Types for Solid Food

Diet Type	Foods
Pureed	*Requires minimal gumming or chewing:* eggs (soft boiled or poached); fruit (baby food, ripe mashed bananas); meats, fish, poultry, cheese (baby food, pureed meats, cottage cheese); potatoes (mashed white or sweet); vegetables (baby food); miscellaneous (gravy, cream sauces, nondairy creamers, butter, margarine); sugar and sweets (jelly, plain pudding, boiled custard); breads and cereals (thick, smooth, hot cereals such as Cream of Wheat or Cream of Rice); avoid all other foods.
Advanced Pureed	*Added pureed foods that require more active gumming:* meat, fish, poultry, cheese, cheese souffle without crust, minced or ground meat; breads and cereals (soft breads without crusts or seeds, oatmeal); avoid all other foods except foods listed in group above.
Mechanical Soft	*Soft, textured foods that are easy to chew, swallow, and digest:* soft cooked fruits and vegetables, including canned, and served whole; breads, soft crackers, dry cereals that become soft in milk; desserts (cream pies and soft cakes without nuts and coconut); meats, soft sandwiches (no crust), soft casseroles, soft meat salads without raw vegetables; potatoes (creamed or baked, without skin), soft noodles, rice; sugars and sweets (soft candies); vegetables (spinach, peas, green beans); avoid toast, coarse cereals, cookies, nuts, bacon, and all other foods not listed in other two groups above.
Soft	*Foods that are easy to chew, swallow, and digest:* slight advancement from mechanical soft breads and cereals (soft bread with crusts, soft dinner rolls, pancakes, hot breads, coffee cakes with nuts); eggs (scrambled or fried, omelettes); meat, diced steaks, chops, meat casseroles, American cheese; vegetables, all cooked (except asparagus) or soft molded, vegetable salads (without lettuce or raw vegetables); avoid hard rolls, nuts, deep-fried foods, popcorn.

Table 1-3   Diet Types for Liquids

Diet Type	Foods
Extra-Thick Liquid	Thick soups that are strained with mashed potatoes; juices thickened with pureed fruit, baby cereal, or gelatin.
Thick Liquids	All liquids thickened as in extra-thick but to a lesser degree
Minimally Thickened Liquids	Strained soups; milkshakes and eggnogs that are not too thin; thick juices or nectars; thick liquids with decreased (or without) thickening agent
Clear and Other Liquids	Unrestricted fluid intake

 DOCUMENTATION

1. Document the patient's progress in any oral intake.
2. Document and report complications.

REFERENCES

Cherney, L.R. (1994) *Clinical Management of Dysphagia in Adults and Children*, 2d ed. Gaithersburg, MD: Aspen Publishers, Inc.

Cherney, L.R. and Souder, T.S. (1996) "Evaluating Swallowing Disorders: The Speech-Language Pathologist's Perspective" *Topics in Stroke Rehabilitation* 3(3):14–26.

Martin-Harris, B. and Cherney, L.R. (1996) "Treating Swallowing Disorders following Stroke" *Topics in Stroke Rehabilitation* 3(3):27–40.

Perlman, A. (1996) "Neuroanatomy and Neurophysiology: Implications for Swallowing" *Topics in Stroke Rehabilitation* 3(3):1–13.

Steffel, J.S. (1981) *Dysphagia Rehabilitation for Neurologically Impaired Adults*. Springfield, IL: Charles C. Thomas.

Feeding Tubes

PURPOSE

To provide fluid and nutrition to patients who are unable to take food/fluids/medication orally

STAFF RESPONSIBLE

EQUIPMENT

No equipment necessary.

 ### GENERAL CONSIDERATIONS

1. It is strongly recommended that insertion of small-diameter flexible polyurethane tubes (e.g., Nutriflex or Dobbhoff) be done by the physician and that radiologic visualization be used initially and thereafter as the only method of confirmation whenever placement is questioned. The small-diameter tubes have an unquestioned advantage in reducing trauma and esophageal-gastric sphincter compromise. Nevertheless, they may also present increased risk of asymptomatic pulmonary intubation, especially in poorly responsive patients. Aspiration of gastric contents is not recommended because negative pressure may collapse or kink the tube. Injected air may be audible on auscultation in the epigastric area even with bronchial placement. This technique is unreliable for assessment of placement. The pH method is more accurate for testing placement.

2. A further advantage of flexible tubes is the transpyloric feeding, which bypasses stomach distention and reduces reflux risk for the patient whose airway is unprotected by reflexes or who must remain recumbent. Disadvantages to transpyloric feeding include bypassing the antibacterial barrier of hydrochloric acid and the loss of intrinsic factor, which may lead to pernicious anemia.

3. Feeding the patient with a small-diameter tube requires the use of a volumetric pump and feedings of low osmolality and rate. These present disadvantages of inconvenience in mobility and expense.

4. Gastric reflux and tube displacement are still real possibilities, especially during strong coughing or gagging.

5. Large-bore, stiff nasogastric tubes present a greater risk of irritation and esophageal sphincter compromise. They are used for short periods of time in alert patients who can protect their airways by gag and cough. Placement is more easily confirmed by gastric secretion pH testing of the aspirate. Feedings may be delivered by gravity boluses when tolerated.

6. If enteric feeding is anticipated for more than a few weeks, the patient should be evaluated for a more direct enteric route and more practical management to normalize his or her care.

7. Because aspiration is a major risk, bedside access to suction and airway equipment is a requirement.

8. Modifications in tube placement technique should reflect the individual patient's needs with regard to age, position limits, level of consciousness, and psychological reaction.

9. Tables 1-4 to 1-6 offer the enteric tube options related to patient characteristics. It is recognized that additional procedures will be required to supplement patients requiring intravenous or total parenteral nutrition.

Table 1-4 Enteric Tube Options for Patients with Functional Gastrointestinal Tract Who Are Alert and Have Protected Airway and Short-Term Need

Delivery Site	Route	Advantages	Disadvantages	Complications	Management and Prevention
Stomach (distal to esophageal sphincter)	Nasogastric (#8 to #16 French red rubber or polyvinyl)	Relative ease in insertion, tube change; place-ment verified by aspiration; normalized digestive process; wide variety of meal replacement formulas; temporary, noninvasive supplementation; intermittent use with oral feeding.	Gastric distention; small-bore, requires pump or syringe feeding and skilled placement; red rubber not translucent; may not be radiopaque; noxious stimulus in face and visual field.	Gastric reflux: emesis; aspiration rupture. Tube displacement (removal or migration); mucous membrane or tissue trauma.	Gastric residuals: slow upgrading of feeding rate, concentration; patient positioning upright; metoclopramide for motility; prevent bowel stasis. Patient's hands are mitted or restrained; adequate stabilization of tube; nostril care; taping technique.
	Gastrostomy (surgical)	Viscous, blenderized diet given as bolus; long-term use; economic; cosmetic and comfortable; no compromise of esophageal sphincter.	Surgical procedure with risks; large stoma.	Infection; gastric leakage or ulceration; hypergranulation of stoma tissue; herniation. Tube displacement, removal, or migration.	Aseptic wound care; antacids; ulcer prevention; cauterization (silver nitrate or mechanical); abdominal support. Initially a dressing will be used however, with long-term use a dressing is optional. Careful mobility techniques; adequate stabilization techniques; abdominal binder, clothes.
	Percutaneous endoscopic gastrostomy (PEG)	Small-bore tube (#10 to #14 French); placement with local anesthesia; few complications; minimal wound at site; economic; easy to care for.	Requires variable healing time for tract to develop before tube change; clogs more easily than large tube.	Tube displacement, removal, or migration.	No dressings needed unless drainage is present. Careful mobility techniques; adequate stabilization techniques; abdominal binder, clothes.

Table 1-5   Enteric Tube Options for Patients at High Risk for Aspiration

Delivery Site	Route	Advantages	Disadvantages	Complications	Management and Prevention
Duodenum	Nasoenteric	Radiopaque; minimal compromise of gastric sphincters; bypasses gastric filling; comfortable oral feeding; little tissue trauma; allows variation in patient position.	Loss of gastric electrolytes, intrinsic factor, and normal digestion; volumetric pump required; lengthy feeding times; requires skilled placement; expensive diet and delivery; easily clogged, kinked tubes; noxious stimulus in face.	Tube displacement, removal, or migration; pulmonary intubation; obstruction; dehydration; diarrhea (three to six loose stools per day); nutrient deficiencies; absorption problems.	Patient restrained; radiograph verification of placement; adequate stabilization; monitor lower bowel sounds and elimination; monitor respiratory function; eliminate lactose and complex nutrients; rule out impaction or obstruction; slow rate of and dilute feeding; antidiarrheal medications; fiber-enriched feeding; rule out electrolyte and endocrine problems and vitamin deficiencies; supplement proteins, vitamins, and minerals.
	Gastroenteric (tube may be single- or double-lumen)	Allows for improvement and upgrading to gastric route from duodenal route; allows gastric drainage while feeding; provides gastric route for bulky medications.	Same as those for nasoenteric and gastrostomy (above), plus: skilled technique required for replacement; expensive; relatively new approach.	Same as those for nasoenteric (above), except: pulmonary intubation.	Same as those for nasoenteric (above); upgrade to gastric feeding as soon as patient meets criteria.

Table 1-6   Enteric Tube Options for Patients at High Risk for Aspiration and Permanent Placement

Delivery Site	Route	Advantages	Disadvantages	Complications	Management and Prevention
Jejunum	Jejunostomy	Bypasses all esophageal and gastric sphincters; allows variation in patient position. Permanent, cuffed placement (grows into subcutaneous tissue).	Skilled technique for replacements; surgical risks; limited tolerance to diet preparations.	Same as Table 1-4 plus enhanced problems with absorption, dehydration, bowel regulation, and small bowel obstruction.	Same as Table 1-4 plus free water supplements, flushes, longer infusion times; supplemented by intravenous, parenteral.
	PEJ (percutaneous endoscopic jejunostomy)	Reduced surgical risk with local anesthetic; cosmetic.			
	Gastrojejunal	Can be converted to gastric feeding route as patient improves.	Relatively new approach.		

Nasal-gastric/enteric Tube Insertion

PURPOSE

To provide fluid and nutrition to patients who are unable to take foods/fluids orally.

STAFF RESPONSIBLE

EQUIPMENT

1. Sterile feeding tube
   - Nasal-gastric/enteric tube of appropriate length and diameter
     # 8 French (newborn to 2 years of age)
     # 10 French (2 to 8 years of age)
     # 12 to # 14 French (8 to 10 years)
     # 14 to # 16 French (10 years to adult)
2. Sterile syringe with compatible Luer-Lok or catheter tip
   5 to 10 mL (newborn to 2 years of age)
   20 mL (2 to 8 years of age)
   50 mL (for # 12 French tubes and up)
3. Water-soluble lubricant or water to moisten the coating of small-bore tubes. Consult manufacturer's recommendation for lubrication.
4. Nonsterile gloves

5. Stethoscope
6. Penlight
7. Tape, steri-strips, or small foam skin protection pads
8. Emesis basin and facial tissue
9. Optional: Ice to increase rigidity of tube for easier passage

 GENERAL CONSIDERATIONS

1. Physician order is required for nasal-gastric/enteric tube placement.
2. Amount and frequency of feeding/hydration is based on the patient's age, weight, and caloric requirements.
3. Patients receiving nasal-gastric/enteric feedings are to have ongoing calorie counts, intake and output measurements, and at least weekly weights.
4. Any time a nasal-gastric/enteric tube is used, there is a chance of aspiration of stomach/gastric contents.
5. It is recommended that the tube be changed every 2 weeks. However, it may be changed more or less frequently based on nursing assessment and judgment. The interval and date of change, as well as special instructions for tube change, should be included in the patient's plan of care.

Procedure

Nasoenteric Tube Insertion

 Steps

1. Gather equipment; verify patient identification; provide privacy; wash hands.
2. Prepare tape (3 to 4 pieces cut ½ lengthwise), steri-strips, or foam pad. (Set rubber tube in ice water now.)
3. Position patient in semi-Fowler's position with pillows supporting head.

4. Explain procedure to patient.

Additional Information

Use nonsterile gloves.

Ice water is not necessary for plastic tubes

Head position facilitates epiglottis closure and swallowing to guide tube into esophagus. Hyperextension encourages tracheal intubation.

It is preferable to have assistance for this procedure. However, if inserting tube into a child/infant without assistance, an infant seat is advised. Hand mittens or mummy restraint with sheet, blanket, or pillow case (for small infant) are also options. Adequate personnel and gentle restraint should provide comfort and safety but not provoke alarm.

5. Check the nasal area and throat for secretions and patency, using a penlight.

   Clean nares gently if needed. Note the integrity of the septal wall or any obstruction. Note in patient care plan for future reference.

6. Estimate the distance from patient's nose to stomach. Allow enough length such that tube will be well into stomach (below xyphoid process).

   Hold catheter at tip of nose, bend tube toward and around back of ear and down to stomach area (below xyphoid process).

7. Mark catheter with piece of tape or marker to indicate total length of tubing that can be inserted.

8. Cleanse skin at nasal area to eliminate oils.

   An alcohol wipe may be used for very oily areas.

9. Lubricate catheter from tip to approximately 4 to 5 in. from other end.

10. Infant or small child should be placed in upright position. Older child and adult should bend head slightly forward.

11. Support head by placing one hand on forehead.

12. Insert catheter posteriorly and inferiorly with dominant hand. To ease insertion, direct the tube along the nasal passage toward the ear on the same side. When the tube reaches the pharyngeal junction, turn the tube inward toward the other nostril and advance.

    This action aims the tube down into the esophagus.

13. Instruct the patient to (dry) swallow frequently to aid passage of the tube into stomach.

    An infant cannot swallow on command, thus a swallow may be stimulated by stroking over the cricoid cartilage.

14. Advance the tube 1 to 3 in. (child) or 3 to 5 in. (adult) each time the patient swallows, until premeasured mark on tube reaches the nostril.

    Gagging is not uncommon. If coughing or choking occurs or if voice changes or is lost, STOP and assess placement. Remove if cough continues. Check mouth for coiled or kinked tubing, and remove tube if present.

15. Tape tube into place and check position by injecting a small amount of air with syringe and listening with stethoscope over epigastric area for a swoosh or gurgling sound. Check pH of gastric contents.

    This confirms placement of rubber or stiff plastic tubes. Small-bore tubes must still be radiographed.

16. When position is verified, secure in place with tape, steri-strips, or foam pad. (See method 1, 2, or 3.)

    Bring tape (steri-strip) under the tube at nares and cross over, taping to top of nose. (Do not pull too tightly, as this may cause pressure leading to skin breakdown.) Cover with a second piece of tape or steri-strip across the nose. Secure at a second point, either on the cheek (midway between the nose and ear on same side as tube) or forehead. The forehead is comfortable for most patients and is out of reach of children and infants. Use tincture of benzoin to facilitate tape adherence. Skin preparation should be used under benzoin to prevent irritation of infant/ child's skin. Remove both before reapplying. Thin strips of extra-thin hydrocolloid dressings can serve as an anchor to protect skin when securing tube with tape or steri-strips.

 DOCUMENTATION

1. Difficulties or problems encountered with nasal-gastric/enteric insertion or feedings.

2. Insertion of nasal-gastric/enteric tube and each feeding

REFERENCES

Eisdorfer, R.M. and Weg, A. (1990) "Percutaneous Endoscopic Gastrostomy: A Retrospective" *Journal of Neurologic Rehab* 4:75–77.

Lipman, T.O. (1987) "Nasopulmonary Intubation with Feeding Tubes, Therapeutic Misadventure or Accepted Complication?" *Nutrition in Clinical Practice* 2:45–48.

Procedure

Nasal-gastric/enteric Tube Removal

 Steps

1. Wash hands.
2. Schedule removal well after feeding. Explain procedure to patient and position him or her upright.
3. Clamp or stopper tube firmly.

4. Loosen tape anchoring tube.
5. Remove tube gently but swiftly.
6. Dispose of mercury-weighted tip of tube in designated container.

 Additional Information

Use nonsterile gloves.

This prevents nausea, emesis, and aspiration.

This prevents release of tube contents above gastric sphincters.

This minimizes gag as tube passes through pharynx.

Mercury cannot be incinerated because of release of toxic fumes. Follow infection control procedures for disposal of other soiled materials.

 DOCUMENTATION

1. Document tube removal and observations in the appropriate record.
2. Report unusual events or difficulties to the physician.

Gastrostomy Tube Reinsertion

PURPOSE

To reinsert a gastrostomy tube into the stomach; to prevent trauma or discomfort to the patient.

STAFF RESPONSIBLE

EQUIPMENT

1. Nonsterile gloves (sterile gloves if indicated)
2. Gastrostomy tube or indwelling Foley catheter of specified size
3. Water-soluble lubricant
4. Prefilled syringe of water if balloon is to be inflated
5. Unused syringe to deflate balloon
6. Soap and water
7. Other cleansing or antiseptic solution as ordered

8. Plastic bag for disposal
9. Tube clamp, stopper, or stopcock
10. Dressings and tape for anchoring
11. Irrigation syringe compatible with distal tube end

 GENERAL CONSIDERATIONS

1. Staff should be aware of agency policies regarding the replacement of various types of gastrostomy tubes.
2. The healing time required from original insertion should be specified by the surgeon. Depending on technique, this may be several days to several weeks. During this time, extra caution is taken to prevent trauma or accidental displacement. Proper stabilization of the tube should be continued. It may be necessary to use a soft binder to protect the site from the patient or accidental traction.
3. Prompt replacement is necessary to prevent the tract from rapid closing or shrinking and to prevent leakage into the abdominal cavity.

4. It is recommended that the physician order for routine change include type, size of tube, and size of balloon to be used.

PATIENT AND FAMILY EDUCATION

1. The family caregiver and patient are taught the procedure as appropriate before community pass or discharge.

2. Replacement equipment with appropriate instructions/precautions must accompany them.

Procedure

Gastrostomy Tube Reinsertion

 Steps

 Additional Information

1. Explain procedure to patient and caregiver.

2. Position patient supine, provide privacy, and drape area.

Choose a quiet time before a feeding to prevent discomfort and spillage.

3. Wash hands.

This is usually a clean procedure unless a fresh or open wound is present.

4. Set up equipment next to patient.
   - Lubricate new tube.
   - Open dressings and tear tape.
   - Apply gloves.

Follow the Centers for Disease Control recommendations for protection from body fluid contact.

5. Remove old dressings and tape and cleanse debris from stoma site and skin.

Prevent introduction of debris into stoma. Use plastic bag for disposal.

6. Remove gastrostomy tube.
   - Gently pull on tube to test balloon placement against stomach wall.
   - Mark tube with tape at its exit point from stoma.
   - Deflate old balloon by aspirating with unused syringe.
   - Pull old tube straight out of stoma.
   - Examine tube and stoma for drainage, color, etc.

This is to mark the length of tube inserted once it is removed. If resistance is met, seek physician's assistance. Adhesions or sutures may be unseen. Note marked length of tube and character of drainage and stoma site.

7. Quickly cleanse site and change gloves if contaminated by debris or discharge.

Avoid introduction of debris into stoma or wound site. Use plastic bag for disposal.

8. Insert new tube.
   - Estimate length to be inserted from marked length on old tube.
   - Insert lubricated tube at right angle to stoma.
   - Pass tube 1 in. or more past referenced length.
   - Aspirate stomach contents to verify placement.
   - Inflate balloon with prescribed amount of water. This is a minimum amount to keep tube in place.

Excessive length may pass tube into gastric outlet or duodenum. This prevents undermining or fistula formation at stoma site. This allows room for balloon inflation. If resistance is met, leave tube in place and seek physician's assistance. Tap water is suitable for a clean procedure. Overinflation may provoke gastric motility or production of secretions because it is perceived as gastric content.

9. Gently pull back on tube until balloon rests against stomach wall.

10. Clamp, plug, or stopper tube.

11. Cleanse site per procedure and dress and anchor.

Use minimum amounts of dressing or tape to prevent irritation to skin but adequate to prevent tube migration or traction.

12. Dress and reposition patient for comfort.

13. Remove plastic bag for disposal.

Follow infection control procedures to prevent cross-contamination.

DOCUMENTATION

1. Document the gastrostomy tube change. Include the reason for change, type and size of tube and balloon removed and reinserted, condition of stoma, observed condition of tube, drainage characteristics, observed tolerance of patient, and instructions to patient or caregiver.

2. Report to the physician any unusual observations.

Enteric Tube Stabilization and Dressings

PURPOSE

To provide stabilization of the tube; to prevent erosion of the skin around the tube; to prevent tube migration or removal

STAFF RESPONSIBLE

EQUIPMENT

Equipment options include those appropriate to nasogastric gastrostomy and jejunostomy tubes.

1. 1-in. hypoallergenic tape (cloth or paper) or steri-strips
2. 4 × 4 gauze
3. Fenestrated dressings or 4 × 4 dressings with 2-in. slit
4. Hydrogen peroxide or other prescribed agents
5. Normal saline
6. Plastic bag for disposal
7. NG stabilization device
8. Optional equipment:
   - Skin barrier
   - Thin hydrocolloid dressings
   - Adhesive remover
   - Tincture of benzoin

Nasogastric Tube Stabilization (Applicable to Nasal-gastric/enteric Tubes)

 GENERAL CONSIDERATIONS

1. In the rehabilitation setting, nasogastric feedings are utilized for short-term management of nutritional needs or for long-term management of patients in whom gastric or jejunostomy tubes are contraindicated.
2. Displacement or removal can occur with traction on or loosening of the tape. Migration or kinking can occur during reanchoring or with vigorous coughing, gagging, or emesis.
3. Considerations for choice of method 1, 2, or 3 include patient skin tolerance, need for rotation of tape site, patient preference or behavior, and presence of other equipment (e.g., oxygen nasal cannula).
4. Alternate the sites of taping, evaluate skin tolerance to techniques, and avoid direct pressure of tubing against skin or mucous membranes. Use of thin hydrocolloid dressings is possible over the skin where you wish to tape.
5. When anchoring over hair-covered skin other than the face, avoid shaving. Rather, clip the hair short. Remove tape in the direction of hair growth.
6. Adhesive removers must be thoroughly washed off with soap and water to avoid chemical burns.

PATIENT AND FAMILY EDUCATION

Educate the patient and caregivers of the purpose, the method used to anchor tube, and the need to keep the nursing staff informed of problems with the tube or anchoring.

Procedure

Method 1

 Steps

 Additional Information

1. Wash hands.
2. Cut a piece of 2 × 2 hypoallergenic tape.
3. Secure tube to upper lip or side of nose (Fig. 1-3*A*).

4. Use a second piece of tape to secure tube to forehead or cheek (Fig. 1-3*B*).
5. Secure tube to patient's clothing.

When taping on nose, do not place tape so that it pulls or causes pressure.

Do not obstruct vision with tube position and tape.

Remember to position tube in a way that keeps it out of reach of any patient who might pull it out.

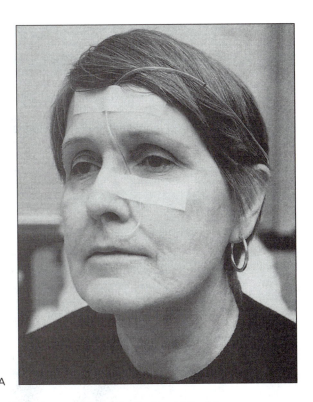

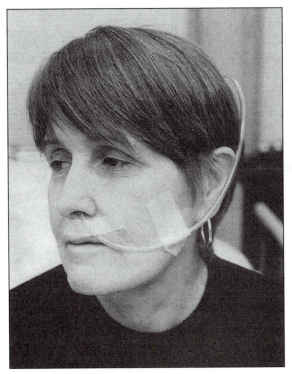

A

B

Figure 1-3 Nasogastric Tube Stabilization, Method 1.

Procedure

Method 2

 Steps

 Additional Information

1. Wash hands.

2. Cut a 1½-in. piece of 1-in. wide hypoallergenic tape or use steri-strip.

3. Split tape about 1 in. lengthwise from one end (Fig. 1-4A).

4. Attach unsplit end to patient's nose, then wrap split ends in opposite direction around tube (Fig. 1-4B to E).

5. If necessary, secure tube to patient's cheek or forehead.

Do not obstruct vision. Keep tube out of reach of patient who may pull it out.

6. With a tincture of benzoin swab, wipe tape on patient's nose or other taped areas.

Tincture of benzoin will absorb through tape and improve adhesion. Use skin barrier as indicated under tape.

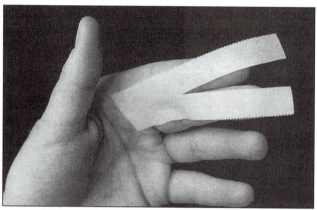

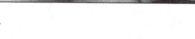

A

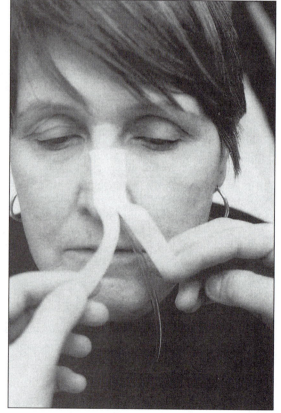

B

Figure 1-4 Nasogastric Tube Stabilization, Method 2.

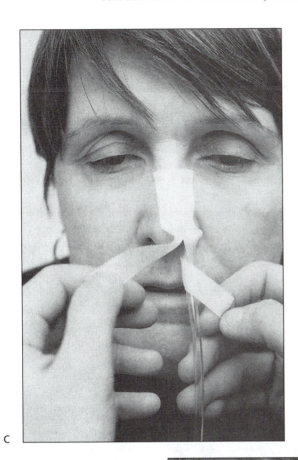

C

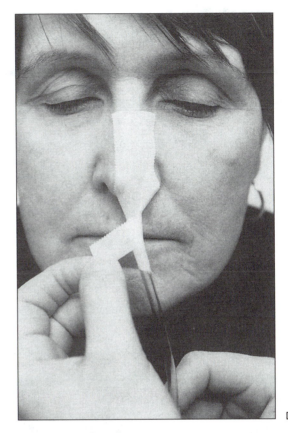

D

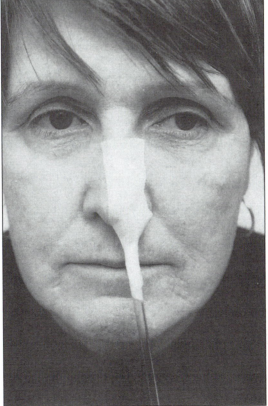

E

Figure 1-4 (continued)

Procedure

Method 3

 Steps

 Additional Information

1. Cleanse patient's nose and cheeks with mild soap and water.

2. Rinse thoroughly and dry completely.

3. Separate the jaws of the device.

4. Peel the release paper from the adhesive skin barrier.

5. Apply the barrier to the patient's nose by pressing down firmly, but gently, across the barrier surface.

6. Secure the tube by closing the clamp around it and snap the device closed (Fig. 1-5).

This will ensure maximum adhesion to the patient's nose. This method can only be used with size 12 to 18 French tubes.

Do not use any lotions or emollients, as the oily residue will interfere with the adhesion of the barrier.

Use two hands.

This will ensure proper adhesion.

REFERENCES

Product information for Suction Tube Attachment Device #9785. Hollister Incorporated, 2000 Hollister Drive, Libertyville, IL 60048.

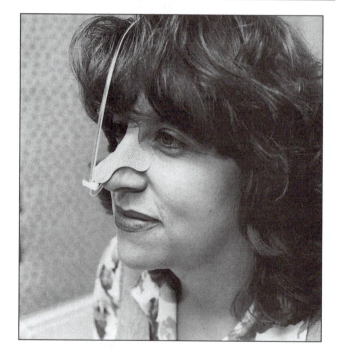

Figure 1-5

Gastric Tube Stabilization and Dressings

GENERAL CONSIDERATIONS

1. Gastrostomy stoma site care for new, infected, or draining wounds requires aseptic cleansing with prescribed agents and rinsing with normal saline. Healed stomas can be cleansed with soap and water and may not need a dressing.

2. One of the problems noted with gastric tube feedings is tube migration. This may cause pyloric or intestinal obstruction, which is prevented by proper anchoring. Tube migration that frequently occurs with traditional gastrostomy tubes (not PEGs) can be prevented with proper anchoring.

3. Excoriation of the stoma edges may occur when lateral traction or taping of the gastric tube is done. Alternate the direction of traction or ease the tension of the traction if this occurs.

4. If gastric tube irrigation or excoriation of stoma edges is a problem, use method 2 for tube stabilization or a similar method that provides vertical traction. If neither of these problems exists, use method 1.

PATIENT AND FAMILY EDUCATION

1. Educate the patient and caregivers of the purpose of the stabilization technique and the care of the stoma site, if appropriate.

2. Inform the patient and caregivers of complications and the need to keep nursing staff informed of problems or anchoring considerations with either method.

Procedure

Method 1

 Steps

1. Wash hands.
2. Remove old dressing.
3. Cleanse around tube.
4. Place a fenestrated dressing (4 × 4 dressing with a slit) around gastric tube. Tab the tape ends. Tape down edges window-frame fashion (Fig. 1-6*A*).
5. If necessary, tape tube down approximately 4 in. from stoma site. Tape straight across or in a V shape, with the base of the V pointing toward the stoma (Fig. 1-6*B*).
6. If desired or necessary, swab the tape with tincture of benzoin.

 Additional Information

Use nonsterile gloves.
Dispose of according to infection control procedures.

This may not be needed if the stoma site is healed.

Use skin barrier or stoma wafer under tape if indicated.

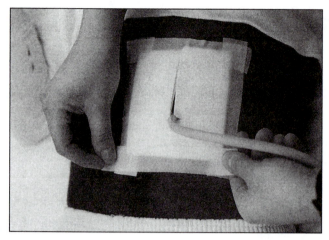
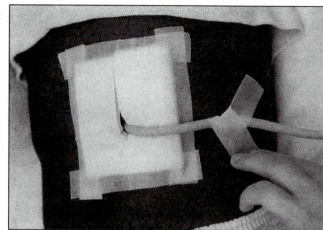

A   B

Figure 1-6   Gastric Tube Stabilization Fenestrated Dressing, Method 1.

Procedure

Method 2 Wu-Tuel Method

 Steps

 Additional Information

1. Wash hands.

Use nonsterile gloves.

2. Remove old dressing.

Dispose of according to infection control procedures.

3. Cleanse around tube.

4. Roll two 4 × 4 dressings together to form a cylinder about 4 in. long by 1 in. in diameter.

5. Place this roll on one side of tube and stoma and wrap tube completely around roll, going over the cylinder first, then under and back over (Fig. 1-7A).

This will provide vertical traction.

6. Place a 4 × 4 dressing over tube and gauze cylinder. Place a piece of tape perpendicular to tube but parallel to gauze roll on opposite side of gauze roll. Then place a piece of tape parallel to and on each side of tube (Fig. 1-7B).

7. Place a piece of tape in a V shape, with the base of the V pointing toward the stoma. Affix this approximately 4 in. from stoma (Fig. 1-7C).

This will prevent retraction of the tube into the stoma.

8. If desired, wipe tape with tincture of benzoin swab to improve adhesion.

Use skin barrier or stoma wafer under tape if indicated.

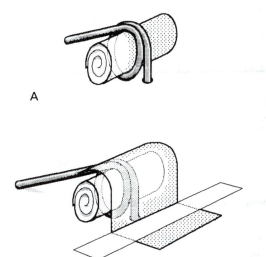

A

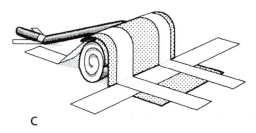

B

C

Figure 1-7

REFERENCES

Tuel, S.M., and Wu, Y. (1986) "A Method for Stabilizing Chronic Gastrostomy or Jejunostomy Tubes." *Archives of Physical Medicine and Rehabilitation* 67, 175–176.

Jejunostomy Tube Stabilization

GENERAL CONSIDERATIONS

1. There are various jejunostomy tubes. Some are anchored internally. The ones that are not have the greatest potential to migrate in or to fall out. Physicians may choose to anchor these tubes by suturing them to the patient's abdomen. Sutures may loosen easily, however, which causes an alteration in skin integrity and comfort for the patient. Therefore, appropriate nursing interventions that include jejunostomy tube stabilization are needed.

2. Jejunostomy stoma site care for new, infected, or draining wounds or suture sites may require cleansing with prescribed agents and rinsing with normal saline. Healed stomas can be cleansed with soap and water.

PATIENT AND FAMILY EDUCATION

Educate the patient and caregivers on tube stabilization procedures, purpose, and potential problems or anchoring issues.

Procedure

Jejunostomy Tube Stabilization

 Steps

1. Wash hands.

2. Remove old dressing.

3. Cleanse around tube.

4. Place fenestrated dressing (4 × 4 dressing with 2-in. slit) around tube. Tape down in window-frame fashion.

5. Take a 4- to 6-in. piece of hypoallergenic tape and make small tabs on each end.

6. Secure tube.
   - Place the piece of tape approximately 4 in. from stoma, perpendicular to tube (Fig. 1-8*A*).
   or
   - Place the piece of tape underneath tube, adhesive side up, approximately 4 in. from stoma. Then cross each piece of tape over top of tube and adhere it to patient's abdomen, forming V shape with base of V pointing away from stoma (Fig. 1-8*B*).

7. With a tincture of benzoin swab, wipe taped areas.

 Additional Information

Use nonsterile gloves.

Discard waste according to infection control procedures.

This may not be needed if stoma site is healed.

Tabs make it easier to remove tape when it needs to be changed.

This provides stabilization to prevent tube from being pulled out.

Tincture of benzoin will absorb through tape and increase tape adhesion. Use skin barrier or stoma wafer as indicated under tape.

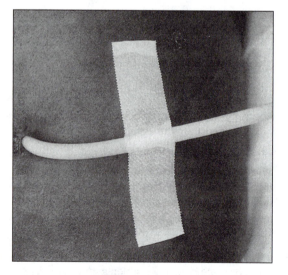

A

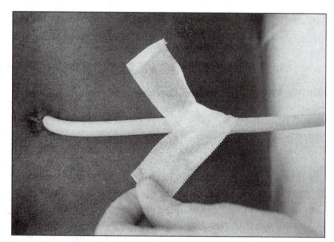

B

Figure 1-8 Jejunostomy Tube Stabilization.

 DOCUMENTATION

1. Record any difficulties with stabilization procedures.

2. Document skin status or other complications.

3. Record the use of special tape/dressings.

Gastric Residual

PURPOSE

To measure gastric contents and, indirectly, gastric motility before, during, or after enteric feeding; to prevent gastroesophageal reflux and potential aspiration

STAFF RESPONSIBLE

EQUIPMENT

1. Syringe (60-mL catheter or Luer-Lok tip compatible with distal tube connection)
2. Clamp, plug, or stopcock
3. Graduated emesis basin or container
4. Nonsterile gloves

 ## GENERAL CONSIDERATIONS

1. Routine measures of gastric residual volume are indicated when:
   - Initiating or upgrading volume, rate, or concentration of enteric feeding solution
   - The patient is identified as at high risk for aspiration
   - Emesis has occurred or is a frequent event
   - Monitoring postoperative recovery from gastrostomy tube insertion or other surgery
   - The patient is febrile or is under other stress that alters metabolic function or state of responsiveness
   - The patient exhibits sudden restlessness, discomfort, or respiratory distress during or after a feeding

2. Measurement of gastric residual is not always an absolute equivalent of gastric content. The proximal end of the gastric tube may access only the upper portion of the gastric volume. Repositioning the patient may be necessary to aspirate contents fully. Astute clinical judgment must guide the nurse's visualization of this procedure and assessment of the patient.

3. In the event of a medical emergency (e.g., seizure, hypotension, or cardiopulmonary arrest) during feeding or soon after feeding, prompt gastric aspiration may prevent reflux and aspiration. For patients at high risk for crisis or whose feeding tolerance is unknown, suction and airway equipment are kept nearby.

4. Gastric contents are usually returned to the stomach because they contain nutrients, digestive enzymes, and perhaps medications. If the contents exceed the ordered amount or if reflux is imminent, however, the contents may be discarded without serious threat of depletion of enzymes or electrolytes. This should be clarified with a physician order. Obvious loss of medication and discarded volume are reported to the physician.

5. Acceptable residual amounts may vary in physician orders. These are determined by consideration of the individual patient, recovery history, risks, or tube placement protocols. As tolerance is demonstrated, residual amounts are based on hourly rate if feeding is continuous or on percentage of feeding volume if feeding is bolused.

6. Metoclopramide is often used as a short-term adjunct to promote gastric motility:
   - To propel an enteric tube into the duodenum
   - To enhance gastric emptying after operative tube placement
   Occasionally, it is used for more persistent problems.

7. The sudden onset of slowed gastric emptying or reflux requires investigation to rule out:
   - Displacement or migration of the gastric tube into the esophageal or pyloric sphincter
   - Severe constipation or other form of intestinal obstruction
   - A patient position (e.g., flexed or left-sided) that delays emptying
   - Febrile or less conscious state

8. Slowed gastric motility may be an anticipated side effect of medications, especially anticholinergics, some antibiotics, preparations in acidic or oil-based solutes, and narcotics. The action of metoclopramide is antagonized by narcotics and anticholinergics. Hypertonic or hypotonic feedings may also slow motility.

9. Jejunostomy tubes and small-diameter polyurethane tubes (nasogastric tubes) are not aspirated routinely because the proximal end is located within the intestine, which is emptied by gravity and peristalsis rather than by the sphincters. Aspiration is also likely to clog or kink a small tube. Gastric reflux can still occur but cannot be measured without placement of a gastric tube. On occasion, a gastric tube may be placed for decompression.

10. The following are common interventions that enhance or promote gastric motility:

- Administering metoclopramide
- Discontinuing medications that decrease gastric motility
- Emptying the lower bowel
- Positioning the patient upright, with trunk extension or right-side lying (or both)
- Diluting the feeding and slowing the rate until tolerance is reestablished
- Correcting metabolic problems
- Instituting olfactory and oral sensory stimulation

PATIENT AND FAMILY EDUCATION

1. Educate the patient and caregivers of the complications and risks that may indicate signs of gastric residual problems.
2. Advise that they report these to the appropriate medical or nursing staff (inpatient or outpatient).

Procedure

Gastric Residual

 Steps

 Additional Information

1. Wash hands and don gloves.

2. Prepare patient with explanation. Include family or caregiver as appropriate.

3. Stop feeding at prescribed time. Pinch tube while disconnecting or unclamping.

4. Insert syringe snugly into tube and aspirate stomach contents gently.

5. Return aspirated contents to stomach.

6. Pinch tube, withdraw syringe, and clamp or reconnect tubing.

7. Resume feeding only when residual amount is acceptable or when modifications are made in feeding program as ordered.

This is a clean procedure. Apply nonsterile gloves.

Caregivers must be able to evaluate gastric emptying if tube is used long term.

Introduction of air can increase distention.

Vigorous aspiration may traumatize mucosa.

Check patient position and comfort to verify reliability of gastric residual.

Observe patient closely for increased distress. Report to physician.

 DOCUMENTATION

1. Document the amount of residual, any unusual appearance, and subsequent actions or interventions.

2. Note whether the physician was notified and the reasons for notification.

Gastric Occult Blood and pH Testing

PURPOSE

To detect the presence of occult blood and to determine the pH of gastric aspirate or vomitus

STAFF RESPONSIBLE

EQUIPMENT

1. "Gastroccult" brand slide
2. "Gastroccult" brand developer
3. Applicator stick/ tongue depressor
4. Nonsterile gloves
5. 20- or 60-cc Luer-Lok or catheter tip syringe
6. Specimen cup or emesis basin
7. Watch with second hand

 GENERAL CONSIDERATIONS

1. The Gastroccult slide test is used to aid in the diagnosis and management of various traumatic or deteriorating gastric conditions, while the pH test may be of use in evaluating antacid therapy. Testing for gastric occult blood is indicated in patients whose clinical symptoms and preliminary blood studies suggest gastrointestinal (GI) bleeding. This test is also used to monitor patients at risk for gastric occult blood.

2. The Gastroccult test cannot be considered conclusive evidence of the presence or absence of upper GI bleeding or pathology. It is designed as a preliminary screening aid and is not intended to replace other diagnostic procedures.

3. Do not use Hemoccult slides or developer to test gastric secretions as they may yield erroneous results. The gastric occult blood test is not affected by low pH. Gastroccult is free from interference by normal therapeutic concentrations of cimetidine (Tagamet), iron or copper salts.

4. Gastric secretions should be tested no sooner than 60 min after the last antacid administration or last stomach irrigation.

5. Many food components (e.g., incompletely cooked meat, raw fruit and vegetables) have peroxidase activity that can produce a (false) positive Gastroccult test result. Thus, a positive result does not always indicate the presence of human blood, and further workup may be indicated per physician.

6. The frequency of testing is determined by physician order. The nurse can also initiate gastric occult blood testing based on nursing assessment; the physician should be notified when this occurs.

7. Store the developer away from heat and light. Keep the lid tightly capped. Do not refrigerate the developer.

8. Do not use the Gastroccult slide or developer after the expiration date or if the paper on the slide has turned green or blue.

9. As with all gastrointestinal-related procedures, adhere to infection control practices and guidelines.

Procedure

Gastric Occult Blood and pH Testing

 Steps

 Additional Information

1. Gather equipment and check expiration date. Identify correct patient. Explain the procedure to the patient. Wash hands. Don nonsterile gloves.

2. Collect a small sample of gastric aspirate or vomitus from syringe or emesis basin.

   Preschoolers may fear the removal of their body secretions. Explain to children that the small drop from their stomach or tummy will be put onto a special card (slide) to make sure that there is no problem inside.

3. Open Gastroccult slide and apply one drop of the gastric sample to the occult blood test area using applicator stick or tongue depressor.

4. Apply two (2) drops of Gastroccult developer directly over the sample and one (1) drop between the positive and negative Performance Monitor areas.

   Any blue originating from the Performance Monitor area should be ignored in the interpretation of the specimen test results.

5. Read occult blood results within 60 s. The development of any blue color in the occult blood test area AFTER ADDITION OF DEVELOPER is regarded as a positive result.

6. Interpret the Performance Monitor results. A blue color will appear in the positive Performance Monitor area within 10 s and will remain stable for at least 60 s. No blue should appear in the negative Performance Monitor area.

   The Performance Monitor feature provides assurance that the slide and developer are functional. In the event that the Performance Monitor areas do not react as expected after application of the developer, the test results should be regarded as invalid. Repeat the test using another slide.

7. Apply one drop of gastric sample to pH test area circle to determine pH results. Interpret the results within 30 s after applying sample. Visually compare the pH test area to the pH color comparators.

   The pH test is an OPTIONAL feature of the Gastroccult slide. The pH test need not be performed unless specifically ordered.

 DOCUMENTATION

1. Notifying the physician of any positive gastric occult blood test results immediately.

2. Documenting the result of gastric occult blood testing.

3. Writing a progress note reflecting a positive result and/or any pertinent nursing assessments made during the procedure or concerning any adverse signs and/or symptoms which the patient may have displayed.

REFERENCES

Gastroccult Slides Product Instructions (1988) San Jose, CA: SmithKline Diagnostics, Inc.

Metheny, N., Wehrle, M.A., Wiersema, L., and Clark, J. (1998) "Testing Feeding Tube Placement: Auscultation vs. pH Method" *American Journal of Nursing* 98(5):37–42.

Potts, R.G., Zaroukian, M.H., Guerrero, P.A. and Baker, C.D. (1993) "Comparison of Blue Dye Visualization and Glucose Oxidase Test Strip Methods for Detecting Pulmonary Aspiration of Enteral Feedings in Intubated Adults" *Chest* 103(1):117–121.

Enteric Feeding Administration

PURPOSE

To meet nutritional and hydration requirements by delivery through nasogastric, gastric, or intestinal routes; to prevent enteral or respiratory complications

STAFF RESPONSIBLE

EQUIPMENT

1. Gastric feeding unit
2. Bottle, bag, or syringe compatible with tubing and pump
3. Volumetric pump as indicated
4. Prescribed feeding
5. Flush solution (usually water)
6. IV pole or hook
7. Clamp or stopper
8. Optional equipment
   - Gastric secretion testing device
   - Nonsterile gloves

GENERAL CONSIDERATIONS

1. Prior to feeding with NG tubes on admission, after insertion, reinsertion, or manipulation of the tube, an x-ray must be performed and read confirming tube placement. No medications or fluids should be given until placement is confirmed.

2. All food should be at room temperature when administered. Never hang more than 4 h of feeding at any time as it can spoil when exposed to room air for prolonged periods.

3. Cans of food are to be opened at time of feeding. Partially filled cans may be stored if covered with lids. Once the opening is securely covered with a lid, the can should be labeled with patient's name, date, and time the can was opened. The can may be stored a maximum of 24 h at which time, if not used, it must be discarded.

4. Wash hands before preparing feedings.

5. Patients on enteral feedings should be weighed twice a week to evaluate feeding program effectiveness.

6. Oral hygiene is essential for patients on enteral feedings and is recommended every 4 h. Oral hygiene prior to administering a feeding can help reduce the incidence of gag-induced emesis and can help stimulate digestion.

7. If diarrhea occurs with tube feedings, consider the following and discuss changes with the physician:
   - Decrease rate of feeding
   - Dilute feeding to promote absorption
   - Change feeding formula
   - Administer small frequent feedings
   - Assess antibiotic usage and other medications
   - Provide frequent perianal care

8. Careful consideration must be given to proper selection of the tube used. Factors to consider include: anticipated length of use, mental status of the patient, nutritional needs, medication route, ability of patient to do oral feedings.

9. The patient should be maintained at a 60-degree angle or higher during the feeding and for 1 h after the feeding.

10. Treatment which can induce emesis (postural drainage, percussion and vibration, oral hygiene, etc.) should be planned not to coincide with feedings if possible. Retraction of the PEG or gastrostomy tube may also cause emesis. Retraction can be reduced with the use of a Wu-Tuel fixation roll.

PATIENT AND FAMILY EDUCATION

1. Educate the patient and caregivers of the proper procedure.

2. Inform the patient and caregivers of the potential problems and risks of this procedure that are to be reported to available medical or nursing staff (inpatient or outpatient).

Procedure

Enteral Feeding Administration

 Steps

1. Position patient sitting or at inclined angle of 60 degrees or more.

2. Place patient in environment that promotes optimal relaxation and contains tolerable stimulation. Support or cradle infants and small children.

3. Complete oral hygiene, toileting, and suctioning before feeding.

4. Wash hands and don gloves.

5. Check for feeding tube placement:
   - By aspirating gastric contents with a syringe, checking pH of contents
   - By observing length of exposed tubing and security of anchoring
   - By gently pulling gastrostomy tube to ensure balloon or mushroom placement at stomach wall

6. Check for feeding tube patency by flushing with water, especially with small-diameter tubes.

7. Set up gastric feeding unit and related equipment. Label equipment with patient name, date, and time. Change disposable equipment at least every 24 h according to CDC guidelines while in the hospital. In the community, cleanse and reuse until _____. Check pump for operation, cleanliness, and a working manual alarm. Set volume rate as ordered.

8. Pour and measure feeding at patient location. Deliver room-temperature or cool fluids at slow rates until tolerance is well established by checking gastric residuals.

9. Deliver feeding at prescribed rate with periodic supervision for:
   - Gastric distention
   - Restlessness
   - Respiratory difficulty
   - Tube displacement
   - Pump malfunctioning

10. Check patient positioning for trunk alignment and extension, especially for those in bed.

11. If movement or turning is necessary, do so slowly with feeding turned off.

12. Maintain patient elevation for at least 60 min after feeding. Prolong this period as necessary. Interrupt continuous

 Additional Information

The supine position is to be avoided for patients at high risk for emesis and aspiration. Gastric emptying is facilitated by upright or right-side lying.

Feeding is normally a social activity. Olfactory, visual, and auditory stimulation are regular components of feeding and may aid gastric motility.

Relaxation of the stomach muscle is necessary for gastric filling. Patients distressed by nonoral intake may need privacy and decreased distraction during normal mealtimes.

Apply nonsterile gloves.

Aspirated gastric contents and checking pH or radiographs are the only certain methods of verifying placement. Abnormally short or long exposed tubing indicates need for further placement checks by physician.

Aspiration is not recommended with small-diameter nasogastric or jejunostomy tubes.

Residual food is a culture medium for bacterial growth. Residue may interfere with equipment operation.

Gastric motility is not affected by fluids at cool temperatures, but subjective discomfort may be reported by patient. Some patients may experience cramping with cold fluids.

Patients with poor arousal or hyperarousal are at high risk for aspiration. Alternatives are slower rates, smaller amounts, or frequent small feedings by syringe.

Patients who slide down in bed or assume a flexed position lose elevation and compress abdominal contents, which may encourage regurgitation.

Vestibular stimulation may trigger emesis.

Verify emptying with gastric residuals.

feedings as necessary for recumbent periods or vestibular activity.

13. Follow feeding with flush solution (usually water). Continuous feedings may be flushed at intervals. Clamp or plug feeding tube.

14. Rinse gastric feeding unit with cool water. Cover delivery end or tuck it securely into unit.

Tube patency is assured. Free water requirement is met. Saline or electrolyte solutions may be used for replacement instead of water.

Cool water will prevent coagulation of protein material. Soap is avoided because of the uncertainty of its complete removal.

DOCUMENTATION

1. Document the delivery of feeding, including type of feeding, tolerance/endurance of the patient, and difficulties in administration.

2. Record intake and calorie count as indicated.

3. Record twice-weekly weights.

4. Document tube placement and length and gastric residuals.

REFERENCES

Broom, J., and Jones, K. (1981) "Causes and Prevention of Diarrhea in Patients Receiving Enteral Nutritional Support." *Journal of Human Nutrition* 35:123–127.

Cataldi-Betcher, E.L., Seltzer, M.H., Slocum, B.A., and Jones, K.W. (1983) "Complications Occurring during Enteral Nutrition Support: A Prospective Study." *Journal of Parenteral and Enteral Nutrition* 7:546–552.

DelRio, D., Williams, K., and Esvelt, B.M. (1982) *Handbook of Enteral Nutrition: A Practical Guide to Tube Feeding.* El Segundo, CA: Medical Specifics.

Flynn, K.T., Norton, L.C., and Fisher, R.L. (1987) "Enteral Tube Feeding: Indications, Practices, and Outcomes." *Image: Journal of Nursing Scholarship* 1(2):16–19.

Griggs, B.A., and Hoppe, M.C. (1979) "Nasogastric Tube Feeding." *American Journal of Nursing* 79:481–485.

Kaminski, M.V., and Freed, B.A. (1981) "Enteral Hyperalimentation: Prevention and Treatment of Complications." *Nutritional Support Services* 1:29–40.

Mamel, J.T. (1987) "Percutaneous Endoscopic Gastrostomy: A Review." *Nutrition in Clinical Practice* 2:65–75.

McGee, L. (1987) "Feeding Gastrostomy: Part 1. Indications and Complications." *Journal of Enterostomal Therapy* 14:73–78.

Metheny, N. (1988) "Measures to Test Placement of Nasogastric and Nasointestinal Feeding Tubes: A Review." *Nursing Research* 37:324–329.

Newmark, S.R., Simpson, M.S., Beskitt, M.P., et al. (1981) "Home Tube Feeding for Long-Term Nutritional Support." *Journal of Parenteral and Enteral Nutrition* 5:76–79.

Rombeau, J.L., and Caldwell, M.D. (1984) *Clinical Nutrition*: Vol. 1. *Enteral and Tube Feeding.* Philadelphia, PA: W.B. Saunders.

Ryan, J.A., and McFadden, M.C. (1982) *Practical Aspects of Jejunal Feeding.* Silver Spring, MD: American Society for Parenteral and Enteral Nutrition (ASPEN); 1–6. Monograph.

Starkey, J.F., Jefferson, P.A., and Kirby, D.F. (1988) "Taking Care of Percutaneous Endoscopic Gastrostomy". *American Journal of Nursing* 88:42–45.

Administration of Enteral Medications

PURPOSE

To administer precise doses of prescribed medication; to prevent obstruction of an enteral tube

STAFF RESPONSIBLE

EQUIPMENT

1. Graduated medicine cups
2. Mortar and pestle or suitable substitute for crushing medications
3. Administration syringe with catheter or syringe tip compatible with enteral tube connector
4. Labeled medication containers
5. Medication order, record, and flow sheet

 GENERAL CONSIDERATIONS

1. As with oral medication, verify the compatibility of drugs with each other and with feeding components.
2. Obtain liquid forms and dose-volume equivalents by physician order. Discuss with the physician the substitution of drugs with like products available in liquid, chewable, or injectable forms. All solid medications must be finely crushed; chewable forms may be easier to crush.
3. Open capsules and empty contents into administration syringe. Do not instill any capsule or particles of capsules into an enteral tube. Consult with physician if any time-release capsules were prescribed, if they can be safely administered.
4. Use enteric-coated tablets with precaution and physician awareness. Destroying the coating by crushing may affect patient tolerance of the drug. Enteric coatings are difficult to crush.
5. Note the volume-required compatibility with fluid requirements or restrictions.
6. Note the content of liquid solutes for calories, alcohol content, or allergens.
7. Ensure clear labeling of suspensions that require thorough shaking to deliver an accurate dose.
8. Avoid thickened solutions, fiber, or bulk formers because these expand in liquid and may obstruct tubes quickly.
9. Administer medications with sufficient liquid (usually water) to
   - Enhance the utilization of the drug as recommended by the product literature
   - Dissolve or finely suspend particles of tablets
   - Flush the tube of residue
   - Reduce the thickness of concentrated medications
   - Avoid overdistention of stomach or intestinal contents
10. Simplify procedures for home and community use for practicality, limitations of the caregiver, and accessibility and economy of the equipment.

PATIENT AND FAMILY EDUCATION

If appropriate, educate the patient and caregivers as to the safe administration of enteral medications including potential problems or risks and side effects.

Procedure

Administration of Enteral Medications

 Steps

1. Wash hands.
2. Pour or draw up each liquid medication separately.

 Additional Information

Apply nonsterile gloves.

This prevents errors in administration and minimizes waste if discarding a medication is necessary.

3. Crush tablets into fine powder and remove thoroughly from container. Avoid pounding or splattering particles outside container. If this occurs, discard thoroughly and begin again.

Dose may be affected by residue left on pestle or in mortar or spilled.

4. Ensure placement and patency of enteral tube. Check gastric residual if appropriate.

Aspirated gastric secretions may be useful for dissolving some medications; see "Gastric Residual" procedure.
Air can cause gastric distention.

5. Fit administration syringe to tube before unclamping tube and fill syringe partially with water.

6. Administer liquid medications first and follow them with water. Use gravity flow or minimum pressure by syringe plunger.

Vigorous syringe pressure may rupture tube, especially small-diameter tubes.

7. Mix crushed medications in syringe, which is partially filled with water. Gently agitate mixture while administering quickly.

Premixing in separate container may lose some dosage. Agitation prevents particles from settling or clinging to syringe or plunger.

8. Flush contents of syringe and tube.

9. Reclamp, plug, or reconnect tube to feeding.

10. Rinse syringes, mortar, and pestle and wipe free of medication traces.

11. Syringes may be reused for same patient only. They are labeled, dated, stored, and discarded according to reuse protocol and infection control precautions. A mortar and pestle are usually used for more than one patient unless they must be confined to the patient. They must not be in contact with patients if multiple patient use is common.

DOCUMENTATION

1. Follow medication documentation protocol.

2. Document and report unusual circumstances or reactions to the administration of enteral medication.

REFERENCES

Holtz, L., Milton, J., and Sturek, J.K. (1987) "Compatibility of Medications with Enteral Feedings." *Journal of Parenteral and Enteral Nutrition* 1:183–186.

Lehmann, S., Barber, J.R. (1991) "Giving Medications by Feeding Tube: How to Avoid Problems" *Nursing91* November 58–61.

Metheny, N. (1988) "Measures to Test Placement of Nasogastric and Nasointestinal Feeding Tubes: A Review." *Nursing Research* 37:324–329.

Oral Care

PURPOSE

To clean the teeth, tongue, and oral mucosa of debris and bacteria; to prevent mucosal bleeding and breakdown; to promote patient comfort

STAFF RESPONSIBLE

EQUIPMENT

1. Warm water
2. Toothpaste or tooth powder
3. Emesis basin
4. Toweling
5. Adequate lighting
6. Soft-bristle toothbrush
7. Optional equipment:
   - Bite block
   - Half-strength peroxide
   - Baking soda
   - Mouth swabs
   - Water-pick
   - Moisturizers
   - Suction equipment
   - Dental floss on a handled device

 GENERAL CONSIDERATIONS

1. Thorough oral hygiene is necessary at least twice a day for any dependent patient. For patients who are to receive nothing by mouth, who are mouth breathers, or who keep their mouths closed, frequency is increased to three or four times a day.

2. Dental examination and cleaning should be scheduled in the post-acute period. Patients with dental injury or previous dentition problems require repairs to prevent pain or loss of teeth. Loose teeth present a risk for aspiration. Patients who grind their teeth require mouth guards to protect their teeth and to inhibit grinding or chewing behaviors.

3. Oral hygiene provides sensory stimulation for arousal and comfort and promotes digestive stimulation and saliva production. It may also induce gagging or coughing. As such, it should precede feedings whenever possible.

4. Oral hygiene is vital to the promotion of personal interactions with staff or family. Poor hygiene can present a real social obstacle that deprives a patient of contact.

5. Avoid the use of acidic preparations, such as lemon, for stimulation or care because they promote deterioration of tooth enamel and can be noxious to tender tissue. Likewise, avoid sweetened or alcohol-based preparations.

6. Cold is also noxious to sensitive teeth and is a stimulant to swallow. Warm water is recommended.

7. Baking soda is an effective cleaner, deodorizer, and antiplaque agent recommended by some dentists. Water-picks are also useful.

8. Mouth moisturizers are used in adjunct to routine hygiene, especially for extreme dryness or accumulations. These include artificial saliva and lip balms. Glycerin and peroxide are drying agents but may be effective for cleansing accumulations; their use should be followed by rinsing and moisturizers.

9. Suction equipment and oral catheters must be available for patients at risk for aspiration or who cooperate poorly.

PATIENT AND FAMILY EDUCATION

Educate the patient and caregivers of the importance of oral hygiene, the procedure as appropriate, and the need for reporting problems or difficulties in performing the procedure.

Procedure

Oral Care

 Steps

 Additional Information

1. Wash hands.

   Use nonsterile gloves, mask, and eye protectors.

2. Explain procedure to patient. Include family or caregiver as appropriate.

3. Position patient upright with head flexed or in elevated side-lying position.

   This promotes ready drainage of oral contents and prevents aspiration.

4. Arrange emesis basin and sufficient toweling. Set up equipment, suction, and supplies in reach and ensure adequate lighting.

5. Open patient's mouth and visualize teeth, tongue, and mucosa. Mouth opening is elicited by gentle head tilt, chin pressure, and jaw massage. Place bite block between back teeth if necessary. Remove mouth guard if present.

   Bite blocks are not to be forced between teeth. It may be necessary to wait for relaxation or to elicit a yawn for mouth opening.

6. Gently brush all surfaces of teeth and top of tongue. Remove debris and excess fluid as it accumulates. If patient bites down on brush or swab, wait for relaxation and then remove.

   Brush tongue lightly and avoid provoking gag if possible. Never put fingers into patient's mouth between teeth! Yanking out brush or swab may cause injury or break handle, leaving a piece of brush in mouth.

7. Rinse with warm water or half-strength peroxide (or both). Wipe or suction excess.

8. Reexamine mouth and teeth.

   Open areas and dental abnormalities may be masked by secretions.

9. Floss teeth if patient is cooperative, or floss can be attached to handled device for patient to use.

   Broken floss can become trapped in mouth and aspirated.

10. Apply medication if ordered or moisturizers to oral mucosa and tongue.

11. Insert mouth guard, if indicated, after cleansing.

12. Remove bite block.

13. Apply lip moisturizer.

 DOCUMENTATION

1. Document care and observations.

2. Report to the physician any signs of breakdown, disrepair, or unstable dentition.

3. Discuss modifications in care as required.

REFERENCES

Daeffler, R.J. (1986) "Oral Care." *The Hospice Journal* 2:81–103.

Nostril Care

PURPOSE

To preserve integrity of nasal mucosa by lubricating mucosa and removing debris; to prevent mucosal bleeding and breakdown; to promote patient comfort; to improve airway patency

STAFF RESPONSIBLE

EQUIPMENT

1. Soap and water
2. Wash cloth
3. Tissues
4. Cotton swabs
5. Flashlight
6. Water-soluble lubricant
7. Optional equipment:
   - Half-strength peroxide

- Tape (hypoallergenic)
- Skin barrier
- Saline nasal spray
- Nonsterile gloves

 ## GENERAL CONSIDERATIONS

1. Particular attention to nasal mucosa is due when
   - Nasoenteric tubes are in place
   - Nasal breathing is the primary route of respiration (if patient keeps mouth tightly closed)
   - Decannulation of tracheostomy has occurred, rerouting intake of air
   - Secretions are obvious and audible and patient cannot clear them on command
2. Nostril care is performed at least daily and more often as indicated by patient characteristics, as above.
3. Schedule the procedure when the patient is relaxed and in an upright position and before feeding.
4. Do not use petrolatum-based products or ointments. Oil droplet aspiration is possible.

Procedure

Nostril Care

 Steps

1. Wash hands.
2. Explain procedure to patient and elicit cooperation. Include caregiver as indicated.
3. If nasogastric tube is in place, remove tape and temporarily anchor it close to nose.
4. Cleanse external nares of tape, debris, oil, and perspiration.
5. Examine internal nares with flashlight for signs of trauma.
6. Lubricate several swabs and wipe nostrils clear from back to front while visualizing with light. Use halfstrength peroxide sparingly for crusted, adherent secretions. Rinse peroxide off with saline or water.

 Additional Information

Apply nonsterile gloves.

Caregiver or other staff can anchor tube and assist.

Adhesive removers must be thoroughly removed by soap and water to avoid irritation.
Nasogastric tubes can cause pressure necrosis.

Dried secretions may mask pressure areas, bleeding, or septal defects. Probing with swabs from front to back can drive secretions into pharyngeal airway to become aspirants or obstructions.

7. Avoid probing beyond length of nostril.

Vigorous sneezing or gagging can dislodge a nasogastric tube or provoke emesis. Deep probing cannot be visualized and may cause trauma to pharynx.

8. Minimize procedure if patient is uncooperative or cannot be controlled.

Gentle head control may be required. If so, another person should assist with this.

9. If ordered, use saline nasal spray at this point on dry internal areas.

Saline spray used two to four times a day maintains mucosal moisture.

10. Clean and dry nasogastric tube.

11. Reposition nasogastric tube to avoid contact with nasal mucosa.

Tubing placed against mucosa causes pressure and possible necrosis.

12. Apply tape securely to tube, tab it for easy removal, and apply it to new site on nose, below nostril, or nearby on cheek.

Alternate tape sites to prevent irritation to skin.

DOCUMENTATION

1. Document nasal care, observations, and interventions.

2. Report to the physician any unusual occurrence and request a change in care as indicated.

Unclogging Enteral Tubes

PURPOSE

To reestablish patency of an enteral feeding tube; to prevent the necessity of tube reinsertion

STAFF RESPONSIBLE

EQUIPMENT

1. Syringes with compatible Luer-Lok or catheter tip
   - 5 to 20 ml for small-diameter tube
   - 20 to 60 ml for tubes larger than # 10 French
2. Optional Equipment
   - Warm water
   - Carbonated beverage
   - Acidic juice
   - Meat tenderizer
   - Nonsterile gloves

 GENERAL CONSIDERATIONS

1. The optimal approach to maintain patency of enteral feeding tubes is to follow procedures for administration of feeding and medications. Nevertheless, obstruction may be anticipated as a common problem when:
   - Small-diameter feeding tubes are used (#10 French or smaller)
   - Viscous formulas are delivered at a slow rate
   - Gastric retention causes stasis of gastric contents
   - Nonliquid medication or supplements are administered
   - Fluid administration is restricted
   - Gastric content includes the residue of oral feeding
2. Attempts to unclog enteral tubes carry risks of tube displacement, tube rupture, and therefore, patient injury. To minimize the risks:
   - Assess the patient's recent history of tube-related complications and their resolutions
   - Use the most conservative, simple approaches first
   - Consult the physician for discussion of options available in unclogging the tube and for eliminating options that are contraindicated
   - Assess the relative risks of unclogging the tube compared to the disadvantages of removing and reinserting the tube.
3. Discuss with the physician modifications in care that minimize the recurrence of clogging
   - Choice of feeding formula or delivery method
   - Alternate choice of tube
   - Form of, or substitute for, medication
   - Frequency, amount, and type of tube flush

Procedure

Unclogging Enteral Tubes

 Steps

1. Wash hands.
2. Explain procedure to patient and position him or her as if for feeding.
3. Examine tube for external signs of displacement
   - Disturbed stabilization
   - Abnormal length of tube (shorter or longer than previously observed)
4. Disconnect and unclamp tube.

 Additional Information

Apply nonsterile gloves.

Attempts to unclog a displaced tube could result in aspiration or tissue trauma. Proximal end of tube may also be located against internal mucosa or kinked or coiled.

5. Gently milk tube from point of insertion to distal end and allow passive gravity drainage.

6. Fill a small syringe with warm water. Inject and withdraw water with gentle plunging action.

7. After a few minutes, wait for water to dissolve plug, then withdraw water from tube.

8. Gently milk tube again as in step 5.

9. Instill acidic, strained juice or fresh, cold, carbonated beverage into tube and clamp for 10 to 15 min.

10. Monitor patient for signs of discomfort or distress. Observe abdominal insertion sites.

11. Withdraw juice or carbonated beverage with gentle plunging.

12. As final approach, mix 1 tbs meat tenderizer with 1 oz water. Draw up in syringe, inject into tube, and clamp tube for 30 min.

13. Gently aspirate tenderizer solution from tube. Use warm water for gentle plunging as in step 6.

14. Discard tenderizer solution and any material unclogged from tube.

15. Flush tube thoroughly with water and resume feeding as appropriate.

16. If attempts to unclog tube are unsuccessful, report to physician for further intervention.

Milking may move a small plug and create mild negative pressure.

Water may dissolve a thin plug of particles. Vigorous plunging may further solidify plug or rupture tube.

Milk from proximal to distal end of tube.

Cranberry and citrus juices approximate acidity of gastric secretions. Carbonated beverages may be acidic or base. Carbonation is most concentrated from a chilled, freshly opened container. Carbonation may work by loosening particles from a mass or by creating pressure in tube. Acidic solutions may be more effective with plugs of medication. With feedings, acidic solutions coagulate protein and form a more solid plug.

Tube rupture may or may not be perceived by patient. Fluid in tube will be released at site of rupture and may leak at insertion site or compromise patient's airway.

Papain has been demonstrated as the effective ingredient of meat tenderizers that is enzymatic in action. Papain is derived from papaya, which is an allergen for some people. Check other ingredients as well for contraindications.

Vigorous plunging may further solidify plug or rupture tube.

 ## DOCUMENTATION

1. Document the problem, the approaches used, and the outcome.

2. Make any necessary modifications in nursing care to prevent its recurrence.

REFERENCES

Nicholson, L.J. (1987) "Declogging Small-Bore Feeding Tubes." *Journal of Parenteral and Enteral Nutrition* 11:594–597.

Webber-Jones, J., Sweeney, K., Winterbottom, A., et al. (1992) "Unclogging a Feeding Tube" *Nursing92* April, 63–64.

CHAPTER 2

Procedures to Maintain Mobility

Introduction

Mobility, or moving easily and freely without restrictions, is an integral part of life. Throughout our lives, we develop skills to learn to control and promote our mobility.

A loss in mobility results in both physical and psychological effects. Jacobs and Geels (1984) identified problems that may result in impaired mobility (Table 2-1).

Table 2-1	Problems That May Result in Impaired Mobility
Problem	**Condition**
Activity intolerance, diminished strength or endurance	Acute conditions: Myocardial Infarctions, Gastrointestinal Disorders Chronic conditions: Cancer, Congestive Heart Failure, Chronic Obstructive Pulmonary Disease, Autoimmune Deficiency Syndromes
Pain or discomfort	Burns, Chronic Pain, Postoperative Pain
Perceptual impairment	Visual Disorders, Tumor, Stroke, Brain Injury or Trauma
Cognitive impairment	Brain Injury or Trauma, Stroke, Tumor
Neuromuscular impairment	Multiple Sclerosis, Parkinson's Disease, Spinal Cord Injury, Myelitis, Amylotrophic Lateral Sclerosis
Musculoskeletal impairment	Arthritis, Fractures, Scoliosis, Muscular Dystrophy
Psychological impairment	Neurosis, Schizophrenia

The effects of immobility on the human body are well documented (Browse, 1965; Olson, 1967; Carnevali and Brueckner, 1970; Hart, Reese, and Fearing, 1981). Various sections of this book present specific interventions to prevent or minimize the effects of immobility on other body systems. For example, Chapter 3 includes procedures to prevent constipation or impaction and Chapter 4 includes procedures to prevent pressure sores.

In using the procedures in this chapter, basic patient safety should be the first concern. Therefore, with any newly admitted patient with potential or actual spinal column instability, it must first be ensured that the entire spine column is stable. Stability is generally determined by the physician on the basis of radiologic and neurologic examinations. If stability of the spinal column in the patient with potential or actual spinal injuries has not been determined, the patient must be placed on spinal precautions.

Stabilization of the spine can be accomplished through surgery or with the use of orthoses. If orthoses are used, it is imperative that those who apply them or work with patients who have them know exactly how they are applied, how they are to fit, how to adjust the orthosis, and who may make such adjustments. If a spinal orthosis is used, the patient must be placed on spinal precautions when the orthosis is removed or adjusted. Clarification of roles of various health workers in regard to maintaining spinal stability is vital.

The second area of concern is positioning. Some patients may be prone to or actually have contractures as a result of abnormal muscle tone or improper posturing. Appropriate positioning and frequent range of motion (ROM) can help prevent further limitations or promote functional ROM. To ensure optimal positioning in some patients, splints can be used. Casts (dropout, serial, and so forth) may be prescribed to stretch out contractures already present. The physical or occupational therapist should be consulted when planning interventions to minimize abnormal tone or to stretch out contractures.

Pain relief can improve mobility skills. Timely administration of pain medications; slow, rhythmic movements; transcutaneous electrical nerve stimulation (TENS); and the like may provide relief and relaxation so that maximum mobility can be achieved. Nevertheless, pain should be considered an important sign when intervening— ROM should only be done to the point of pain that can be detected by the patient's comments and behaviors.

Transfer techniques built on neurodevelopmental techniques as taught by Bobath (1978) and Gee and Passarella (1985) have been integrated into the procedures on mobility. The best transfers are ones that minimize any lifting and optimize the patient's own abilities. When determining how best to transfer any patient, the overview in Fig. 2-1 will lead to the most appropriate type of transfer.

The nurse should always encourage the patient to assist in the transfer to the maximum positive extent possible. Patients should *never* be allowed to put their arms around the nurse's neck. The nurse must use good body mechanics to protect himself or herself from potential back or other injury. A gait belt and simple one-step commands should be used. These

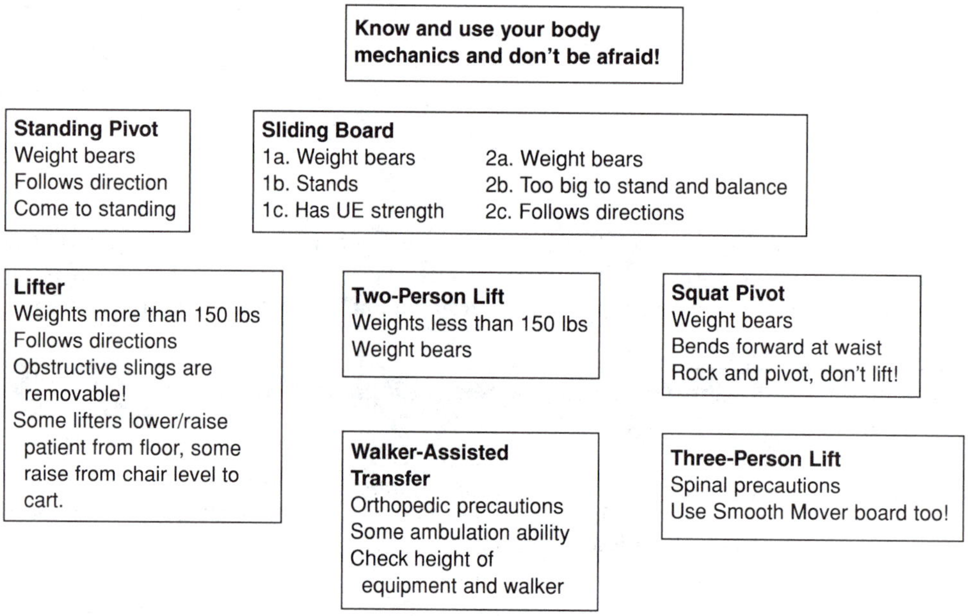

```
┌──────────────────────────────────┐
│         Know and use your body    │
│     mechanics and don't be afraid!│
└──────────────────────────────────┘
```

Standing Pivot
Weight bears
Follows direction
Come to standing

Sliding Board
1a. Weight bears
1b. Stands
1c. Has UE strength

2a. Weight bears
2b. Too big to stand and balance
2c. Follows directions

Lifter
Weights more than 150 lbs
Follows directions
Obstructive slings are
  removable!
Some lifters lower/raise
  patient from floor, some
  raise from chair level to
  cart.

Two-Person Lift
Weights less than 150 lbs
Weight bears

Squat Pivot
Weight bears
Bends forward at waist
Rock and pivot, don't lift!

**Walker-Assisted
Transfer**
Orthopedic precautions
Some ambulation ability
Check height of
  equipment and walker

Three-Person Lift
Spinal precautions
Use Smooth Mover board too!

Figure 2-1   Overview for determining best transfer techniques

help communicate clearly to the patient what is happening or going to happen in the transfer and establish a routine. When trying new transfer methods, the nurse should practice first on staff members to learn the steps and to identify potential problems. When the nurse is transferring a patient for the first time, someone should stand by for assistance and afterwards give feedback on the performance, use of body mechanics, and so forth.

Ambulation, with and without assistive devices, improves self-esteem. Suggestions for safe ambulation and correct use of assistive devices is presented. Community mobility skills are also important for safe care at home and the surrounding community.

Amputations may be the result of disease or trauma. They severely impair the individual's body image and restrict mobility. Early postoperative treatment and remobilization speeds emotional readjustment and resumption of everyday life skills.

REFERENCES

Bobath, B. (1978) *Adult Hemiplegia: Evaluation and Treatment* (2nd ed.) London: Heinemann Medical Books.

Browse, N.L. (1965) *The Physiology and Pathology of Bedrest.* Springfield, IL: Thomas.

Carnevali, D. and Brueckner, S. (1970) "Immobilization: Reassessment of a Concept" *American Journal of Nursing* 70:1502–1507.

Gee, Z.L. and Passarella, P.M. (1985) *Nursing Care of the Stroke Patient: A Therapeutic Approach* Pittsburgh, PA: AREN-Publications.

Jacobs, M.M. and Geels, W. (1984) *Signs and Symptoms in Nursing* Philadelphia: Lippincott.

Olson, E.V. (1967) "The Hazards of Immobility" *American Journal of Nursing* 67:780.

Spinal Column Stability Management

Assessment and Management of Spinal Column

PURPOSE

To identify patients at high risk for spinal column instability; to ensure and maintain spinal stability of all high-risk patients

STAFF RESPONSIBLE

GENERAL CONSIDERATIONS

1. Any nursing staff member may institute spinal precautions when admitting a patient if the patient meets any of the following criteria:

   - A spinal cord injury within the last 6 months
   - Spinal stabilization surgery within the last 6 months
   - An unstable spine due to disease process (cancer, osteoporosis, or the like), spinal surgery (except laminectomy without fracture), or immediately after a fall

2. Spinal precautions are clarified, further defined, or discontinued only by written physician prescription.

3. Determination of spinal stability is based on examination of full-spine roentgenograms to ensure skeletal alignment and stability with or without spinal orthoses and on sensory and motor examination.

4. Spinal orthoses are applied, adjusted, and removed only by trained personnel in accordance with specific orthosis procedures or specific physician order.

5. Whenever an orthosis is removed, spinal precautions will be followed until the orthosis is reapplied.

6. Definition of Terms
   - "Spinal precautions" mean that:
     - The patient is to be kept supine, lying flat in bed, without a pillow under the head, with appropriate periodic repositioning by staff
     - The head and lower section of the bed are not to be elevated
     - Logroll methods are to be used for all turning of the patient
     - Patient may not be positioned prone or ¾ prone unless specifically ordered

- "Stable with orthosis on" means that:
  - If prescribed orthosis is fitted securely in place, the patient may engage in the following activities:
    - One- or two-person turns
    - Head-of-bed elevated to 90 degrees
    - Wheelchair to 90 degrees (as tolerated)
    - Transfers by Trans-aid, sliding board, Surgilift, dependent pivot
    - Long sitting
    - Ambulation, if appropriate
    - Activities of daily living (as able)
    - Weekend passes when medically stable
    - Showers (sitting position)
    - Pool, only if specifically ordered
    - ROM and manual muscle test of all joints except the spine unless specifically contraindicated
  - If prescribed orthosis is not securely in place, spinal precautions as described above are to be observed.
- "Remove brace for hygiene" means that orthosis may only be removed after bathing/showering and skin care and that, while removed, spinal precautions should be observed. (Orthosis is not removed during showering, but removed afterwards to dry it.)
- "D/C spinal orthosis" means that the spine is stable and that restrictions to activity are discontinued unless otherwise specifically designated by the physician.
- "Stable without orthosis" means that the spine is stable and that activities functionally consistent with the condition or level of the lesion, including those listed in (6), are permitted.

7. Spinal precautions can be individualized according to physician prescription. Some patients may have their orthosis (or some part) removed while in bed and sit at varying degrees.

8. Spinal precautions used in radiology include: The Knight-Taylor orthosis is unclipped to place the metal clips aside in the anteroposterior view of the thoracolumbar spine after the patient is positioned supine on the table. For all other views, the orthosis remains intact. A transfer board is used to transfer the patient from cart to x-ray table. Views such as flexion-extension that necessitate complete removal of any orthosis or any part of a sternal occipital mandibular immobilizer (SOMI) require the presence of a physician. The technologist will remove the orthosis while the physician stabilizes the spine. If a patient is

admitted without orthosis, the same precautions as described previously are followed.

9. In the event of life-threatening emergencies, the need for life-support measures transcends spinal stability considerations. Although every reasonable effort to continue spinal stability should be employed, maintaining patency of airway and adequacy of ventilation and circulation are the first priorities. Jaw thrust with simultaneous cervical spine immobilization and other required maneuvers should be carried out with every possible precaution.

PATIENT AND FAMILY EDUCATION

1. Initial teaching should include spinal precautions, patient's and family's role in spinal precautions, function of orthosis, and patient's and family's role in orthosis management (cooperation with protocols).
2. If the patient will be discharged or on a pass with an orthosis, obtain written permission from the physician before teaching the application or removal of the orthosis.

Procedure

Methods to Establish Presence of Spinal Column Stability

 Steps

 Additional Information

1. Position patient supine

Bed should be flat, no elevation. No pillows under patient's head or trunk.

2. Assess correct body alignment by drawing an imaginary line from the patient's chin through the suprasternal notch to the symphysis pubis (Fig. 2-2).

This line will be straight if the patient is in correct alignment with the head in midline. If the patient has deformities, such as those caused by scoliosis or contractures, this line may never be straight.

3. Second, draw an imaginary line (from one side of the body to the other) through the shoulders and then through the hips.

These two lines will be parallel if the patient is in correct alignment. This ensures that both sides of the body are symmetric from the midline.

4. Make a judgment as to the degree of misalignment and the effect on the patient.

If the misalignment is minute, the patient should be logrolled into correct alignment. If the misalignment is severe or if there is loss of sensation or motor function, or if the patient complains of paresthesia, the physician should be called to see the patient. Subsequent prescriptions are carried out and documented.

 DOCUMENTATION

1. Record the need for spinal precautions.
2. Document patient and family education.
3. Document follow-through and any problems.

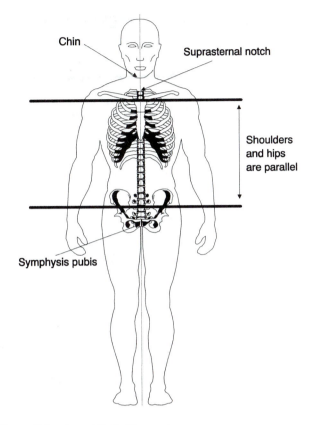

Figure 2-2 Correct Body Alignment

Logroll

PURPOSE

To maintain vertebral alignment during position change

STAFF RESPONSIBLE

EQUIPMENT

1. Three or more regular pillows
2. One firm head pillow of compact thickness equal to shoulder width or folded sheepskin, rolled sheepskin, rolled towel, or blanket
3. Bed, cart, or mat

 GENERAL CONSIDERATIONS

1. To logroll is to turn the patient so that the vertebral column moves as one unit.

2. Logrolling is required as follows:
   • For all spinal cord–injured patients who are admitted for the first time or who are readmitted within 6 months of injury or spinal stabilization until physician authorizes spinal stability prescriptions
   • As prescribed by physician
   • For all patients on spinal precautions (see procedure for managing spinal cord instability)

3. Spinal precautions mean that the patient is to be kept supine, lying flat in bed, with appropriate periodic repositioning and pressure relief supports. The head and lower foot section of the bed are not to be elevated. Logroll methods are to be used for all turning of the patient.

4. To assess for correct vertebral alignment in supine or side lying, the nurse must ensure that the chin is in line with the suprasternal notch and the symphysis pubis. The head must be in midline, both sides of the body symmetric from the midline, and the shoulders aligned with the hips.

5. The frequency of turning and positioning is determined by the nurse on assessing:
   • The patient's skin tolerance
   • The patient's respiratory condition
   • The patient's comfort

6. When the patient is designated by the physician as stable with orthosis on, logrolling is not required while the orthosis is on.

PATIENT AND FAMILY EDUCATION

1. The patient and family are taught the importance of logrolling to gain their cooperation in maintaining vertebral alignment.
2. The family members may participate in the procedure only after proper instruction and supervision by a nurse.

Procedure

Logroll

 Steps

Preparation

1. Assemble at least three staff members on same side of bed.
2. Wash hands, and remove any watches, bracelets, or rings.
3. Remove glasses and neck chains from patient.
4. Provide privacy.
5. Have pillows ready and available for final positioning.
6. All staff stand on same side of bed (Fig. 2-3A):
   • Tallest and strongest person (1) stands at head of patient, opposite to side that patient will face after turn.
   • Second tallest person (2) stands at patient's waist.
   • Third tallest person (3) stands between patient's buttocks and knees.

SUPINE TO SIDE LYING

 Steps

1. Each person consecutively places arms under patient by placing palms up and pressing down on mattress (Fig. 2-3B).
2. Position head pillow:
   • Head pillow is placed next to patient's head on side away from positioned staff.
   • Person 1 counts to three. On "three" all lift patient toward them to side of bed. Pillow may need re-adjustment (Fig. 2-3C).
3. Again, person 1 counts to three. On "three" all roll the patient away from them, onto his or her side in one coordinated movement (Fig. 2-3D).
4. Persons 1 and 2 stay in position and stabilize patient at head, shoulders, and hips to maintain alignment.

Additional Information

If patient's head is unsupported or uncontrolled, an additional staff member is needed to hold the head.
These may scratch the patient or cause pain.

They may be accidentally tugged on or pulled.

(1) This person controls head, shoulders, and chest area.

(2) This person controls chest to buttocks.
(3) This person controls buttocks and thighs.

 Additional Information

This is the only lifting that should occur during this procedure.

As patient reaches 90-degree angle to bed, each person places one arm in front of patient to block further rolling. Patient's head should roll onto head pillow.

Chin should be in line with suprasternal notch and symphysis pubis, head in midline, shoulders aligned with hips.

5. Person 3 steps to foot or head of bed and checks alignment.

6. Person 3 adjusts head pillow under patient's head and places one regular pillow behind patient's back and two regular pillows between legs.

7. Person 1 gently pulls own arms out from under patient, one arm at a time. Person 2 then does same.

8. Externally rotate and protract shoulder that patient is lying on, and place patient's arms in functional position (Fig. 2-3*E*).

If patient is slightly out of alignment, person 3 should return to position, and all should realign patient by logrolling again. If patient is severely out of alignment or exhibiting changes in sensation or motor function, contact physician. Do not move patient.

Legs are positioned so that top leg is slightly in front of or in back of bottom leg and ankle, knee and hip of top leg are in same horizontal plane.

Opposite arm of patient is placed in front or back of hip in functional position. If patient has upper extremity edema, support hand and arm on pillows, splints, foam blocks, or patient's hip.

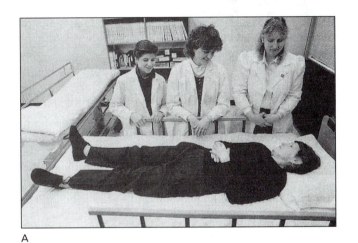

A

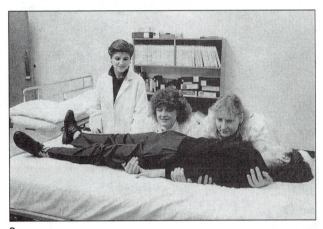

B

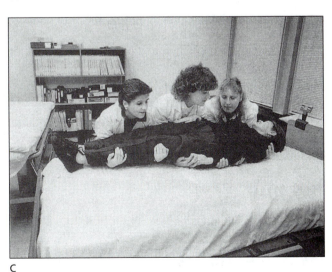

C

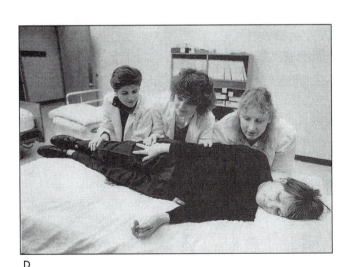

D

Figure 2-3 Logrolling

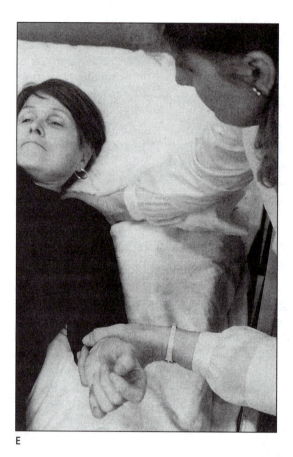

E

Figure 2-3 Logrolling (continued)

SIDE LYING TO SUPINE

 Steps

 Additional Information

1. Repeat steps 1 through 6 in preparation.

2. Persons 1 and 2 stabilize patient at shoulders and hips while person 3 removes back and leg pillows and adjusts head pillow.

   Head pillow should be adjusted so that when patient is rolled supine head is flat on bed.

3. Person 3 returns to previous position.

4. All staff place their hands palms up under patient's side and against patient's back.

   Consecutively place arms under patient by placing palms up and pressing down on mattress.

5. Person 1 counts to three. On "three" all roll patient toward them onto back in one coordinated movement.

6. Pull arms gently out from under patient, one arm at a time.

7. Person 3 checks alignment.

   Chin should be in line with suprasternal notch and symphysis pubis, head in midline, shoulders aligned with hips.

8. Put up side rails, move to opposite side of bed, and take up previous positions.

9. Person 1 counts to three. On "three" all lift patient to middle of bed.

   This should be the only lifting of patient.

10. Person 3 moves to foot of bed and checks alignment.

11. One person places patient's arms at sides in functional position.

If hand edema is a problem, that hand should be propped up on patient's hip or leg or with pillows, splints, or foam blocks.

 DOCUMENTATION

1. Document routine repositioning.
2. Note any unusual occurrences during the procedure (e.g., pain, positioning problems, poor tolerance, signs and symptoms of neurologic changes, and so forth).
3. Post "Patient Alert" signs at the bedside.

REFERENCES

Agee, B.L. and Herman, C. (1984) "Cervical Logrolling on a Standard Hospital Bed" *American Journal of Nursing* 84, 314–318.

Application, Removal, and Care of Spinal Orthoses

PURPOSE

To correctly apply, adjust, and remove spinal orthoses to maintain orthotic support of the spinal column

STAFF RESPONSIBLE

EQUIPMENT

No equipment necessary.

 GENERAL CONSIDERATIONS

1. The physician will write prescriptions specifying:
   • Which orthosis is to be worn
   • When the orthosis is to be worn
   • When the orthosis can be removed
   • How the patient is to be handled with and without the orthosis
   • Limits to mobility and activities (transfers and exercise); see "Assessment and Management of Spinal Cord Mobility"

2. The nurse and physical therapist determine:
   • Sitting angle
   • Type of wheelchair

3. Orthoses are prescribed depending on factors such as type, extent, and location of injury; patient's general health, healing history, and cooperation; anticipated duration of healing; allowance for maximum mobility; and the desired position for healing to occur.

4. Most orthoses do not provide total immobility (Table 2-2) but rather consist of specific components that limit movement detrimental to healing. A clear understanding of

Table 2-2	Limitations of ROM		
Type of Brace	**Limits Flexion**	**Limits Flexion, Extension, and Lateral Movements**	**Limits Flexion, Extension, Lateral Movements, and Rotation**
Cervical Orthosis (CO) (Fig. 2-4, *A, B*)		Soft cervical collars	SOMI, Philadelphia, Aspen, Newport
Cervical Thoracic Orthosis (Fig. 2-5)			Halo Jacket
Cervical Thoracolumbar Sacral Orthosis (CTLSO) (Fig. 2-6)			Halo Jacket, TLSO with SOMI attachment
Thoracolumbar Sacral Orthosis (TLSO) (Fig. 2-7 *A, B*)	Jewett	Knight-Taylor	TLSO/body jacket
Lumbar Sacral Orthosis (LSO) (Fig. 2-8)			Corset, TLSO, body jacket

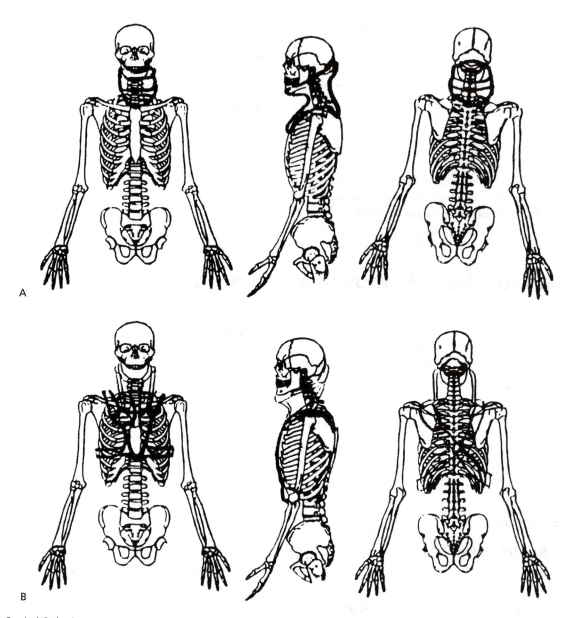

A

B

Figure 2-4   Cervical Orthosis

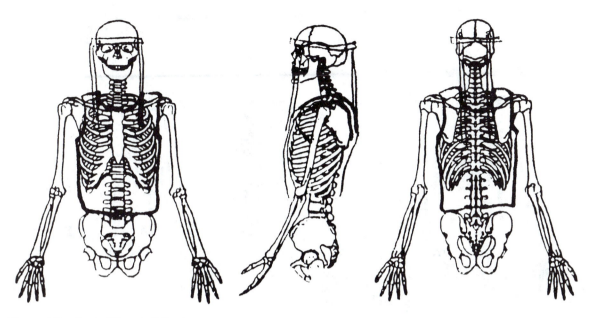

Figure 2-5 Cervical Thoracic Orthosis

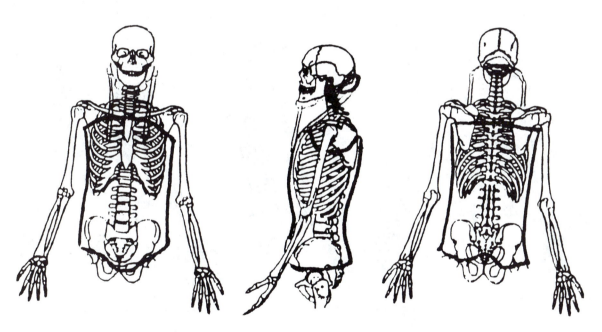

Figure 2-6 Cervical Thoracolumbar Sacral Orthosis

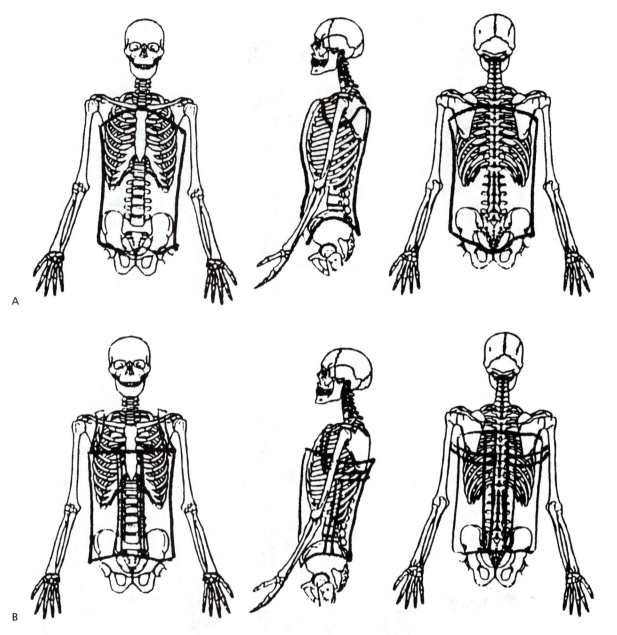

A

B

Figure 2-7 Thoracolumbar Sacral Orthosis

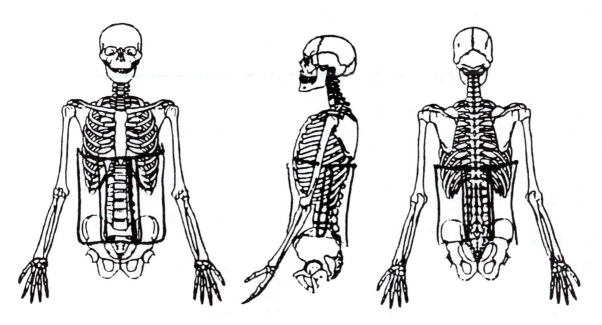

Figure 2-8 Lumbar Sacral Orthosis

these principles and the position to be maintained (neutral, flexion, or extension) is essential to the type of brace worn, patient assessment, interventions, decision making, and teaching.

5. Maximum orthotic support is provided by applying and maintaining the orthosis position at approximate anatomic landmarks (Fig. 2-9) and by molding the orthotic components to the individual patient's body contour. Additional padding to fill contours and to relieve pressure areas is only a temporary measure. No substantial padding (more than ½ in.) is permitted without the physician's prescription. An orthotist should be consulted.

6. Notify the physician concerning problems with orthotic fit or complaints of pain. If an orthotist is consulted, assist with patient position during adjustment and check for fit and problems in all usual patient positions while orthotist is present. Restrict patient movement and activity until adjustments are made.

7. Major orthotic adjustments (e.g., remolding, affixing pads, and disassembling components) are to be done only by a physician or an orthotist under physician prescription.

8. Minor orthotic adjustments (e.g., tightening or loosening straps and changing the level of the chin piece) are to be performed and anticipated by a nurse whenever a patient's position is changed. The shifting of body mass within some orthoses requires minor adjustments to maintain desired position and support. Other personnel are directed to stabilize the position until the adjustment is completed.

9. Routine skin checks, hygiene, and application or removal of clothing are important adjuncts to the care of a patient in an orthosis and must be planned for in response to individual patient problems and tolerance, in accordance with

physician prescription, and with assistance from nursing resource personnel. Patient weight gain or loss must be monitored at least weekly because it can affect orthotic fit.

PATIENT AND FAMILY EDUCATION

1. The patient and family are to be carefully instructed regarding the purpose of the orthosis and mobility restrictions, the importance of full cooperation for maintenance of spinal stability, and the necessity of seeking out the nurse's assistance for needed adjustments.

2. The patient and family may be instructed and supervised in the application, removal, and adjustment of an orthosis by a nurse only with a written prescription by the attending physician.

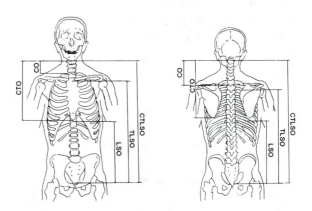

Figure 2-9 Characteristic Fitting Patterns of Spinal Orthoses to Bony Landmarks. *Source:* From "Clinical Applications in Spinal Orthotics" by D.G. Mueller, 1987, *Topics in Acute Care and Trauma Rehabilitation, 1*(3), p. 60. Copyright January 1987 by Aspen Publishers, Inc. Reprinted by permission of Glenn Case, illustrator.

Procedures

Cervical Orthoses: Soft Cervical Collar

GENERAL CONSIDERATIONS FOR SOFT CERVICAL COLLAR

1. Soft cervical collars restrict some degree of anterior flexion, posterior extension, and lateral movement of the cervical spine.

2. They are seldom restrictive enough if the injury or condition requires bony immobilization of the cervical spine.

3. They are helpful, after other cervical orthoses have been used, to support weak neck muscles until strength and endurance have developed.

4. Questions regarding adequate spinal stabilization should be discussed with the physician.

TO APPLY CERVICAL COLLAR

 Steps

1. Position patient supine.

2. Position collar so that Velcro closure is posterior and collar rests on inner crest of clavicle.

3. Fasten Velcro closure.

 Additional Information

Observe spinal precautions when collar is off, if collar is prescribed for spinal column stability.

Collar should fit snugly around patient's neck, yet not so tightly that it restricts respirations or is uncomfortable.

TO REMOVE SOFT CERVICAL COLLAR

 Steps

1. Position patient supine.
2. Unfasten Velcro closure.
3. Remove collar.

 Additional Information

Observe spinal precautions when collar is off.

CARE OF PATIENT USING SOFT CERVICAL COLLAR

 Steps

1. Wash patient's neck and chin.
2. Rub in a light layer of cornstarch or powder if collar is dirty or developing an odor.
3. Perform routine skin checks twice a day and as necessary.

4. Tee shirts may be worn under cervical collar.

5. Remove collar to take off tee shirt before hygiene procedures.

6. Shower or bathe patient (on flat-surface cart) without collar.

 Additional Information

This minimizes dirt buildup.

Powder should be lightly applied and rubbed in thoroughly before applying collar.

Special attention should be given to neck, cervical incision areas, and clavicles. Notify physician regarding problems with collar fit and complaints of pain.

Button-front shirts or V-neck tee shirts are easiest to manage.

A prescription to remove collar for hygiene must be written. Observe spinal precautions with collar off.

Clean and reapply collar after hygiene. Collar should be in place during transfers.

Procedures

Cervical Orthoses: Hard/Molded Cervical Collar
(Philadelphia, Aspen, Newport, and Others)

 GENERAL CONSIDERATIONS FOR HARD/MOLDED CERVICAL COLLAR

1. Hard/molded cervical collars restrict to a moderate degree anterior flexion, posterior extension, and lateral and rotating movements of the cervical spine.

2. They may be used to stabilize the cervical spine, to facilitate healing and to prevent further neurologic damage.

3. The collar is composed of two pieces of rigid foam or plastic reinforced anteriorly and posteriorly. Two Velcro closures are located laterally.

TO APPLY HARD/MOLDED CERVICAL COLLAR

 Steps

1. Position patient supine, without pillow under head.
2. Position posterior piece behind patient's head and neck with minimal head and neck movements.
3. Position anterior piece beneath patient's chin, and rest lower edge of collar on inner crest of clavicles.
4. Tuck anterior piece's lateral edges into posterior piece's lateral edges.
5. Secure Velcro closures on both lateral sides.

 Additional Information

Observe spinal precautions when collar is off.

Collar should fit snugly around patient's neck, yet not so tightly that it restricts respirations or is uncomfortable.

TO REMOVE HARD/MOLDED CERVICAL COLLAR

 Steps

1. Position patient supine, without pillow under the head.
2. Unfasten Velcro closures.
3. Remove anterior piece of collar.
4. Remove posterior piece of collar by pressing down on bed to minimize head and neck movement.

 Additional Information

Observe spinal precautions when collar is off.

CARE OF PATIENT USING HARD/MOLDED CERVICAL COLLAR

 Steps

1. Wash patient's neck and chin daily and as needed.
2. Routine skin checks are to be performed daily and as needed.

3. Tee shirts may be worn under Hard/Molded Cervical Collar.
4. Shower patient normally with collar on.

5. Remove collar, implementing spinal precautions, dry collar and patient, then reapply collar.

 Additional Information

This minimizes dirt buildup.

Special attention should be given to neck, cervical incision areas, clavicles, and chin. Notify physician regarding problems with collar fit and complaints of pain.

Button-front shirts or V-neck tee shirts are easiest to manage.

A prescription to remove collar for hygiene must be written, even though it's only to dry the collar.

Observe spinal precautions with collar off.

Procedures

Cervical Orthoses: Sternal Occipital Mandibular Immobilizer (SOMI) Orthosis

GENERAL CONSIDERATIONS FOR SOMI

1. The SOMI restricts to a moderate degree anterior flexion, posterior extension, and lateral and rotating movements of the cervical spine.

2. Maximum orthotic support is provided by applying and maintaining the SOMI orthosis in the following positions:
   - Sternal piece, ½ to 1 in. below the suprasternal notch
   - Occipital piece, just under the projection of the occiput
   - Mandibular piece, so that the patient can open his or her mouth wide enough to chew but not as wide as possible

3. The chin piece will need adjustment with position change (sitting, lying, or standing).

4. Tee shirts worn under a SOMI should have a loose neck opening and be one to two sizes larger than usual.

TO APPLY OR REMOVE SOMI

 Steps

1. Position patient supine, head neutral, no pillow under head.

2. Put on sternal piece with shoulder supports.

3. Feed shoulder straps under neck to opposite side.

4. Pull straps down past scapulae and fasten to front of sternal piece.

5. Turn occipital piece, and slide it under posterior aspect of neck just under projection of occiput.

6. Turn occipital piece so that prongs fit in sternal piece, and lock it in place.

7. Place mandibular support under chin and set in proper hole.

8. Lock mandibular support in place.

9. Buckle lateral chin straps beneath projection of occipital piece.

10. Reverse procedure to remove.

Additional Information

Neutral is when a straight plane passing under chin will be perpendicular to plane of bed with patient in supine position and parallel to floor in 90-degree angle with patient in sitting position.

The middle of the sternal piece should be 1 in. below sternal notch.

Be careful because patient may have increased sensitivity in posterior neck due to healing cervical incision.

Cup and lift each shoulder slightly to facilitate movement of strap over scapulae.

Put pressure on bed when sliding piece through to avoid pulling hair, touching stitches, and chilling neck from cold metal.

Position so that patient can open mouth enough to chew but not as wide as possible. Patient should see only distal one-third to one-half of lap when sitting and only toes when supine.

TO APPLY OR REMOVE TEE SHIRT UNDER SOMI

 Steps

1. Position patient in supine position.

2. Put one arm in tee shirt.

 Additional Information

If patient has pain or limited range in one shoulder, pull this arm through first.

3. Pull tee shirt over patient's head from front to back. Do not move head.

4. Slide tee shirt behind head with minimal head movement.

5. Pull other arm through sleeve.

6. Pull shirt down over chest.

7. Apply brace per above instructions.

8. Remove shirt by reversing procedure.

CARE OF PATIENT USING SOMI

 Steps

1. Perform routine skin checks.

2. No substantial padding (more than ½ in.) of orthosis is permitted without physician's order.

3. Remove brace to take off tee shirt before hygiene procedures.

4. Reapply brace before showering.

5. Remove brace, dry, and reapply after showering.

6. Mark horizontal and vertical chin support adjustments.

 Additional Information

Special attention should be given to occiput, scapula, chin, and clavicles. Notify physician of reddened areas and plan for pressure relief.

Tee shirts should be worn under SOMI brace. These shirts should have a large neck opening and be one to two sizes larger than regularly worn so as to avoid excessive movement of neck during application or removal.

A prescription to remove brace for hygiene must be written if patient is to be on spinal precautions when brace is off.

Do not transport patient with a mechanical lifter when SOMI brace is off. These devices do not provide enough support.

Two people are to be available when adjusting chin piece with patient in sitting or standing position (one to hold patient's head).

Procedures

Cervical Thoracic Orthoses: Halo Jacket

 GENERAL CONSIDERATIONS FOR HALO JACKET

1. There are several different types of halo jackets; one is shown in Fig. 2-10. Regardless of type, there are certain common characteristics:
   - The halo is stabilized by pins that are inserted into the patient's skull. This results in maximal limitations in head and neck (cervical spine) flexion, extension, hyperextension, rotation, and lateral movements.
   - The halo is usually applied by a physician in surgery after a fusion or other surgical procedure has been performed.
   - The halo usually remains in place for at least 3 months.

2. Do not use rods, head support bars, or any other metal hardware to turn, lift, or transfer patient.

3. Daily care should include:
   - Checking all bolts and skull pins for tightness, change in pin position, or movement of the pin
   - Inspecting skin surfaces for pressure areas
   - Inspecting skull pins for inflammation or drainage and signs of infection, including pain, tenderness, redness, heat, edema, odor, and skin adhesions
   - Cleaning all pin sites with soap and water

4. Weekly tightening of bolts by means of a torque screwdriver should be performed by a physician.

5. Inform physician immediately of:
   - Any pressure areas around or under halo brace

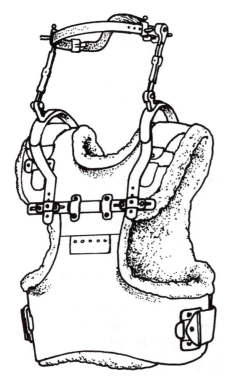

Figure 2-10   Halo Jacket

- Suspected infection at or around pin sites
- Patient complaints of pin site pain
- Patient complaints of clicking noises or buzzing

BATHING PATIENT WITH HALO JACKET

 Steps

1. Position patient supine.
2. Test anterior vest, hardware bolts, and skull pins with your fingers for tightness.
3. Inspect skull pin sites for any sign of infection or adhesions.
4. Cleanse skin surrounding skull pins with soap and water.
5. Open straps at bottom of vest and inspect skin surface for pressure.
6. Cleanse skin surface without soap under vest padding.
7. Dry skin surfaces thoroughly.
8. Refasten straps at bottom of vest.
9. Position patient on each side, and repeat steps 5 through 8.

- Slight movement of patient's head or neck (head rocks in halo) (could indicate loose pin)
- Pins loose or unscrewed when checked
- Patient complaints of paresthesia
- Changes in patient's motor abilities or sensation

6. The vest lining should be kept clean and dry. A physician's prescription is necessary to remove the liner to shower the patient. Do not shower the patient with the liner in place, unless a replacement is available. When showering a patient with a halo jacket, protect the liner by removing it. The patient's hair may be washed carefully. After drying the inside and outside of the jacket, replace the liner. The sheepskin liner may be removed for pool therapy.
7. Halo vests usually have a crease or removable plate for cardiopulmonary emergencies. A cardiac board is not necessary if the patient remains in the posterior shell of the brace.
8. All patients with a halo brace should have a complete wrench set attached to their wheelchair or nearby (e.g., taped to the front vest plate) at all times. A complete wrench set should be available on the nursing floor for emergency use.
9. The halo ring should ride 1 cm above the patient's eyebrows and ears and at least 1.5 cm away from the head. Skull pins should be at 90-degree angles to the skull. All bolts should be tight. The physician may tighten the bolts on a regular basis (weekly).

 Additional Information

If bolts are loose, institute spinal precautions and notify physician.

Hair surrounding pin sites should be kept short to aid in inspection and to prevent infection.

If crusts need to be removed, use ½ saline to ½ hydrogen peroxide to remove crusts.

Feel with your hands. Use flashlight if needed.

Use damp cloth to clean surfaces under vest.

Wet or damp vest padding can lead to skin breakdown or infection and will need to be changed.

Patient should be supported in side-lying position by another caregiver, so nurse can provide care with both hands.

HALO JACKET WITH VELCRO SHEEPSKIN LINER

 Steps

1. Position patient for liner removal.
2. Detach sheepskin liner, starting at shoulders and working downward.
3. Remove liner pieces.

4. If in bed, position in shower chair.
5. Shower patient.
6. Dry patient's exposed skin.
7. Use dry washcloth to dry inside of halo jacket and patient's trunk.
8. Replace sheepskin liner, starting at shoulders and working downward.

 Additional Information

Either sitting in shower chair or lying in bed.

Liner is usually in two pieces, an anterior and a posterior piece.

Side straps may need to be opened to facilitate smooth reinsertion of the liner.

Carefully transfer patient from bed to shower chair.

May transfer patient to bed to dry thoroughly.

Procedures

Thoracolumbar Sacral Orthoses: Knight-Taylor Orthosis with Pectoral Horns

 GENERAL CONSIDERATIONS FOR KNIGHT-TAYLOR ORTHOSIS

1. The Knight-Taylor orthosis restricts anterior flexion, posterior extension, and lateral movements of the thoracolumbosacral spine. The addition of a chin piece can result in limitations of the cervical spine.

2. Maximum orthotic support is provided by applying and maintaining the Knight-Taylor orthosis in the following positions:
   - Vertebral spinal process should lie between the paraspinal bars or along the main bar
   - Lateral lower edge of the orthosis should lie above the head of the femur and below the iliac crest

   - Shoulders should be slightly retracted
   - If a chin piece is used the head should be maintained in a neutral position

3. Minor orthotic adjustments (e.g., tightening or loosening straps and changing the level of the chin cup) are to be anticipated and performed by a nurse whenever a patient's position is changed. Shifting of body mass requires adjustment to maintain desired position and support.

4. Patient weight gain or loss must be monitored weekly because it can affect the orthotic fit.

5. The Knight-Taylor orthosis provides support to the abdomen. When the orthosis is removed, monitor for orthostatic hypotension, trunk instability, and changes in the patient's voiding pattern.

TO APPLY KNIGHT-TAYLOR ORTHOSIS

 Steps

1. Logroll patient to side-lying position. Two people should stabilize patient.

2. Center posterior of orthosis on back.

3. Align lower edge of orthosis so that lateral sides are centered between trochanter and iliac crest.

4. Feed lateral side of orthosis and corset under patient.

 Additional Information

Observe spinal precautions. When orthosis is applied, the detachable pectoral horn should be bottom-most and removed.

If paraspinal bars are present, be sure that the vertebral spinal processes lie between them.

5. Tighten and fasten straps of anterior corset from bottom up.

6. Feed loose pectoral horn under patient's axilla that is against bed (feed shoulder strap over shoulders if present).

7. Screw pectoral horn into place as noted previously.

8. Turn patient to supine position, holding posterior orthosis firmly against patient.

9. Fasten chin piece if present.

10. Adjust shoulder straps if present to position shoulders in retraction and external rotation.

11. Assess fit.

Make sure it is snug so as to prevent sliding up when patient sits.

Screw tightly. Note if thread becomes stripped and screw slips.

No need to logroll if corset and pectoral horns are in place.

Orthosis should restrict anterior flexion, posterior extension, and lateral movements of thoracolumbosacral spine. Chin piece limits cervical spine movement.

TO REMOVE KNIGHT-TAYLOR ORTHOSIS

 Steps

1. Position patient side lying.

2. Unfasten shoulder strap, or unscrew and remove pectoral horn on which patient is lying.

3. Undo all straps on corset (and chin piece if applicable).

4. Roll corset back under patient.

5. Standing behind patient, gently pull off brace.

6. Carefully raise patient's uppermost arm so that other pectoral horn does not catch or scratch arm.

7. Logroll patient to desired position in correct alignment.

 Additional Information

Detachable pectoral horn should be bottom-most.

At this time, patient begins on spinal precautions. Two people should stabilize patient. Note and mark holes from which screws were removed when removing pectoral horn.

So corset will not scrape patient's skin when removed, press brace against mattress to facilitate its removal and to prevent injury to patient.

Transfers are not performed without orthosis applied.

CARE OF PATIENT USING KNIGHT-TAYLOR ORTHOSIS

 Steps

1. Perform routine skin checks.

2. No substantial padding of orthosis is permitted without physician's prescription.

3. Remove brace to take off tee shirt before hygiene procedures.

4. Reapply brace before showering.

 Additional Information

Special attention should be given to chin, scapulae, vertebrae, and anterior pectorals.

Tee shirts should be worn under Knight-Taylor brace and should be one to two sizes larger than regularly worn so as to avoid excessive movement when dressing or undressing.

A prescription to remove brace for hygiene must be written if patient is to be on spinal precautions when brace is off. Do not transport patient with mechanical lifter when Knight-Taylor brace is off. These devices do not provide enough support.

An extra corset will allow for increased independence because patient will be able to shower when sitting up with brace on. Remove wet corset and apply dry corset after showering with patient supine or on spinal precautions. Allow wet corset to air dry. Use of a dryer may damage metal stays in corset.

Procedures

Thoracolumbar Sacral Orthoses: TLSO/Body Jacket

GENERAL CONSIDERATIONS FOR TLSO/BODY JACKET

1. TLSO/body jackets restrict anterior flexion, posterior extension, lateral and rotating movements of the thoraco-lumbosacral and lumbosacral spine.

2. The TLSO/body jacket may or may not indicate spinal instability. It may be used as a preventive measure for spinal deformities and respiratory compromise. It is important to ascertain the purpose of the TLSO/body jacket.

3. When a TLSO/body jacket is used as a preventive measure, spinal precautions are not necessary when the patient is not wearing the TLSO/body jacket or when applying the TLSO/body jacket. The patient may apply and remove the TLSO/body jacket.

4. When the TLSO/body jacket is used for spinal stability, the patient should be logrolled to one side for the nurse to position the posterior shell and then logrolled supine. The anterior shell should be positioned correctly and the straps secured.

5. TLSO/body jackets are individually created for each patient to fit his or her body. Weight gain and loss should be monitored at least weekly. A child's growth also needs to be monitored to ensure proper fit.

6. Notify the physician if the patient complains of pain after TLSO/body jacket application or if weight gain or loss or growth occurs rapidly.

TO APPLY TLSO/BODY JACKET

 Steps

1. Logroll to side lying.
2. Place posterior shell behind patient, feeding lateral edge underneath side on which patient is lying.
3. Logroll supine into posterior shell.
4. Apply anterior shell.
5. Secure closures.

TO REMOVE TLSO/BODY JACKET

 Steps

1. Position patient supine.
2. Disengage side closures.
3. Remove anterior shell of TLSO/body jacket.
4. Logroll to side.
5. Remove posterior shell from patient.

 Additional Information

If on spinal precautions.

TLSO/body jacket should fit properly across chest and under arms to iliac crests.
Patient is now off spinal precautions.

 Additional Information

Logroll patient to side if TLSO/body jacket is used for spinal stability.

Procedure

TLSO with SOMI

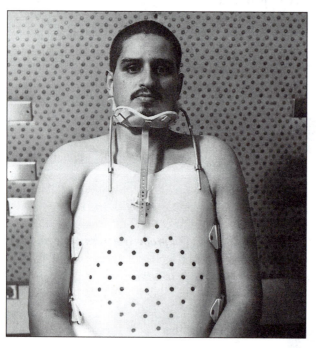

Figure 2-11

 GENERAL CONSIDERATIONS FOR TLSO WITH SOMI

1. The SOMI portion restricts to a moderate degree anterior flexion, posterior extension, lateral and rotating movements of the cervical spine (Fig. 2-11). The TLSO/body jacket portion restricts anterior flexion, posterior extension, lateral and rotating movements of the thoracolumbosacral and lumbosacral spine.

2. Maximum orthotic support is provided by applying and maintaining the SOMI portion of the orthosis in the following positions:
   - Occipital piece, just under the projection of the occiput
   - Mandibular piece, so that the patient can open his or her mouth wide enough to chew but not as wide as possible

3. The chin piece will need adjustment with position change (sitting, lying, or standing).

4. Tee shirts should be worn under TLSO with SOMI. These shirts should have a large neck opening and be one to two sizes larger than regularly worn so as to avoid excessive movement of neck during application or removal. Remove orthosis for changing the tee shirt and to dry after showering only.

5. When applying the TLSO portion, the patient should be logrolled to one side for the nurse to position the posterior shell and then logrolled supine. The anterior shell should be positioned correctly. The occipital portion of the SOMI should be attached. The mandibular portion of the SOMI should be attached. Then the buckles of the TLSO should be secured.

6. TLSO/body jackets are individually created for each patient to fit his or her body. Weight gain and loss should be monitored at least weekly. A child's growth also needs to be monitored to ensure proper fit.

7. Notify the physician if the patient complains of pain after TLSO with SOMI application or if weight gain or loss or growth occurs rapidly.

8. Check occiput area for skin problems especially.

TO APPLY TLSO WITH SOMI

Steps

1. Logroll to side lying.
2. Place posterior shell behind patient, feeding lateral edge underneath side on which patient is lying.
3. Logroll to supine in posterior shell. Position patient supine, head neutral, no pillow under head.
4. Apply anterior shell.
5. Turn occipital piece of SOMI, and slide it under posterior aspect of neck just under projection of occiput.

 Additional Information

TLSO/body jacket should fit properly across chest and under arms to iliac crests.

Be careful because patient may have increased sensitivity in posterior neck due to healing cervical incision.

6. Turn occipital piece so that prongs fit in TLSO, and lock it in place.

7. Place mandibular support under chin and set in proper hole.

Put pressure on bed when sliding piece through to avoid pulling hair, touching stitches, and chilling neck from cold metal.

Position so that patient can open mouth enough to chew but not as wide as possible. Patient should see only distal one-third to one-half of lap when sitting and only toes when supine.

8. Lock mandibular support in place.

9. Buckle lateral chin straps beneath projection of occipital piece.

10. Secure side straps on TLSO.

TO REMOVE TLSO WITH SOMI ATTACHMENT

 Steps

1. Position patient supine

2. Remove mandibular piece of SOMI.

3. Loosen occipital piece of SOMI and turn it sideways to remove.

4. Disengage side closures.

5. Remove anterior shell of TLSO/body jacket.

6. Logroll to side.

7. Remove posterior shell from patient.

 Additional Information

TO APPLY OR REMOVE TEE SHIRT UNDER SOMI

 Steps

1. Position patient in supine position.

2. Put one arm in tee shirt.

3. Pull tee shirt over patient's head from front to back. Do not move head.

4. Slide tee shirt behind head with minimal head movement.

5. Pull other arm through sleeve.

6. Pull shirt down over chest.

7. Logroll to side to put tee shirt down in back and apply posterior shell of TLSO.

8. Apply brace as instructed.

9. Remove shirt by reversing procedure.

 Additional Information

If patient has pain or limited range in one shoulder, pull this arm through first.

CARE OF PATIENT USING TLSO WITH SOMI ATTACHMENT

 Steps

1. Perform routine skin checks.

2. No substantial padding (more than ½ in.) of orthosis is permitted without physician's order.

 Additional Information

Special attention should be given to occiput, scapula, and chin. Notify physician of reddened areas and plan for pressure relief.

3. Remove brace to take off tee shirt before hygiene procedures.

4. Reapply brace before showering.

5. Remove brace, dry, and reapply after showering.

6. Mark horizontal and vertical chin support adjustments.

A prescription to remove brace for hygiene must be written if patient is to be on spinal precautions when brace is off.

Do not transport patient with a mechanical lifter when TLSO with SOMI is off. These devices do not provide enough support.

Two people are to be available when adjusting chin piece with patient in sitting or standing position (one to hold patient's head).

Procedures

Thoracolumbar Sacral Orthoses: Corset

GENERAL CONSIDERATIONS FOR CORSET

1. Corsets restrict anterior flexion, posterior extension, and lateral and rotating movements of the thoracolumbosacral and lumbosacral spine.

2. A corset may or may not indicate spinal instability. It may be used as a support to relieve back pain. It is important to ascertain the purpose of the corset.

3. When a corset is used as a support, spinal precautions are not necessary when the patient is not wearing the corset or when applying the corset. The patient may apply and remove it himself or herself.

4. When the corset is used for spinal stability, the patient should be supine for the nurse to position the posterior portion of the corset correctly.

5. Notify the physician if weight gain or loss or periods of rapid growth occur because these will alter fit.

TO APPLY CORSET

 Steps

1. Position patient supine.
2. Roll up far side of corset to facilitate easy pull through once patient is lying on corset.
3. Tuck corset under patient.
4. Gently pull out far side of corset.

5. Approximate edges of corset.

6. Latch both edges of corset together.

TO REMOVE CORSET

 Steps

1. Position patient supine.
2. Disengage corset latches.
3. Roll sides of corset distal to patient.
4. Tuck one side of corset under patient's far posterior side.
5. Gently pull corset out from underneath patient.

 Additional Information

Watch that clips do not scrape patient's skin.

Center posterior portion of corset so that metal stays are symmetrically placed.

Anterior portion of corset should lie above anterior iliac crest. If LSO corset, top anterior edge should lie below ribs. If TLSO corset, top anterior edge should lie over the ribs.

 Additional Information

DOCUMENTATION

1. Document the physician's prescriptions and related measures regarding the specific spinal orthosis.
2. Note any problems in the fit of the orthosis.
3. Note any problems that the patient is experiencing during adjustment to the orthosis.
4. Note the patient's tolerance and compliance.
5. Document any actions taken to remedy any problems.
6. Note the nursing measures that are currently in effect.

REFERENCES

Hanak, M. and Scott, A. (1983) *Spinal Cord Injury: An Illustrated Guide for Health Care Professionals* New York: Springer.

Matthews, P.J. and Carlson, C.E. (1987) *Spinal Cord Injury: A Guide to Rehabilitation Nursing* Rockville, MD: Aspen.

Mueller, D.G. (1987) "Clinical Applications in Spinal Orthotics" *Topics in Acute Care and Trauma Rehabilitation* 1:48–61.

Olson, R.S. (1996) "Halo Skeletal Traction Pin Site Care: Towards Developing a Standard of Care" *Rehabilitation Nursing* 21(5):243–6, 257, 284.

Styrcula, L. (1994) "Traction Basics: Part III. Types of Traction" *Orthopaedic Nursing* 13(4):34–44.

Zejdlik, C.M. (1983) *Management of Spinal Cord Injury* Belmont, CA: Wadsworth.

Maintenance of Range of Motion

Straight-Plane Range of Motion (ROM)

PURPOSE

To achieve safely the fullest range of functional motion possible within joints that have been affected by the consequences of disease, trauma, or immobility

STAFF RESPONSIBLE

 GENERAL CONSIDERATIONS

1. Decisions regarding the frequency and type of ROM to be used on selected joints are to be made by the nurse in conjunction with the physician, physical therapist, and occupational therapist. The specifics are to be recorded in the patient's nursing care plan.

2. ROM may be of the active, active assistive, or passive types as indicated.

3. Each joint being ranged is to be cupped in one hand to monitor it for resistance, pain, increased tone, or crepitus. Pain is the limiting factor. Resistance and tone can be overcome by proper movements. The joint is ranged no farther than its limits. Report changes in the limits to the physician and therapists.

4. Each joint is to be ranged singularly, slowly, and rhythmically, with each motion being repeated only as directed, usually three or more times.

5. Combine motions at wrist and hand and at ankle and foot, unless directed otherwise by the physician and/or therapists.

6. Encourage the patient to deep breathe and to relax during ROM. A relaxing environment is therapeutic.

7. ROM can and should be combined with routine care and activities of daily living.

8. Periodically document the frequency of ROM, the patient's tolerance, and the effects of ROM.

9. Upper extremity spasticity and pain can interfere with the rehabilitation process. One area which is often overlooked when performing PROM with an individual with hemi-

plegia is the presence of spasticity and movement ability in the scapula. When the arm is raised in flexion or abduction, the scapula must glide and rotate upwardly in a 2:1 ratio. In the hemiplegic shoulder, the muscles which move the scapula downward are often spastic. This makes it difficult for the scapula to glide upwards, which is necessary for pain-free movement. Scapular mobilization techniques are used to reduce spasticity and to passively assist with the gliding motion of the scapula.

10. Definitions of terms (Table 2-3):
    - Range of motion or range of joint motion (ROJM): the extent of movement within a given joint
    - Median: pertaining to or toward the middle or midline
    - Flexion: the bending of a joint in which the two adjacent parts approach each other
    - Extension: the straightening of a joint in which two adjacent parts are brought into straight alignment
    - Hyperextension: moving the joint in the direction of extension beyond a straight line
    - Abduction: movement away from the midline of the body
    - Adduction: movement toward the midline of the body
    - Internal rotation: turning toward the midline
    - Rotation: turning a joint on its own axis
    - External rotation: turning away from the midline
    - Pronation: turning the forearm so that the palmar surface of the hand is facing downward
    - Supination: turning the forearm so that the palmar surface of the hand is facing upward (also referred to as radial-ulna articulation)
    - Deviation: used to describe abduction or adduction of the wrist
    - Opposition: placing the palmar surface of the thumb so that it touches the base of the fingers
    - Dorsiflexion: ankle movement in which the upper surface of the foot approaches the anterior surface of the lower leg
    - Plantar flexion: the movement of the ankle in which the foot is bent down in the direction of the sole
    - Inversion: the turning of the foot so that the sole tends to face inward
    - Eversion: the turning of the foot so that the sole tends to face outward
    - Active ROM: those exercises in which the contraction of the person's muscle accomplishes the movement

within the free range, entirely or in part, without the aid or opposition of some external force

- Active assistive ROM: those exercises in which the contraction of the person's muscles accomplishes the movement within the free range with the aid of some external force
- Passive ROM: those movements within the free range of motion that are produced entirely by an external force without active contraction of the person's muscles
- Resistive ROM: those movements possible at the joint that are produced entirely by an external force producing muscle stretching or contraction

PATIENT AND FAMILY EDUCATION

1. Teach the patient and family to perform ROM as soon as possible, with special attention to the limiting factor of pain, following their own individualized program.

2. Teach the patient and family to report any pain, changes in joints and movements, concerns, and complications to the nurse, therapist, or physician immediately.

Table 2-3   Movements Possible at Each Joint with Patient Supine

Neck	Shoulder	Elbow	Wrist	Fingers and Thumb	Forearm	Hip	Knee	Ankle	Toes
Forward flexion	Flexion	Flexion	Flexion	Flexion	Supination	Flexion	Flexion	Dorsiflexion (heel cord stretch)	Flexion
Extension	Extension	Extension	Extension	Extension	Pronation (radial-ulna articulation)	Extension	Extension	Plantar flexion	Extension
Lateral flexion	Abduction		Abduction (ulna deviation)	Abduction		Abduction		Inversion (in dorsiflexion)	Abduction
Rotation	Adduction		Adduction (radial deviation)	Adduction		Adduction		Eversion (in plantar flexion)	Adduction
Hyper-extension	Ext. rotation			Opposition (thumb)		Ext. rotation			
	Int. rotation					Int. rotation			
	Protraction								
	Retraction								

Procedures

Range of motion sequence includes movements to be done and verbal cues to patient, family, or staff.

Neck

To be done only by patient, sitting or supine without pillow, with cues from staff. Movements are contraindicated in patients with cervical orthoses.

Movement

1. Flexion (Fig. 2-12*A*)
2. Extension (Fig. 2-12*B*)
3. Hyperextension (Fig. 2-12*C*)

4. Lateral flexion (Fig. 2-12*D*)
5. Rotation (Fig. 2-12*E*)

Patient Directions

"Chin on chest"

"Chin up"

"Look at ceiling" (may be contraindicated in elderly patients; extreme ranges should be avoided)

"Ear to shoulder" (right and left)

"Look over shoulder" (right and left; may be contraindicated in elderly patients; extreme ranges should be avoided)

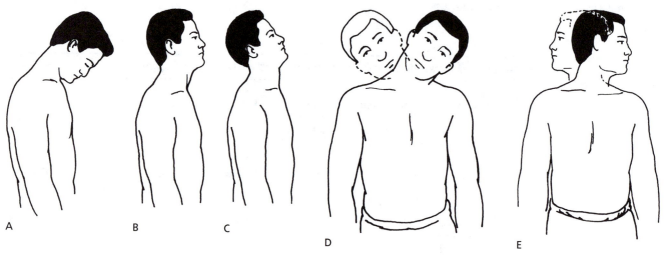

Figure 2-12   Neck ROM. (**A**) Flexion, (**B**) Extension, (**C**) Hyperextension, (**D**) Lateral Flexion, (**E**) Rotation.

Scapular Mobilization

Cup the inferior angle of the scapula with one hand and support upper arm with other. As you flex the shoulder, gently move the inferior angle of the scapula horizontal away from the spine (Fig. 2-13).

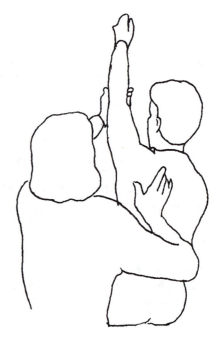

Figure 2-13

Shoulder

Start by protracting shoulder, arm pronated. Nurse places one hand over scapula to check movements as shoulder exercises are performed. Upward and outward movement of scapula accompanies shoulder movement. (Fig. 2-14).

Movement

1. Flexion-extension (Fig. 2-14*A*)

2. Abduction-adduction (Fig. 2-14*B*)

3. External and internal rotation (Fig. 2-14*C*)

Patient Directions

"Reach for headboard; down at side" or "Reach up to the sky; down at side"

"Move arm out and in" or "Move arm away from you, then back"

First position arm out to side at shoulder level with elbow bent at right angle, "Thumb a ride over same shoulder, move arm forward while turning thumb in at side"

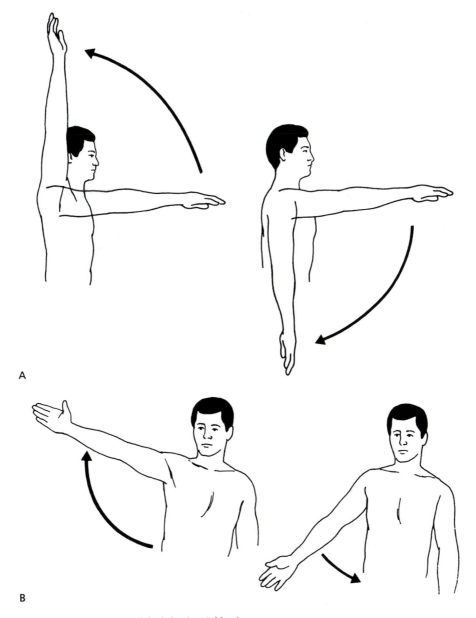

Figure 2-14   Shoulder ROM. (**A**) Flexion-Extension, (**B**) Abduction-Adduction.

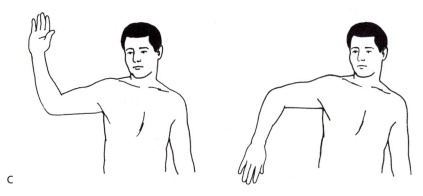

Figure 2-14 (continued) (**C**) External and Internal Rotation.

Elbow and Forearm

Start with arm in supination.

Movement

1. Flexion-extension (Fig. 2-15*A*)
2. Supination-pronation (Fig. 2-15*B*)

Patient Directions

"Bend and straighten"
With elbow fixed, "Turn palm up, palm down"

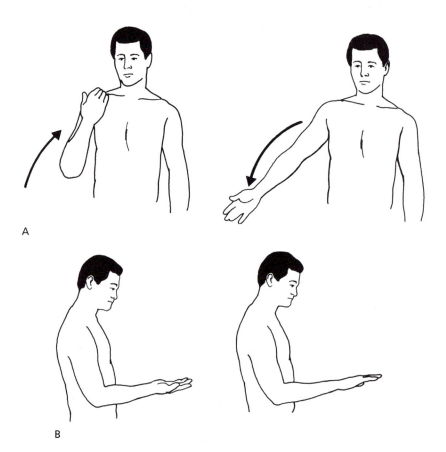

Figure 2-15 Elbow and Forearm ROM. (**A**) Flexion-Extension, (**B**) Supination-Pronation.

Wrist and Hand

Start by propping arm up on elbow, forearm pronated; one hand on wrist and thumb, other hand around fingers to facilitate natural tenodesis in hands.

Movement

1. Wrist flexion and finger extension, abduction (Fig. 2-16*A*)
2. Wrist extension and finger flexion, thumb opposed (Fig. 2-16*B*)

Patient Directions

"Down and out"

"Up and in"

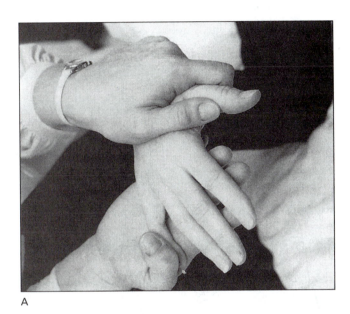 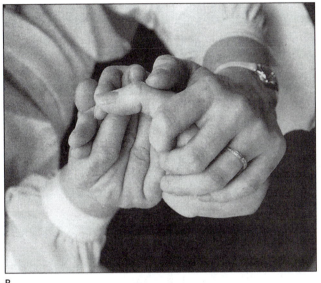

A   B

Figure 2-16   Wrist and Hand ROM. (**A**) Wrist Flexion and Finger Extension, Abduction; (**B**) Wrist Extension and Finger Flexion, Thumb Opposed.

Wrist

Start with arm straight and pronated.

Movement

1. Ulnar and radial deviation (Fig. 2-17)

Patient Directions

"Turn wrist in and out in flat plane"

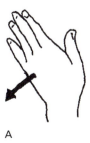   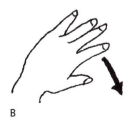

A   B

Figure 2-17   Wrist ROM. (**A**) Ulnar Deviation, (**B**) Radial Deviation.

Hip

Start by protracting hip. Find trochanter with cupped hand, place other hand on back of calf.

Movement

1. Flexion-extension (Fig. 2-18*A*)
2. Abduction-adduction (Fig. 2-18*B*)
3. External and internal rotation (Fig. 2-18*C*)

4. Hyperextension (position patient prone or side lying) (Fig. 2-18*D*)

Patient Directions

"Sole of foot to ceiling and down"

"Move leg out and in"

"Use palms of hands only on thighs and shins, roll back and forth like a rolling pin"

Prone: "Lift straight leg toward ceiling (30 to 45 degrees hyperextension)" Side lying: "Move top straight leg back toward side of bed"

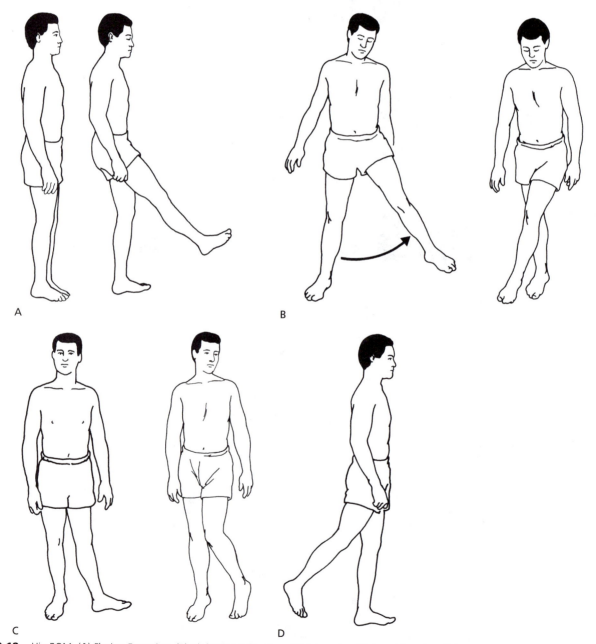

A   B

C   D

Figure 2-18   Hip ROM. (**A**) Flexion-Extension, (**B**) Abduction-Adduction, (**C**) External and Internal Rotation, (**D**) Hyperextension.

Scapular Mobilization with Trunk Rotation

Position side lying. Place your hands at scapula and pelvis. Stretch and rotate top side of trunk in diagonal to elongate trunk so upper body rotates separately from lower body (Fig. 2-19). Then bring the scapula back and pelvis forward, so hand hold is reversed.

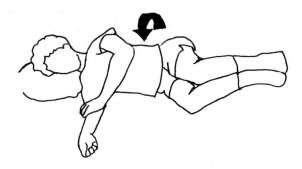

Figure 2-19

Knee

Movement

1. Flexion (Fig. 2-20*A*)
2. Extension (Fig. 2-20*B*)

Patient Directions

"Bend your knee and raise toward your head"

"With leg in bent position, straighten your leg"

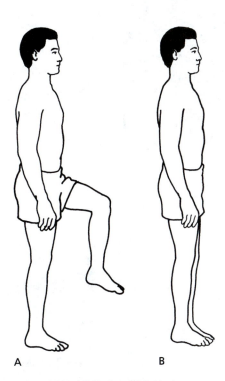

A   B

Figure 2-20   Knee ROM. (**A**) Flexion, (**B**) Extension.

Ankle and Foot

Start with one hand cupping heel, the other around midsection of foot. Besides dorsiflexion and inversion, a good stretch of the heel cords must be done by helper to decrease risk of tightening or fixation.

Movement

1. Dorsiflexion and inversion (Fig. 2-21)
2. Plantar flexion and eversion (Fig. 2-22)

Patient Directions

Toes up, sole in: "Up and in"

Toes down, sole out: "Down and out"

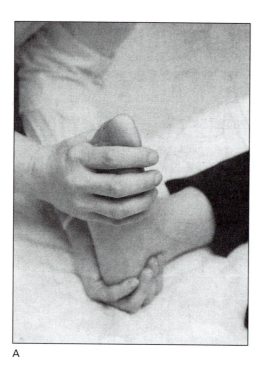 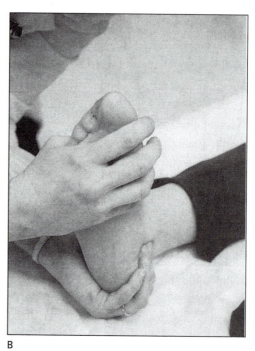

Figure 2-21 Dorsiflexion and Inversion. (**A**) View 1, (**B**) View 2.

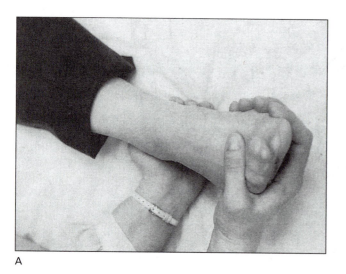 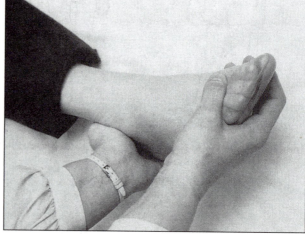

Figure 2-22 Plantar Flexion and Eversion. (**A**) View 1, (**B**) View 2.

DOCUMENTATION

1. Specify frequency, type, position, and times of ROM.
2. Document any complications, patient complaints, and therapeutic effects noted.
3. Note effectiveness of patient and family teaching.

Upper Extremity Self-Range of Motion for the Patient with Hemiplegia

PURPOSE

To maintain and/or increase the functional ROM of the affected extremity; to prevent deformities or contractures in the affected extremity; to promote awareness of the affected side of the body; to aid in decreasing edema in an affected hand; to provide some sensation to an affected extremity; to enhance strength and quality of movement when there is a return of voluntary motion

STAFF RESPONSIBLE

 GENERAL CONSIDERATIONS

1. ROM exercises are contraindicated in a "hot" joint, that is, a joint that is inflamed, red, warm, or swollen.
2. The following exercises should be carried out daily; each exercise is to be performed five to ten times.
3. Because the exercises may cause pain to the patient, movements should be carried out only to the point of pain.
4. Some patients may tend to overrange or inaccurately range themselves, thus producing pain or joint deformity (subluxation). Such patients should be guided to remain within the specific range and number of repetitions.
5. The patient should perform exercises while sitting down unless otherwise instructed.

PATIENT AND FAMILY EDUCATION

1. Teach the patient to self-range as soon as possible, to follow his or her own individualized ROM program, and to report pain or other complications to the nurse.
2. Patient should maintain good posture while performing exercises, breathe normally, move slowly, and allow joints to be stretched gradually.
3. Patient should hold the movements for several counts, moving only to the joint's limits and not pushing too hard to increase ROM.
4. Patient may enjoy listening to music while performing exercises.
5. Patient may substitute or change exercises from day to day. The first 11 exercises should consistently make up the core of daily exercises, or they can be used as a shortened exercise program.
6. Teach the patient to avoid pain by beginning with midrange movements and gradually increasing the range over time. The extremes of the range should be avoided.
7. Teach the patient to avoid shoulder pain by doing shoulder exercises while lying supine, which will support the shoulder blade.
8. Patient should avoid excessive overhead stretches.
9. Hand or finger edema can make movement of joints difficult. Teach the patient to minimize edema during rest periods by keeping the affected arm elevated when possible and massaging the affected arm in long, one-way strokes from finger tips to elbow.

Procedures

1. Side stretch (Fig. 2-23): "Shift weight over to right side as you look to ceiling on right side. Then reverse, shift weight over to left side, looking to ceiling on left side. As you do this you should feel your trunk stretching out."

2. Drop it (Fig. 2-24): "Clasp hands together, hunch shoulders forward, and hang arms down between legs as close to ankles as possible. Then bring arms up into lap and sit up as straight as possible."

3. Head diagonals (Fig. 2-25): "Look up and over right shoulder, then down to left hip. Then reverse. Look up over left shoulder, then down to right hip. Remember to twist waist as you move."

4. Shoulder shrugs (Fig. 2-26): "Rest affected arm on top of strong arm. Push up to shrug right shoulder, then left. Now try to shrug both shoulders at the same time."

5. Open the door (Fig. 2-27): "Keeping weaker elbow in at side (inside of armrest of wheelchair), hold weaker forearm at wrist. Push forearm away from body, then back in."

6. Reach for the sky (Fig. 2-28): "Clasp hands together and raise arms up, then down to lap. Keep arms even. Avoid raising arms over head if painful or difficult to do."

7. Stir the pudding (Fig. 2-29): "Clasp hands together, reach arms out to right, in front, then out to left. Repeat in opposite direction."

8. Chopping wood (Fig. 2-30): "Clasp hands together and bend and straighten elbows by touching right shoulder and left knee. Repeat in opposite direction, bend and straighten elbows, touching left shoulder and right knee."

9. Push-pull (Fig. 2-31): "Clasp hands together with thumbs facing up. Push affected wrist away (bend it out), then pull it back (bend it in). Thumbs should remain facing up."

10. Finger bends (Fig. 2-32): "Rest affected hand in other hand. Bend all three joints of all affected fingers into a fist. Straighten fingers out."

11. Armflip (Fig. 2-33): "Clasp hands together, then touch back of right hand to right knee. Then reverse by touching back of left hand to left knee."

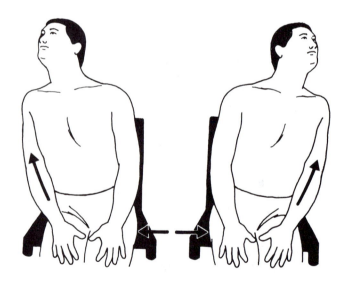

Figure 2-23 Side Stretch.

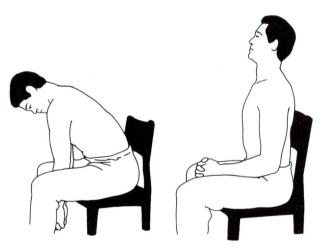

Figure 2-24 Drop It.

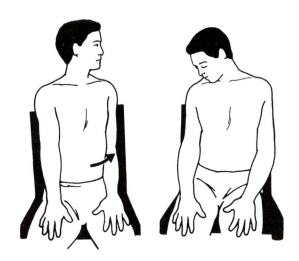

Figure 2-25 Head Diagonals.

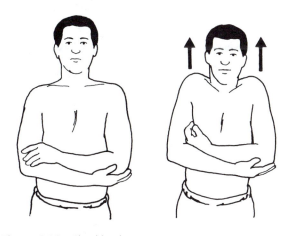

Figure 2-26 Shoulder shrugs.

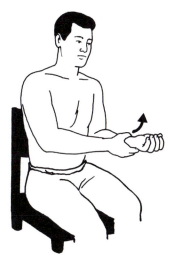

Figure 2-27 Open the Door.

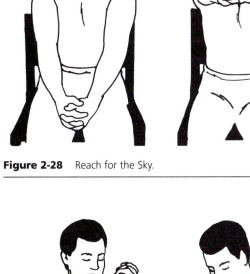

Figure 2-28 Reach for the Sky.

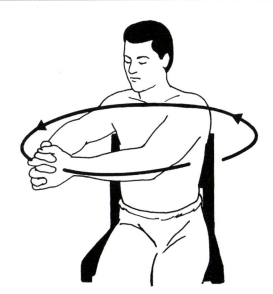

Figure 2-29 Stir the Pudding.

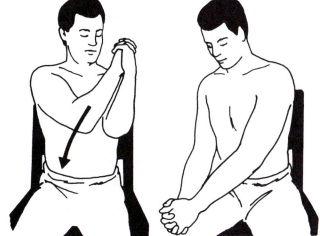

Figure 2-30 Chopping Wood.

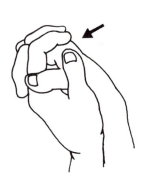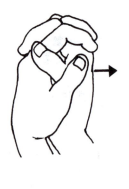

Figure 2-31 Push-Pull.

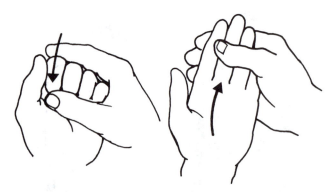

Figure 2-32 Finger Bends.

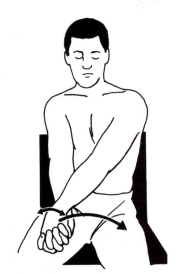

Figure 2-33 Arm Flip.

OPTIONAL OR ADDITIONAL EXERCISES

1. Body slump (Fig. 2-34): "Slump back in chair, then sit forward with back straight and head up."

2. Side-by-side (Fig. 2-35): "Look down toward floor on right side as you shift weight onto right side (buttock). Then reverse. Look down to floor on left side as you shift weight to left side."

3. Head up (Fig. 2-36): "Look up toward ceiling, then down to floor. Attempt to arch your back as you look up."

4. Head turn (Fig. 2-37): "Turn head to right, twisting waist as you look behind right shoulder. Then reverse, turn head to left, twisting waist as you look behind your left shoulder."

5. Ear touch (Fig. 2-38): "Looking straight ahead, touch right ear to right shoulder and attempt to shrug shoulder to meet ear. Reverse."

6. Chin tuck (Fig. 2-39): "Rest affected arm on top of other arm. Raise arms up to chin level. Then lower them. Keep elbows and arms even."

7. Rock the baby (Fig. 2-40): "Rest affected arm on top of strong arm. Rock arms to right and left. Attempt to lift right buttock off chair while shifting weight from side to side."

8. Thumb circles and hitch a ride (Figs. 2-41 and 2-42): "Hold tip of affected thumb with fingers of other hand. Turn in slow, large circles. Bend affected thumb across palm to touch little finger, then straighten thumb out."

9. Weight-bearing (Fig. 2-43): "Position affected arm on table straight in front with palm down. Do a reaching task over affected arm, moving items from side to side with other arm so that affected arm accepts light weight shifts."

10. Two-arm grasp (Fig. 2-44): "Clasp hands together. Reach for an object on one side, and move it over to other side. May also work high to low: reach for high object placed on unaffected side, and place it across and low on affected side."

11. Two-arm towel stretch (Fig. 2-45): "Clasp hands together and place arms on a towel, which is laid out on table. Move arms in figure-of-eight pattern and diagonals and circle right and left."

DOCUMENTATION

1. Specify frequency, type, position, and times of ROM.
2. Note any complications, patient complaints, and therapeutic effects noted.
3. Note effectiveness of patient and family teaching.

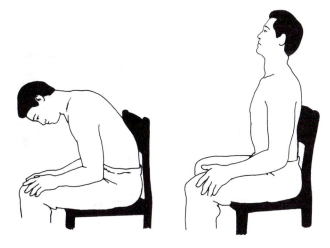

Figure 2-34   Body Slump.

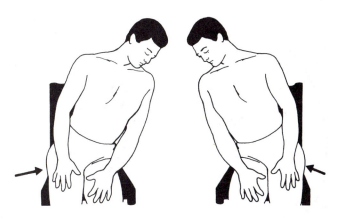

Figure 2-35   Side-to-Side.

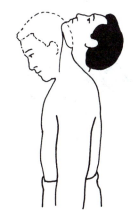

Figure 2-36   Head Up.

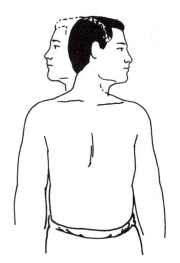

Figure 2-37   Head Turn.

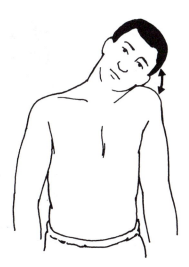

Figure 2-38   Ear Touch.

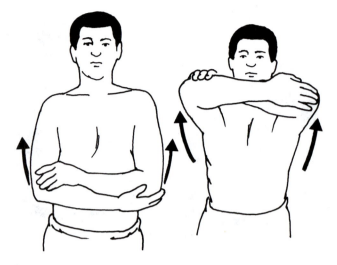

Figure 2-39 Chin Tuck.

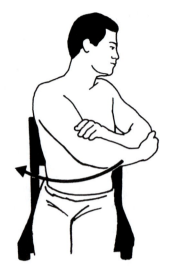

Figure 2-40 Rock the Baby.

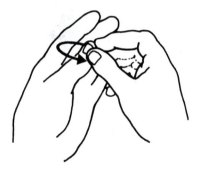

Figure 2-41 Thumb Circles.

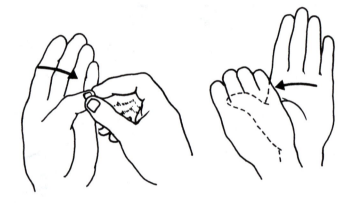

Figure 2-42 Hitch a Ride.

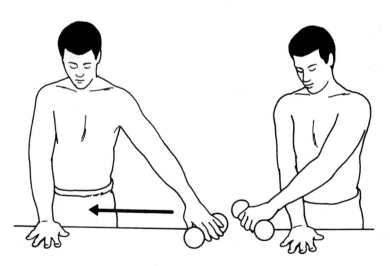

Figure 2-43 Weight-Bearing.

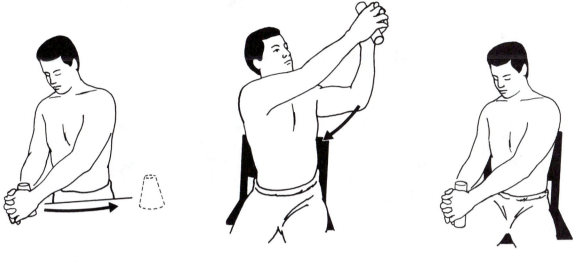

Figure 2-44   Two-Arm Grasp.

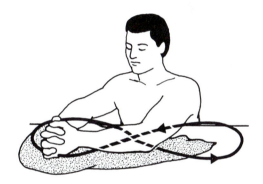

Figure 2-45   Two-Arm Towel Stretch.

Continuous Passive Range of Motion

PURPOSE

To promote maximal ROM of the knee, wrist, or hand through slow, progressive motion using a mechanical device

STAFF RESPONSIBLE

EQUIPMENT

1. Continuous passive range of motion (CPM) machine (Figs. 2-46 and 2-47). (See local/national manufacturer product information.)
2. Disposable padding to support the extremity.

 ## GENERAL CONSIDERATIONS

1. A physician's prescription is required for the use of the CPM machine. The prescription should include the flexion-extension setting, frequency, and speed. The machine may be set to run on automatic or manual mode (depending on the unit).
2. CPM is indicated to increase and maintain knee, wrist, and/or hand ROM to prevent joint stiffness, especially during the postoperative period, and to reduce pain, throbbing sensation, and edema.
3. The body part (hip and knee, wrist, or hand and fingers) should be in the extended position when the device is turned on and off.
4. The flexion-extension setting should be checked before starting the device.

5. Discontinue use of the machine if the patient complains of increased pain or discomfort.

6. Do not raise the head of the bed above 30 degrees from the horizontal when using the CPM for hip and knee.

7. When installing or removing the device, always set the device on its lowest setting.

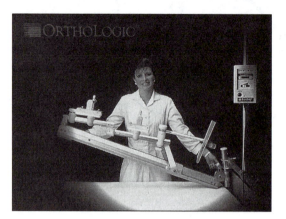

Figure 2-46 LiteLift™ Hospital CPM. Reproduced with permission from OrthoLogic, Tempe, AZ.

PATIENT AND FAMILY EDUCATION

1. Teach the patient and family the purpose of the machine, its benefits, and how to use it.

2. Assess issues of noncompliance in using the device and notify physician if appropriate.

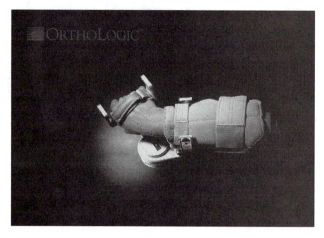

Figure 2-47 W2 Wrist CPM. Reproduced with permission from OrthoLogic, Tempe, AZ.

Procedures

Knee CPM

MEASUREMENTS

 Steps

1. Measure patient's leg (in in.) from greater trochanter to knee axis.
2. Adjust thigh bar (if present) to equal this measurement.

3. Measure patient's leg (in in.) from knee axis to lateral malleolus.
4. Adjust calf bar (if present) to equal this measurement.

5. Add thigh and calf measurements together.
6. Set hip extension bar to this number, to nearest whole inch.
7. Use up and down arrows to increase or decrease parameters.

 Additional Information

Number on thigh bar should line up with proximal end of latch.

Number on calf bar should line up with distal end of each latch.

Measurements of total leg length should line up with end of device.

Whatever is flashing on screen can be changed with arrows.

PROGRAMMING THE DEVICE

 Steps

1. Press limit button. Use up and down arrows to adjust desired degree of extension.
2. Press limit button again. Use up and down arrows to adjust desired degree of flexion.
3. Press rate button. Use up and down arrows to adjust desired rate.
4. Press time button.

 Additional Information

"Extension" will flash on screen.

"Flexion" will flash on screen.

"Rate" will flash on screen.

Panel should read "Continuous Time." If it does not, press up arrow until it does.

STARTING CPM

 Steps

1. Place padding on calf and foot.
2. Place machine on bed.
3. Angle machine slightly toward outside corner of bed.

4. Place leg in device so that knee is centered with white knee hinge.
5. Press start-stop button.

 Additional Information

New padding is used for each patient.
Attach to footboard.
This slight abduction will maintain proper anatomic alignment.
Leg should be extended.

Make sure device is plugged in and that green power switch is turned on.

DISCONTINUING CPM

 Steps

1. Press start-stop button.
2. Remove leg from device.
3. Turn off green power switch.
4. Unplug machine.

 Additional Information

Stop device when leg is extended straight.

Procedures

Wrist and Hand CPM

PROGRAMMING THE DEVICE

 Steps

1. Press limit button. Use up and down arrows to adjust desired degree of extension.
2. Press limit button again. Use up and down arrows to adjust desired degree of flexion.
3. Press rate button. Use up and down arrows to adjust desired rate.
4. Press time button.

Additional Information

"Extension" will flash on screen.

"Flexion" will flash on screen.

"Rate" will flash on screen.

Panel should read "Continuous Time." If it does not, press up arrow until it does.

STARTING CPM

 Steps

1. Place padding on wrist, or gloves and finger attachments on patient.
2. Place machine on flat surface.
3. Place arm or hand in device so that it is centered.
4. Press start-stop button.

 Additional Information

New padding gloves and/or finger attachments are used for each patient.

Attach to table or bed for additional support.

Make sure device is plugged in and that green power switch is turned on.

DISCONTINUING CPM

 Steps

1. Press start-stop button.
2. Remove arm or hand from device.
3. Turn off green power switch.
4. Unplug machine.

 Additional Information

Stop device when arm or hand is extended straight.

 DOCUMENTATION

1. Record flexion-extension settings.
2. Note patient compliance, tolerance, effects of treatment, use of pain medication.
3. Note effectiveness of patient and family teaching.
4. Note length of time of the treatment.

REFERENCES

Brander, V.A., Stulberg, S.D., and Chang, R.W. (1994) "Rehabilitation Following Hip and Knee Arthroplasty" *Physical Medicine and Rehabilitation Clinics of North America* 5(4):815–836.

OrthoLogic product information. Courtesy of OrthoLogic, 1275 W. Washington Street, Tempe, AZ 85281; 1-800-rent-cpm; *www.orthologic.com.*

Care of the Patient in a Solid or Bivalve Cast

PURPOSE

To immobilize a bony structure to promote healing of a fracture, dislocation, or surgical site; to maintain or increase ROM through serial application or use of dropout casting; to facilitate positioning through use of bivalve casts; to preserve circulation and skin integrity under the casted area

STAFF RESPONSIBLE

EQUIPMENT

1. Flashlight.
2. Waterproof cast tape.

 GENERAL CONSIDERATIONS

1. Keep the cast clean and dry at all times. When a cast gets wet, it may soften and crack.
2. Nursing assessments of a casted extremity include:
   - Neurologic and vascular status
   - Presence, amount, color, and change in drainage
   - Skin characteristics

   Any impairment should be reported to the physician immediately.
3. Impaired circulation can be identified by:
   - Patient complaints of localized pain
   - Absence of pulse under the cast
   - Symptoms of coldness, pallor, duskiness, or cyanosis
   - Edema
   - Loss of movement

- Numbness
- Slow capillary refill with blanching

In unresponsive or cognitively impaired patients, increased agitation or restlessness after cast application should be investigated.

4. Any drainage noted should be circled with a ball-point pen and labeled with the date and time.

5. Any unexplained, offensive odors from beneath the cast should be reported immediately because these may be evidence of skin breakdown.

6. A window may be cut in the cast by the physician to allow for:
   - Removal of pressure from a bony prominence
   - Checking of circulation and pulse
   - Changing of dressing
   - Checking of surgical site

7. The cast may be bivalved in such a manner as to make it removable when it is no longer necessary for constant wear. The bivalved cast is held together by Velcro straps or elastic wrap and is used for positioning as prescribed. Increased circulation and decreased tone can result from the use of a bivalved cast.

8. No showers or tub baths are given unless you have a cast guard or are able to cover the cast tightly with plastic bags and tape. Give sponge baths. Bivalved casts can be removed for hygiene purposes if specifically prescribed by a physician.

9. Do not allow weight-bearing on a casted extremity unless prescribed by the physician.

10. Any writing on the cast must be done with materials that will not seal the cast and prevent it from "breathing." Color crayons, Magic Markers, and pens are acceptable; paint and other oil-based materials are not to be used.

11. A cast cutter for emergency removal of a cast should be available at all times.

12. Stains (food, dirt, grime, or excrement) can be removed with the use of a damp (not wet) cloth, kitchen cleanser, and gentle rubbing.

13. To protect the cast from incontinence:
    - Cover perineal area of cast with plastic sterile drape or plastic wrap, and check skin frequently for moisture buildup or irritation
    - Use Pampers or small diapers tucked into the groin area, and change them frequently
    - Place the patient in a prone position with the head higher than the feet to facilitate drainage when in a hip spica cast

PATIENT AND FAMILY EDUCATION

Teach the patient and family the purpose and benefits of the cast, how to care for the cast (if it will be used at home), and how to assess circulation and signs and symptoms of cast problems or emergency situations.

Procedures

Care of Wet or Damp Cast

 Steps

 Additional Information

1. Leave cast exposed to air until dry.

Fiberglass cast dries immediately. Plaster cast dries in 24 to 48 h, depending on size. Plaster hip spica or body cast dries in 48 to 72 h.

2. Place pillows to support cast (lengthwise), especially under hips and knees.

Cast will flatten over bony prominence, causing tissue damage if wet or damp and unsupported on hard surfaces. Use foam pillows, not feather pillows.

3. Position properly to prevent depressions in cast.

Depressed areas can cause tissue breakdown, dependent edema, and impaired circulation.

4. Lift cast with palms of hands, not fingers.

Do not use abduction bar, if present, as a handle when lifting or turning patients.

5. If necessary, turn patient with two staff members.

This ensures patient comfort and prevents cast destruction. Turn to uncasted side as much as possible.

6. Elevate casted extremity.

This decreases or prevents edema in extremity.

7. Assess neurologic and vascular status, drainage patterns, skin, and odor every 4 h and as needed.

Skin Care of Casted Extremity

 Steps

1. Check skin around all edges of cast with flashlight.
2. Wash exposed part of extremity with soap and water, rinse well, and dry.
3. Apply lotion sparingly around cast edges if skin is dry and cracking. Do not put inside cast.
4. Check for any signs of complications.

 Additional Information

Observe for redness, any change in color, broken skin areas, or offensive odor.

Do not get cast wet.

Lotions and moisture may cause skin breakdown in an enclosed area.

Check for discomfort, pulses, edema, skin temperatures, and color below casted area.

 DOCUMENTATION

1. Note any changes in neurovascular status, presence and amount of drainage, presence of odor, and any complications of immobility.
2. Note the use of bivalve casts, wearing times, positioning recommendations, and routine cast care.

Positioning to Facilitate Function

Bed Positioning in the Presence of Increased Tone (Spasticity)

PURPOSE

To normalize muscle tone, while in bed, for patients with increased tone or spasticity; to prevent contractures or deformities in patients prone to increased tone or spasticity; to maintain functional ROM with bed positioning; to improve gastrointestinal and respiratory function (secondary effect of trunk extension)

STAFF RESPONSIBLE

EQUIPMENT

1. Foam blocks (18 to 20 in. long × 6 to 8 in. wide × 4 in. high)
2. Pillows (not down or feather)
3. Pillow cases

 GENERAL CONSIDERATIONS

1. Normal muscle tone is defined as enough muscle contraction to allow for movement against gravity and full ROM of the joints. Increased tone results in positions against gravity, which occur in patterns (synergies), leading to nonfunctional and fixed postures in the trunk and extremities and possibly decreased ROM.

2. Patients exhibiting mild to severe increases in tone with synergy should have their trunk, head, and affected limbs positioned in opposite patterns to normalize tone. Always begin by assessing and positioning the trunk, then the head, and then the extremities (proximal to distal). Consult the physical therapist and occupational therapist for assistance.

3. Increased tone patterns may be unilateral (as in the hemiplegic patient) or bilateral (as in the head trauma patient). With unilateral tone patterns, the affected side is to be considered the weaker or shortened side in the rest of these procedures. These procedures are to be used with patients whose increased tone patterns are primarily flexion, extension, or mixed.

4. Identify shortening of the trunk with the patient supine or sitting. Consider the shortened side the weaker or affected side. Instead of positioning the patient side lying, position him or her three-quarters prone with the affected side up and three-quarters supine with the affected side up or down. Position the patient supine and prone. Difficulties in the prone position (discomfort, increased tone, or respiratory distress) need to be closely monitored and the position discontinued if necessary. The most common contraindication to prone positioning is obstruction of the airway (i.e., if the patient has a tracheostomy or buries his or her face in the pillow).

5. Some patients with abnormal tone may exhibit the asymmetric tonic neck reflex (fencing reflex), in which the head turns away from the flexed side of the body. Carefully position such a patient's head in neutral and midline with foam blocks or a pillow to prevent activation of this reflex. Some patients have increased flexion of the neck. These patients respond well to a flat pillow or no pillow under their head, which actually encourages hyperextension but results in neutral and midline positioning.

6. Patients with increased tone tend to adduct their shoulders and hips, resulting in contractures. Position their extremities with the shoulder and hip abducted. Protract and flatten the scapula before abducting and externally rotating the shoulder. Externally rotate and abduct the hip in slight flexion.

7. Weight-bearing or placement in a weight-bearing position decreases spasticity.

8. When handling patients, use firm, palmar pressure. Avoid fingertip and light touch. Use two hands. Movements are to be slow and smooth. Use your whole body (i.e., your voice, body, and movement).

9. Try to combine or maximize relaxation techniques: showering, warm towels, partial bathing, room temperature, fluids, soothing music, fan for cooling, and removal or reduction of noxious stimuli (full bladder, infection, fever, skin problems, bowel problems, orthopedic problems, or deep vein thrombus).

10. Position the patient on a firm surface (exception: patients with predominant extensor tone need to sag) and select an appropriate mattress topper. Use small, firm positioning aids such as foam blocks, pillows, towel rolls, bolsters, and wedges. Blankets and towels have smooth, soft surfaces and thus will decrease tone. Many patients have an increase in autonomic response with resulting diaphoresis, so that absorbent material will aid in patient comfort. If the patient has low tone (flaccid), use rough surfaces to increase tone. Close monitoring is necessary to validate the response and objective of increasing or decreasing tone. Coordinate use of splints, bivalved casts, and the like with the therapists and devise a positioning schedule.

11. Facilitate follow-through with optimal positioning by drawing or taking pictures of the patient in these positions. Post the picture or drawing over the patient's bed or in the room. Practice placing the patient in these positions with staff members.

12. Monitor the patient after positioning for discomfort, restlessness, and increased diaphoresis which would indicate the patient's tolerance or response.

13. If you have a patient with a combination of flexion and extension patterns (which is often the case), remember to position the patient out of those patterns to increase normal tone and movement.

Table 2-4 Medications Used to Manage Spasticity

Generic and Common Trade Names	Mechanism of Action	Specific Uses	Dosages	Toxicity, Side Effects, Interactions
Baclofen/Lioresal	Decreases frequency and amplitude of muscle spasm in response to muscle stretching	Generalized spasticity	PO: Initially, 5 mg BID, to 20–30 mg QID Intrathecally by pump, 2× test dose, then adjust	Sedation, fatigue, nausea, vertigo, hypotonia, muscle weakness, mental depression, headache, hypotension, seizures.
Botulinum toxin/ Botox	Inhibits release of acetylcholine from the presynaptic membrane	Focal dystonia, selected spasticity in stroke, cerebral palsy and spinal cord injury	Localized injection, of up to 400 units, works in 2–3 days, up to 2–3 weeks; wears off in 6 weeks to 2 months Injections need repeating every 3–4 months	Flulike symptoms and excessive weakness of injected muscle or spread of toxin to adjacent muscles.
Dantrolene/Dantrium	Decreases skeletal muscle strength by interfering with excitation-contraction coupling in muscle groups; interferes with release of activator calcium	Spasticity associated with spinal cord injury, stroke, cerebral palsy, or multiple sclerosis	PO: 25 mg daily, increasing to max of 100 mg QID	Cardiac and smooth muscle are only slightly depressed. Liver function changes, generalized muscle weakness, sedation, and hepatitis may result.
Diazepam/Valium	Potentiates action of GABA, acts at spinal cord level	Treatment of muscle spasms	PO: 2 mg BID, then increase to 60 mg daily	Sedation, fatigue, memory impairment, headache, constipation, dry mouth, hepatic dysfunction.
Tizanidine/Zanaflex	α-2 adrenergic agonist properties at spinal and supra-spinal receptor sites	Centrally acting, useful in multiple sclerosis, spinal cord injury	PO: 4 mg TID, and increase in 2 to 4 mg steps to 36 mg/day (lasts 3–5 h, clinically)	Drowsiness, weakness, dry mouth, fatigue, insomnia, mild hypertension.

Procedures

Supine Position to Minimize Flexion Spasticity on Affected Side

 Steps

 Additional Information

1. Position patient supine in middle of bed.

    Start with bed flat and no pillows or blocks under patient.

2. Turn patient on unaffected side to place positioning props.

    Make sure that side rail is up. Some patients may not have to be turned to place towels.

3. Place folded towel under affected scapula and hip.

    This will facilitate shoulder and hip protraction. For severe spasticity, a foam block placed lengthwise below the affected scapula down to the hip may be necessary.

4. Roll patient back to supine position.

5. Place small, firm pillow under or next to patient's head to keep it in midline.

    This is to facilitate positioning of head in neutral and midline; no pillow may be needed.

6. Position upper and lower extremities in abduction and extension as much as possible with towels, small pillows, or foam blocks.

    Start with shoulder and work down arm to hand. Then start at hip and work down to foot.

Supine Position to Minimize Extension Spasticity on Affected Side

 Steps

 Additional Information

1. Position patient supine in middle of bed.

    Start with bed flat and no pillows or blocks under patient. Patients who have severe rigidity may require elevation of head of bed to 30 degrees. This facilitates trunk flexion.

2. Place small pillow under occiput.

    To flex head forward to neutral, midline.

3. Place small, folded towel under scapula and put upper extremity in slight flexion.

    This protracts shoulder, producing relaxation of arm. Slight flexion of elbow will break up extension synergy. Pillow under affected arm may be used to prevent edema.

4. Place small, folded towel or foam block under hip.

    This protracts hip, which relaxes extremity. Patients with severe rigidity may require elevation of knee Gatch to 15 to 20 degrees. This is to facilitate slight flexion of hips and knees.

5. Place small roll under leg slightly above knee.

    This facilitates flexion of knee and at same time prevents occlusion of popliteal artery.

6. Place pillow between feet and foot of bed.

    Firm-surfaced footboard should be avoided because it may increase extension. Do not place anything under ball of foot because this will increase tone.

Three-Quarters Supine Position to Minimize Flexion Spasticity on Affected Side

 Steps

 Additional Information

1. Position patient supine in center of bed.

Start with bed flat and no pillows or blocks under patient.

2. Roll patient onto either side.

3. Place pillows or foam blocks across back at subscapular level or at small of back (or both) or one foam block above small of back.

Number and position of pillows or foam blocks is dependent on amount of tone and size of patient.

4. Roll patient back over these blocks to three-quarters supine position and pull blocks through.

This will encourage extension of head, shoulder protraction, and scapular flattening on affected side.

5. Position head in neutral, midline position.

Place small, rolled towel or pillow under head to block rotation in patients with severely increased tone.

6. Gently abduct both arms:
   - Affected arm in bottom position: position this arm in extension and forearm in supination (or neutral).
   - Affected arm in top position: position this arm in extension with pillow supporting arm in horizontal plane. Forearm is slightly supinated or neutral.

Use pillows or foam blocks to facilitate abduction and support arms. Place small pillow under forearm or hand to minimize edema.

7. Gently abduct both legs:
   - Affected leg in bottom position: position leg forward and in slight flexion. Hip is protracted.
   - Affected leg in top position: position leg in slight flexion behind bottom leg. Support leg in a horizontal plane with pillows.

8. Use foam blocks to bridge any bony areas as needed.

Three-Quarters Prone Position to Minimize Flexion Spasticity on Affected Side

 Steps

 Additional Information

1. Position patient supine in center of bed.

Start with bed flat and no pillows or blocks under patient.

2. Move patient to side of bed closest to unaffected side.

3. Place trunk roll, foam blocks, or firm pillow next to affected side of trunk below axilla level.

4. Roll patient forward over roll, foam blocks, or firm pillow.

This will stretch both sides of the trunk. Pad side rail closest to affected side.

5. Position affected upper extremity behind trunk.

This encourages shoulder abduction and protraction.

6. Turn head toward unaffected side.

Place small pillow under head to facilitate neutral positioning if needed.

7. Position topmost upper extremity to front, rolling shoulder forward.

8. Position affected lower extremity in back of lower extremity on bottom, extending hip and bending knee slightly.

This will promote hip extension, abduction, and protraction.

DOCUMENTATION

1. Record the response to positioning (i.e., increased or decreased tone).
2. Document patient and family teaching.

REFERENCES

American Nurses Association (1996) "Facts and Comparisons" *Nurses Drug Facts* St. Louis, MO; pp. 79–81, 263–265, 276–278, 1025, 1046.

Bobath, B. (1978) *Adult Hemiplegia: Evaluation and Treatment* (2d ed.) London: Heinemann Medical Books.

Gee, Z.L. and Passarella, P.M. (1978) "Starting Right" *American Journal of Nursing* 87:802–808.

Gee, Z.L. and Passarella, P.M. (1985) *Nursing Care of the Stroke Patient: A Therapeutic Approach* Pittsburgh, PA: AREN-Publications.

Johnson, K.M.M. ed. (1997) *Advanced Practice Nursing in Rehabilitation* Glenview, IL: Association of Rehabilitation Nurses, pp. 81–82.

Johnstone, M. (1976) *The Stroke Patient: Principals of Rehabilitation* Edinburgh: Churchill-Livingstone.

Kuric, J.L. (1994) "Intrathecal Baclofen Therapy: New Technology for Treating Spasticity" *Rehab Rounds,* Fall 1994:1–2.

Law, M. and Cadman, D. (1988) "Measurement of Spasticity: A Clinician's Guide" *Physical & Occupational Therapy in Pediatrics* 8(2/3):77–95.

Nance, P.W., Sheremata, W.A., Lynch, S.G., et al. (1997) "Relationship of the Antispasticity Effect of Tizanidine to Plasma Concentration in Patients with Multiple Sclerosis" *Archives of Neurology* 54:731–736.

O'Brien, M.T. and Pallett, P.J. (1978) *Total Care of the Stroke Patient* Boston: Little, Brown & Company.

Pallett, P.J. and O'Brien, M.T. (1985) *Textbook of Neurological Nursing* Boston: Little, Brown & Company.

Moving Up in Bed (Scooting)

PURPOSE

To assist the patient to scoot up in bed

STAFF RESPONSIBLE

EQUIPMENT

No equipment necessary.

GENERAL CONSIDERATIONS

1. Many patients find themselves at the bottom of the bed and unable to scoot up in bed themselves. Using neuro-developmental techniques (NDT), most patients can be assisted to scoot up in bed without drawsheets or the assistance of more than one person.
2. The patient must be able to bear weight and bend the knees to lift the pelvis to use this method. It may not be used in patients who cannot weight bear because of pelvic or lower extremity fractures or in patients with post-hip or -knee replacements.
3. Although initially the patient may need maximal assistance, over time the patient should become more independent.
4. Wear nonsterile gloves.

Procedure

Scooting up in Bed

 Steps

 Additional Information

1. Lower head of bed and knee Gatch so patient is supine in flat (180-degree) bed.

   Bed must be flat.

2. Remove pillow(s) from under patient's head or top of bed.

   There should be no obstacles to upward movement on the bed itself.

3. Instruct patient to grab ahold of the side rails to help push self upward.

   An overhead trapeze could be used.

4. Instruct patient to bend both legs at the knees and put feet flat on the bed.

   Assist patient if unable to do so independently.

5. Position yourself on the patient's weaker side, with one knee on the bed, facing toward the head of the bed (Fig. 2-48*A*).

   Your chest should be level with the patient's knees.

6. Place your shoulder against the patient's weaker knee and cup the heel of the same foot in your hand (Fig. 2-48*B*).

   You will be stabilizing the heel, so the foot does not move on the bed.

7. With your other hand open flat, slide your fingers under the patient's buttock to cue them to bridge the pelvis while pushing against the knee and stabilizing the foot.

   Cue the patient to "scoot up," mimicking the same movement on the stronger side, and touching their chin to their chest and/or pushing down into the bed with their elbows.

8. Reposition the weak heel and have the patient reposition the other foot.

   Although it may seem that very little movement occurred, several repetitions are usually sufficient to move the patient to the top of the bed.

9. Repeat steps 5 to 7.

   As patients practice this skill, less assistance is necessary.

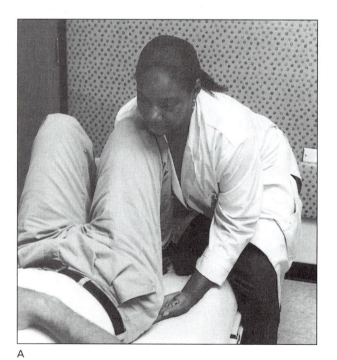

A

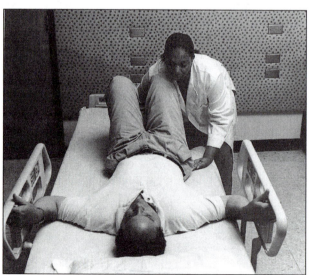

B

Figure 2-48

DOCUMENTATION

1. Patient's improved independence in motor skills.

REFERENCES

Bobath, B. (1978) *Adult Hemiplegia: Evaluation and Treatment* (2d ed.) London: Heinemann Medical Books.

Gee, Z.L. and Passarella, P.M. (1978) "Starting Right" *American Journal of Nursing* 87:802–808.

Gee, Z.L. and Passarella, P.M. (1985) *Nursing Care of the Stroke Patient: A Therapeutic Approach* Pittsburgh, PA: AREN-Publications.

Toileting in Bed

PURPOSE

To assist patient to be more independent when (s)he must use the bedpan in bed

STAFF RESPONSIBLE

EQUIPMENT

1. Nonsterile gloves
2. Bedpan
3. Waterproof bed protector

GENERAL CONSIDERATIONS

1. Many patients find themselves requiring assistance using the bedpan when in bed. Although using a bedpan in bed is not the most desirable way to urinate or defecate, sometimes it is the best option. Every possibility should be explored to avoid using a bedpan in bed (use of bedside commode, female/male urinal at the bedside, etc.). This technique is used to minimize spilling and promote independence.

2. Using NDT techniques, most patients can be assisted to place the bedpan with the assistance of one person. The patient must be able to bear weight and bend their knees to lift their pelvis to use this method. It may not be used in patients who cannot weight bear because of pelvic or lower extremity fractures or in patients post-hip or -knee replacements.

3. Although initially the patient may need maximal assistance, over time the patient should become more independent.

4. Wear nonsterile gloves.

Procedure

Toileting in Bed

 Steps

1. Assist patient to a supine position in bed so once bedpan is placed, the head of the bed can be easily elevated.

2. Instruct patient to bend both legs at the knees and put feet flat on the bed.

3. Position yourself on the patient's weaker side, with one knee on the bed, facing toward the head of the bed.

 Additional Information

Once bedpan is placed, patient should be elevated to a sitting position as close to 90 degrees as possible to increase intraabdominal pressure and facilitate complete bowel and bladder emptying.

Assist patient if unable to do so independently.

Your chest should be level with the patient's knees, and bedpan (and waterproof pad) should be next to patient's hips.

4. Press downward toward the foot of the bed and downward toward the mattress on the patient's weaker knee, while cueing the patient to "lift," use other hand under buttocks to initially help lift (Fig. 2-49*A*).

5. Slide bedpan (and waterproof pad) under bridged buttocks (Fig. 2-49*B*).

6. Assist patient to sitting.

7. Remove bedpan in same manner.

Patient should be performing same movement with other side. Stabilize patient's weaker foot with your body.

Use your upper arm to hold the lower thigh in the desired position. Patient should be expected eventually to help place the bedpan.

Use bed controls and pillows to bring patient to 90 degrees.

Since patient is not rolling to the side, the risk of spilling the bedpan is decreased. The waterproof pad should be removed after pericare is completed.

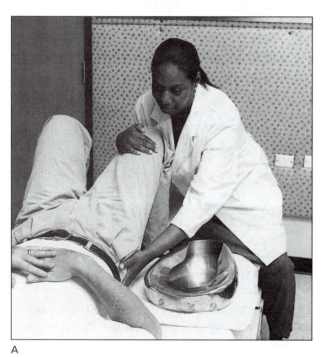

A

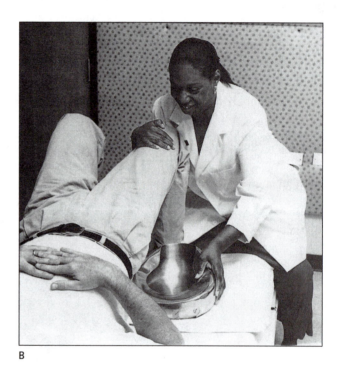

B

Figure 2-49

DOCUMENTATION

1. Patient's improved independence in motor skills.

REFERENCES

Bobath, B. (1978) *Adult Hemiplegia: Evaluation and Treatment* (2d ed.) London: Heinemann Medical Books.

Gee, Z.L. and Passarella, P.M. (1978) "Starting Right" *American Journal of Nursing* 87:802–808.

Gee, Z.L. and Passarella, P.M. (1985) *Nursing Care of the Stroke Patient: A Therapeutic Approach* Pittsburgh, PA: AREN-Publications.

Wheelchair Selection and Positioning

PURPOSE

To aid in selecting a wheelchair that best meets the patient's short-term and long-term needs; to safely position the patient in a wheelchair

STAFF RESPONSIBLE

EQUIPMENT

No equipment necessary

 ## GENERAL CONSIDERATIONS

1. Traditionally, physical therapists have the pivotal role in wheelchair selection. Input from other healthcare clinicians may be helpful, based on the current speed that patients are discharged from acute care to other settings. A basic understanding of the different wheelchair types aids in understanding how to best meet the patient's wheelchair needs. All team members should be using the same terminology (Fig. 2-50).

2. Factors to be considered:
   - Patient's medical diagnosis, including secondary diagnoses
   - Short-term or long-term need, which affects durability, ease of transport, cosmesis
   - Stable or progressive or periods of remission and exacerbation type of disability, which affects patient comfort, balance, stability, change in functional status, progressive loss of independence, and adaptability
   - Associated neurologic deficits, such as sensory and visual disorders, which may require special equipment modifications
   - Precautions or limitations, like weight-bearing precautions, positioning or activity restrictions
   - Significant past medical history that requires special equipment or modifications
   - Current functional status: ability to transfer, move about in bed, propel a wheelchair, ambulate, sitting and standing balance, amount of physical assistance, range of motion, strength, ability to compensate for limitations, gains in function since admission, sitting tolerance
   - Mental status: cognitive deficits, judgment, safety awareness, error awareness, ability to compensate for cognitive deficits, motivation, involvement in care, goal-setting and discharge planning

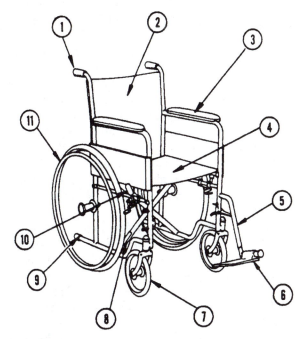

1. Handgrips/Push Handles
2. Back Upholstery
3. Armrests
4. Seat Upholstery
5. Front Rigging
6. Footplate
7. Casters
8. Crossbraces (Serial No.)
9. Tipping Lever
10. Wheel Locks
11. Wheel and Handrim

Figure 2-50 Wheelchair terminology. Taken from Everest and Jennings, Wheelchair Prescriptions Series, Booklet No. 1—Measuring the Patient. Used by permission, Everest and Jennings, Inc.

   - Environment: discharge location/home assessment to include—entrance to home, stairs, presence/absence of a railing, doorway widths (especially bathroom and bedroom)
   - Financial assistance: medical coverage—what is covered, secondary insurance, patient or family supplements, fundraising and charity funds available

3. Wheelchairs come in a variety of shapes, sizes, and costs. There are manual chairs and electric chairs and scooters. Some basic types of wheelchair options include:
   - Wheelchair seat dimensions: standard adult (18-in. seat width), narrow adult (16-in. seat width), extra-large adult (20- to 24-in. seat width), junior (16-in. seat width) and pediatric sizes down to 10 in. wide.
   - Wheelchair backs: standard (90 degrees), semireclining (30 to 90 degrees), full reclining (to horizontal) and hook on head rests to support the head if weak or poor head control.
   - Wheelchair arms: standard, desk arms (shortened to fit under a desk), detachable arms, partial arms (usually detachable or swing out of the way).

- Wheelchair footrests: standard; swinging, detachable, and elevating.
- Wheelchair brakes: toggle brakes, with either push locking action or pull locking action, or lever brakes. Brake extensions are available.
- Wheelchair wheels: standard wheels—24 in. in diameter with separate wheel and hand rim; lightweight wheels—have wheel and hand rim as one; Solid rubber tires are standard, but pneumatic tires are recommended for uneven surfaces, such as grass, gravel, sand. Spoke guards protect the spokes from any items becoming caught in them (hands, fingers, etc.). Standard hand rims are chrome plated. Rubber tipped projections can be added to aid in pushing the hand rims, for those with poor or absent grasp. The projections can be placed horizontal, oblique, or vertical.
- Wheelchair tipping lever: horizontal projections at the bottom and back of the wheelchair. They allow for tipping the wheelchair backwards to overcome curbs, electrical cords, and other items that present an obstacle. Tiny wheels might be used. They are anti-tippers, to prevent the chair from tipping over completely.
- Wheelchair power: manual or electrical, run by battery. The battery needs recharging daily. The electric wheelchair should never be recharged with a person in it. The battery charger should be plugged in to an appropriate electrical outlet. The battery charger should be placed on a flat surface at all times. Some wheelchairs have removable power packs that can be easily reaffixed to a manual wheelchair when the patient's condition deteriorates and a power chair is needed.

4. Any patient with sensory or motor deficits that affect their trunk, lower extremities, and buttocks should have a wheelchair cushion in the wheelchair at all times. The wheelchair cushions vary in price and materials (Table 2-5).

5. Wheelchair accessories are available. Armrests and lapboard (clear and of solid material) may be helpful. Wheelchair gloves aid in manual wheelchair propulsion and keep the hands cleaner, especially if traveling outside.

6. Ideal wheelchair positioning, unless contraindicated by patient's physical condition/precautions/limitations, should start at the lower trunk with an anterior pelvic tilt and strive for symmetry between the right and left sides of the patient's body. Both feet should rest at the same level, with knees level with hips. When not in motion, encourage the patient to rest both feet on the floor in a weight-bearing position and to sit with his or her arms slightly flexed on the table in front of him or her to promote greater trunk extension and better posture. Recognizing deviations from this position allows for prompt correction, increased function by the patient, and safety for all.

Table 2-5   Wheelchair Cushion Options

Cushion	Comments
Roho	Rubber projections, filled with air, has waterproof cover. Comes in variety of styles for varying levels of patient independence in pressure relief activities and transfers and for skin care needs. Needs to be checked for air loss and proper patient flotation.
Jay	Molded urethane base with gel pad, offers seating stability. Accessories are available to customize for individual needs.
Jay Combi	Foam cushion includes lumbar support cushion.
Avanti Contoured Foam Cushion	Light-weight foam contoured for seating stability.
Avanti Standard	Made of varying densities of tempered foam for support.

Procedure

Wheelchair Positioning

 Steps

 Additional Information

1. Direct/assist patient to move backwards in the chair so buttocks are low against the back rest.

This is contraindicated if the patient has hip precautions. If (s)he cannot maintain it, try a lumbar support (towel roll, foam block, commercial products are available too). This will help him or her shift into an anterior pelvic tilt.

2. Place feet on footplates.

This will help stabilize the trunk, especially if the footrests are level and equal. If elevating footrests are required, be sure to use bilateral ones to promote symmetry.

3. Adjust armrests.

Elevating armrests or a lapboard may be used to help control weak or paralyzed upper extremities, to promote proper shoulder/arm/hand placement, and to aid in edema management.

4. Apply any specialized accessories.

Trunk supports may be needed if poor trunk balance, or a towel roll/foam block could be used if patient leans to weak side. Discuss options with therapists.

 DOCUMENTATION

1. Note type of wheelchair and accessories used.
2. Teach patient, family, and caregivers the names, purposes, and care of the wheelchair and parts.

REFERENCES

Gee, Z.L. and Passarella, P.M. (1985) *Nursing Care of the Stroke Patient: A Therapeutic Approach* Pittsburgh, PA: AREN-Publications.

Mattingly, D. (1993). "Wheelchair Selection" *Orthopaedic Nursing* 12(4): 11–16.

Sine, R.D., Holcomb, J.D., Roush, R.E., et al. (1983) *Basic Rehabilitation Techniques: A Self-Instructional Guide* 2d ed. Rockville, MD: Aspen.

Ambulation

PURPOSE

To walk safely

STAFF RESPONSIBLE

EQUIPMENT

No equipment necessary.

 GENERAL CONSIDERATIONS

1. Before attempting ambulation, pre-gait training is imperative. Pre-gait training includes: coming to sitting, sitting balance, coming to standing, and standing balance. The patient must be able to perform these activities safely to progress to ambulation.

2. When assisting a patient to come to sitting, allow the patient to do as much of it as possible. Teach the patient to move as a unit—no twisting, and to roll to the side of the bed, then to push up using the arms. Once the patient is sitting, check for cardiac symptoms, such as dizziness, sustained change in pulse rate, syncope.

3. Check sitting balance. A "short sit" would be sitting with legs dangling, starting with upper extremity support, and then without upper extremity support, and progress to a "long sit," where legs are extended in front of the patient, with and then without upper extremity support. Good sitting balance should include long sitting, even while moving arms, and ability to meet challenges to balance. The ability to come to sitting and long sit is an indication of good trunk control, which is imperative for standing.

4. When assisting a patient to transfer, assess their ability to control their trunk and extremities. Transfers, such as standing pivot transfers, are a good way to teach the patient to come to standing. As their transfer abilities improve, their standing improves. The patient should be able to come to standing from different chair heights. The higher the chair (start with the chair 1½ times the length of the patient's leg from the knee to the foot), the easier it will be for the patient to stand. Lower the height of the chair to normal height as the patient's strength and abilities increase. Once the patient is standing, check standing balance. When standing, the patient must be able to balance without the support of his or her arms and able to meet challenges to balance. Eventually, the patient must stand alone, without any help, to ambulate safely.

5. The patient must safely perform these pre-gait exercises to gain strength, endurance, and balance before attempting ambulation.

6. Once the pre-gait skills have been accomplished, be sure your patient is wearing the right shoes for walking. Tied shoes with rubber heels are the best. "Gym" shoes are readily available and popular. Make sure they fit properly. "High-tops" can provide extra ankle support. Make sure the shoes are not heavy. Shoes that slide off the patient's feet, such as scuffs, slippers without backs, high heels, and slippery soles, can result in falls and sprains and should *not* be used.

7. Use a gait belt and "guard" the patient while walking. "Guarding" is the safest and most appropriate way to prevent falls. Most patients fall toward their weak side, either forward or backward. They fall because their legs are weak and/or their balance is poor. To "guard" a patient from falls while ambulating, stand on his or her weak side and just a little behind him or her. Place your same side hand on the patient's weak side shoulder and your other hand on the patient's gait belt in the small of the back. (Your finger and palm should be up for best support.) This position will allow you to control the patient's shoulders and hips and if (s)he loses balance, support him or her by stepping into his or her body and lowering him or her to the floor. As the patient's walking abilities improve, start to release his or her shoulder and then the belt, but stay on the weak side and a little behind him or her.

8. While walking with your patient, continually monitor for cardiac signs and symptoms. Remember to emphasize safety over speed when walking.

9. During "normal" ambulation, each leg alternates between the stance phase (where the leg is on the ground) and the swing phase (where the leg swings from the behind to the forward position).

10. Follow the directions of the physical therapist when ambulating patients. The physical therapist will instruct the patient on assistive devices and ambulation techniques.

Table 2-6   Assistive Devices for Ambulation

Type	What it Does	Who Should Use	Description
Short leg orthosis	Stabilizes the ankle at 90 degrees and prevents it from moving from side to side.	If drop foot or weak ankles	Made out of metal and attached to the shoe, or made out of plastic and inserted into the shoe.
Knee immobilizer	Keeps the knee extended, doesn't allow for flexion.	Those who cannot extend knee for proper swing in ambulation, or to avoid weight bearing	Heavy metal stays covered with cloth, and strap across the patella.
Standard walker	Provides a firm and stable support for weakness or balance problems.	Has two strong arms, but weak legs or mild balance problems	Made out of metal with rubber tips, adjustable.
Rolling walker	Provides a firm support for weakness or balance problems.	Has two strong arms, but problems with balance (mild) and/or initiating movement	Same as above, with wheels on front legs. The best ones lock when pushed on firmly.
Crutches	Provides support for weak or non-weight-bearing leg/foot.	Has two strong arms and good balance, but cannot weight bear on leg/foot	Made of steel or wood, adjustable, with rubber tips.
Walk cane	Provides firm and stable support for weakness or balance problems.	Has one strong arm, (hemiplegic), lateral instability when moving	Made of metal with four legs, adjustable and rubber tips.
Quad cane	Provides support for weakness and balance problems.	Same as above, but less severe	Made of metal with four legs, wide or narrow base, adjustable with rubber tips.
Cane	Provides support for weakness and mild balance problems.	Same as above, but less severe	Made of metal, wood, or other materials, should have rubber tip.

Procedure

Ambulation

 Steps

 Additional Information

1. Instruct the patient to stand straight with shoulders back and pelvis in an anterior pelvic tilt.

Assist your patient into this position.

2. The patient should push off with his or her toes and the ball of the foot from the ground, bending the knee and hip slightly at the same time.

The patient must shift his or her weight to the other leg for the leg to swing forward.

3. Cue the patient to land his or her foot on the floor with the heel first.

The foot should be pointed straight ahead with feet apart and the knee coming into full extension.

4. The patient should roll onto the ball of the foot and bend slightly at the knee, then fully extend the knee.

This will allow for weight bearing.

5. Repeat as tolerated.

Monitor for fatigue and loss of balance and any signs of cardiac/respiratory problems.

DOCUMENTATION

1. Patient's endurance and distance ambulating.
2. Any changes in pulse or blood pressure and complaints during ambulation.
3. Any problems during ambulation.

REFERENCES

Brander, V.A., Stulberg, S.D., Chang, R.W. (1994) "Rehabilitation Following Hip and Knee Arthroplasty" *Physical Medicine and Rehabilitation Clinics of North America* 5(4):815–836.

Sine, R.D., Holcomb, J.D., Roush, R.E., et al. (1983) *Basic Rehabilitation Techniques: A Self-Instructional Guide* 2d ed. Rockville, MD: Aspen.

Nursing Care of the Patient with Special Equipment

Nursing Care for the Patient with the Functional Electrical Stimulation or Transcutaneous Electrical Nerve Stimulation Unit

PURPOSE

Functional electrical stimulation (FES): To stimulate contraction of a specific muscle to enhance movement; to increase strength in weak muscles; to decrease spasticity of specific muscles by stimulating the antagonistic muscles; to help resolve shoulder subluxations; to promote sensory motor integration; to increase venous return

Transcutaneous electrical nerve stimulation (TENS): To block specific localized pain or nerve irritation

STAFF RESPONSIBLE

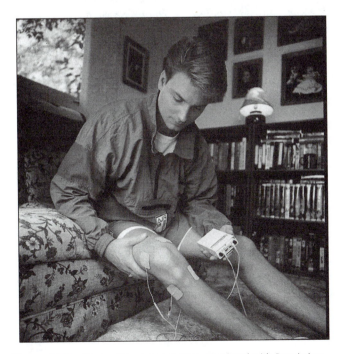

Figure 2-51 Electro Stimulation System. Reprinted with Permission from Rehabilicare, New Brighton, MN.

EQUIPMENT

See local/national manufacturer product information.

1. Electrodes (patches)
2. Lead wires
3. FES or TENS unit (Fig. 2-51)
4. Instructions for prescribed use

 ### GENERAL CONSIDERATIONS

1. The nurse's support and belief in a treatment modality such as FES or TENS may have an effect on the patient's compliance and satisfaction with the treatment. When a device such as TENS is used, the nurse's belief that the patient is in pain, that the pain is real, and that TENS can help alleviate it influences the patient in a positive manner. Other pain relief methods such as massage, imagery, progressive relaxation exercises, cold packs or icing, warm moist packs, and medications should be incorporated in the pain relief program as appropriate and effective.

2. The physical therapist or physician is responsible for placement of electrodes and setting of dials on the FES or TENS unit. Electrodes may be left in place for 1 week, provided that they remain secure.

3. The physical therapist or physician will supply nursing with specific instructions for dial settings, frequency and duration of the treatment, positioning of the patient during treatment, and the patient's level of independence in the treatment.

4. The physical therapist initiates the use of the FES or TENS unit and notifies nursing of the treatment.

5. Nursing requires a physician's prescription to use FES and TENS on the patient unit.

6. Showering is not contraindicated with this treatment. The electrodes can become wet and do not need to be covered, but they should be disconnected from the unit before showering the patient.

7. The TENS or FES unit is kept with the patient or is locked up when not in use.

Procedure

 Steps

 Additional Information

1. Review with physical therapist the individualized patient instructions before initial use of FES or TENS unit on patient unit.

   FES is contraindicated in patients with cardiac pacemakers or orthopedically unstable areas unless they are immobilized.

2. Position patient in specified position as instructed by physical therapist or physician.

3. Check placement of electrodes.

   Check for electrode adherence to skin and proper placement over desired muscle. If electrode has become loose along edges, it can be reinforced with paper tape. If electrode has fallen off completely, ask physical therapist to replace in proper position. Do not continue with treatment.

4. Check lead wires for any fraying that could indicate an electrical hazard.

   If this is found, do not continue with treatment. Notify physical therapist as soon as possible.

5. Check that FES or TENS unit is off.

6. Plug appropriate lead wires into electrodes and into FES or TENS unit per physical therapist's or physician's instructions.

7. Check dials on FES or TENS unit for proper settings.

   Verify with physical therapist's instruction sheet.

8. Check patient's pulse and blood pressure before, during, and after FES.

9. Turn unit on.

   Units vary in that some require that nurse set voltage dial.

10. Check patient comfort.

    If patient complains of burning sensation, check for loosening of electrodes or inadequate gel.

11. After designated treatment time has elapsed, switch unit off.

    Unit is set to shut off automatically after designated treatment time has elapsed (usually 15 to 20 min). Switch is still on, however, and wears out FES or TENS unit batteries.

12. Disconnect all lead wires from electrodes.

 DOCUMENTATION

1. Note the time of treatment and the patient's response.

2. Note any problems or concerns.

REFERENCES

Smith, R. (1998) "Current Trends in Electrotherapy" *Rehab Management* 11(3):30–38.

Nursing Care for the Patient with External Fixator Pins

PURPOSE

To prevent infection, possibly osteomyelitis, and/or other complications due to metal pins surgically inserted into the bone

STAFF RESPONSIBLE

EQUIPMENT

No equipment necessary.

GENERAL CONSIDERATIONS

1. Specific instructions for external fixator pin site care varies from physician to physician and institution to institution. Practice protocol should include assessments and care, sterile versus clean technique, cleansing and debridement, use of ointments and dressings, and patient teaching.
2. Inspection and assessment of pin sites should include:
   - Signs of inflammation or drainage
   - Signs of infection including pain, tenderness, redness, heat, edema, odor, or drainage
   - Any change in pin position or movement of the pin (shifting or bending of the pin)
   - Baseline measurement of the pin on both sides of the extremity
3. Lightly tapping the lateral aspect of the bone adjacent to the pin may be recommenced. If severe pain results, this may indicate the presence of infection (Nichol, 1993).
4. Crusts that form around the pin is the body's normal response to trauma and can provide a barrier to the outside environment (Wallis, 1991).
5. External fixator pins have a greater potential to develop pin reactions than skeletal traction pins. Pin looseness may correlate with an increase in infections (Mahon et al., 1991).

PATIENT AND FAMILY EDUCATION

1. The same protocol followed in the acute care setting should continue in the home setting.
2. Pin site cleaning and dressings may be done with clean, rather than sterile, technique in the home.

Procedure

External Fixator Pin Site Care

 Steps

1. Assess skin around pins on regular basis.
2. Check pins for looseness and any movement or changes.
3. Cleanse in circular motion, from inner aspect to outer aspect with normal saline, if prescribed.
4. Apply dressing, if prescribed.

 Additional Information

Observe for signs of inflammation, drainage, and infection.

Compare to baseline measurements.

Other cleansing agents may damage tissue, affect the metal in the pins, or be absorbed systemically.

Ointments may be prescribed as a barrier. Dressing application should be with sterile technique.

 DOCUMENTATION

1. Pin site protocol components should be clearly identified.
2. Baseline measurements of the pins should be recorded on admission.
3. Any problems or complications (signs of inflammation, infection, loose pins) should be reported to physician.

REFERENCES

Asci, J.A. and Beyea, S.C. (1994) "Orthopaedic Update: External Pinsite Care: An Integrative Review of the Research" *Online Journal of Knowledge Synthesis for Nursing* [online serial] Available: volume number 1, document number 12.

Beeman, J., and Diehl, B. (1995) "A Credentialing Program for Nursing Staff Caring for Pediatric Patients with a Ilizarov Apparatus" *Rehabilitation Nursing* 20(5):278–282.

Hart, K. (1994) "Using the Ilizarov External Fixator in Bone Transport" *Orthopaedic Nursing* 13(1):35–40.

Mahon, J., Seligson, D., Henry, S., et al. (1991) "Factors in Pin Tract Infections" *Orthopedics* 14:305–308.

Miller, M. (1983) "Nursing Care of the Patient with External Fixation Therapy" *Orthopaedic Nursing* 2(1):11–15.

Nichol, D. (1993) "Wound Care. Preventing Infection." *Nursing Times* 89(13):78–79.

Wallis, S. (1991) "An Agenda to Promote Self-Care: Nursing Care of Skeletal Pin Sites" *Professional Nurse* 6(12):715–716, 718–720.

Amputation Care

PURPOSE

To promote physical and psychological healing after amputation of a body part

STAFF RESPONSIBLE

EQUIPMENT

1. Stump socks
2. Rigid dressing (includes molded cast, cover sock, and cuff)
3. Shrinker socks
4. Compressogrip/tubegrip

 GENERAL CONSIDERATIONS

1. Amputation care applies to all clients with an amputated limb. Lower extremity amputations are considered Symes (partial foot), below knee (BK) or transtibial, above knee (AK) or transfemoral, and hip disarticulation. Upper extremity amputations are considered digital, partial hand, wrist disarticulation, below elbow (BE) or transradial, above elbow (AE) or transhumoral, and shoulder disarticulation. In lower extremity amputations, the goals are to promote consistent and uniform stump shrinkage and allow for early weight bearing and ambulation training, as well as protect the residual limb. To meet these goals, for BK amputations, the rigid removable dressing and shrinker socks should be used, and for AK amputations, compressogrip/tubegrip and shrinker socks should be used. The goals for upper extremity amputations are to shrink the stump and shape it for prosthetic fitting. For BE and AE amputations, compressogrip/tubegrip is used.

2. Stump shrinkage is desirable, even for patients who are not candidates for prostheses, to decrease pain and to enhance healing of the residual limb.

3. Skin visual checks of the stump should be performed at least twice a day to assess circulation and skin condition.

4. Skin wound treatments should be continued, as prescribed, underneath the rigid removable dressing or shrinker socks or compressogrip/tubegrip.

5. Common contractures that occur with lower extremity amputation are:
   - Hip flexion
   - Hip abduction
   - Hip external rotation
   - Knee flexion

6. Avoid the use of pillows under the lower extremity residual limb in bed positioning, as this may contribute to joint contractures.

7. Use a padded knee extension board to promote knee extension while sitting in the wheelchair.

8. Ambulation with appropriate ambulation aids and prosthesis (temporary or permanent) should be encouraged if prescribed by the physician, with necessary assistance as indicated by the physical therapist.

9. The patient's weight should be strictly monitored and maintained to ensure proper prosthetic fit.

10. Phantom limb sensations and pain may start at any time after surgery and may be triggered by pressure on other areas. Weight-bearing positioning (early ambulation with temporary prosthesis), deep pressure, and desensitization techniques may help alleviate these sensations. Analgesic medications may be needed. Topical analgesics can also be used.

11. Body image changes occur after an amputation. Anticipate them and provide atmosphere of acceptance, trust, and support. Help to use clothing to minimize body changes and to enhance appearance. Acknowledge and give positive reinforcement when client attempts to improve or accommodate body changes. Teach ways to enhance confidence and abilities.

PATIENT AND FAMILY EDUCATION

1. Patient and family should be clear on the process to obtain a prosthesis to avoid confusion and conflicting goals.

2. Patient and family teaching to include: skin checks—how and when to do them and what to report to the physician/therapist/nurse; how to use shrinker device (rigid removable dressing, shrinker socks, compressogrip/tubegrip), when to increase or decrease number of shrinker socks, how to care for these items; positioning program to prevent contractures and mobility program to increase wearing time, endurance, and strength.

Procedure

Amputation Care

 Steps

 Additional Information

1. Position amputated limb in proper body alignment (Fig. 2-52*A*).

   Assist patient to position amputated limb in neutral position.

2. Position BK and AK patients prone for at least 20 min at least twice a day (Fig. 2-52*B*).

   Hip should be in neutral rotation and neutral abduction-adduction. If BK, add knee extension.

3. Position BK patients with knee extension when sitting.

   Use a padded board to ensure full knee extension with the hip at 90-degree flexion.

4. Ensure proper application and fit of rigid removable dressing for BK amputation (Figs. 2-53 and 2-54).

   The rigid removable dressing (RRD) should be removed every morning and every evening for skin and circulation checks, then reapplied. Change stump socks, replacing same number, unless directed otherwise. Patient may have tube-grip under RRD to increase shrinkage. A red area under the RRD does **not** *mean that it should be left off, but should be reported to the physician and therapist. If the RRD is too loose, additional stump socks may need to be added. Check with the therapist.*

5. Check stump at least twice a day.

   Skin checks should include presence of any reddened, soft, hot areas, pressure ulcers, and wound/incision assessments. Circulation checks should include: misshapen stumps, blisters, changes in temperature, pain, amount of edema, and loss/change in sensation.

6. Administer analgesics as needed.

   Encourage patient to premedicate before painful activities.

7. Assist with range of motion exercises as prescribed by the physician and/or therapist.

8. Assist/cue patient to increase mobility and self-care –activities.

   Aid with sliding board training to increase mobility. Towels or blankets may improve patient's confidence in socializing with others.

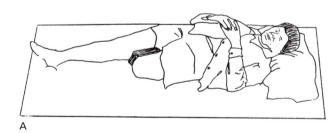
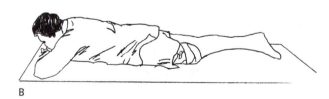

A

B

Figure 2-52

 DOCUMENTATION

1. Document the use of the removable rigid dressing.
2. Note the skin status and the patient's tolerance.
3. Note the patient's and family's education and mastery of application.
4. Note the patient's positioning methods and schedule.
5. Note the patient's tolerance to positioning, presence of joint contracture, or presence of edema in the residual limb.
6. Note the effectiveness of patient and family education.

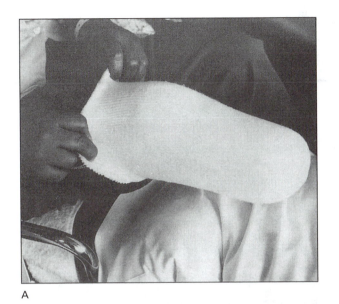

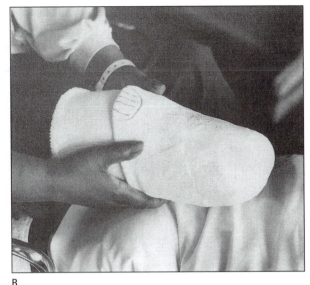

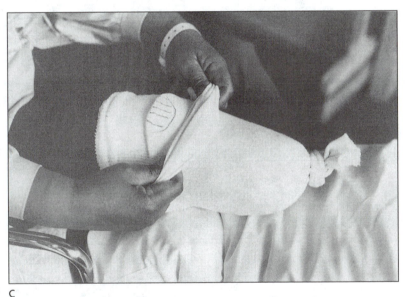

Figure 2-53   Applying Removable Rigid Dressing in Below-Knee Amputation. (**A**) Applying Socks, (**B**) Applying Molded Cast, (**C**) Applying Cover Sock.

REFERENCES

American Academy of Orthopaedic Surgeons (1981) *Atlas of Limb Prosthetics: Surgical and Prosthetic Principles* St. Louis, MO: Mosby.

Banerjee, S.N. (1982) *Rehabilitation Management of Amputees* Baltimore, MD: Williams & Wilkins.

Engstrom, B. and Van De Ven, C. (1985) *Physiotherapy for Amputees* New York: Churchill Livingstone.

Karacoloff, L.A. (1986) *Lower Extremity Amputation: A Guide to Functional Outcomes in Physical Therapy Management* Rockville, MD: Aspen.

Kostiuk, J.P. (1981) *Amputation Surgery and Rehabilitation: The Toronto Experience* New York: Churchill-Livingstone.

Rehabilitation Institute of Chicago (1978) *Pre-Prosthetic Care for Above Knee Amputees* Chicago: Rehabilitation Institute of Chicago.

Rehabilitation Institute of Chicago (1978) *Pre-Prosthetic Care for Below Knee Amputees* Chicago: Rehabilitation Institute of Chicago.

Williams, A.M. and Deaton, S.B. (1997) "Phantom Limb Pain: Elusive, Yet Real" *Rehabilitation Nursing* 22(2):73–77.

Wu, Y. and Krick, H. (1987) "Removable Rigid Dressing for Below-Knee Amputees" *Clinical Prosthetics and Orthotics* 11:33–44.

Yetzer, E.A. (1996) "Helping the Patient through the Experience of an Amputation" *Orthopaedic Nursing* 15(6):45–49.

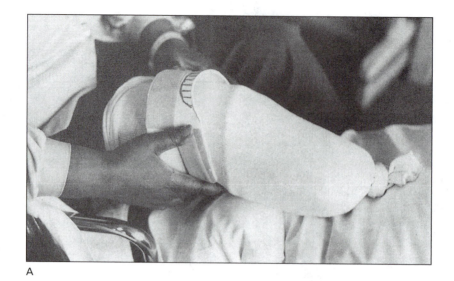

A

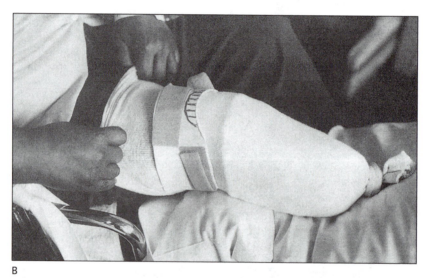

B

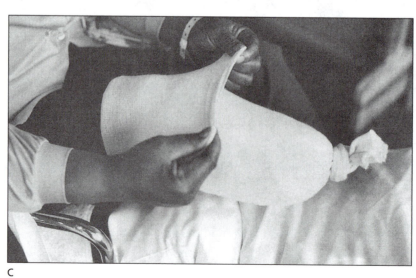

C

Figure 2-54 Applying Removable Rigid Dressing in Below-Knee Amputation. **(A)** Applying Cuff, **(B)** Pulling up Socks, **(C)** Folding over Sock Edges.

Transfer Techniques

Moving Forward and Backward in Wheelchair

PURPOSE

To position patient properly in a wheelchair before or after transfers or to improve posture

STAFF RESPONSIBLE

EQUIPMENT

No equipment necessary.

GENERAL CONSIDERATIONS

1. To facilitate normal movement and tone, the patient should be encouraged to participate as much as possible (for example, a patient with hemiplegia may slide the unaffected side of his or her body forward in the chair to prepare to transfer).

2. Technique 1 should be used with patients who can also do the squat pivot transfer. Contraindications are:
   - Patients with leg casts or body casts
   - Patients with spinal orthoses (CTO, TLSO, CTLSO, or LSO)
   - Patients with trunk extension contractures
   - Patients with labile orthostatic hypotension or chronic obstructive pulmonary disease
   - Patients with arthritis or orther diseases that prohibit flexion of hip and knee joints while weight bearing

3. Technique 2 should be used when contraindications exist for the use of technique 1.

4. When sitting, the patient will be more functional if he or she assumes and maintains an anterior pelvic tilt, symmetric trunk, and head in midline alignment. Recognizing deviations from this position allows for prompt correction, increased function of the patient, and safety for all.

PATIENT AND FAMILY EDUCATION

Teach this technique to the family to facilitate the transfer process. As the procedure is repeated, the patient may be able to assist more.

Procedures

Moving Forward

 Steps

 Additional Information

1. Position wheelchair for transfer (90 degrees to other surface).

2. Remove footrests or swing them out of the way.

3. Lock brakes.

4. Remove armrests.

5. Remove safety strap.

6. Have patient assist as much as possible. Face patient with wide base of support. Bend knees to bring you to or slightly above the same level as the patient's face.

Patient's feet should be securely on floor with wide base of support and toes a little behind knees. If patient's legs do not touch floor, be prepared to brace patient more forcefully; this procedure should move patient forward so that feet will touch floor.

7. Bring the patient's right shoulder forward to lean against your right shoulder (Fig. 2-55A).

8. Encircle patient's trunk with your arms and cup patient's left scapula with your right hand (Fig. 2-55*B*).

9. Place your left hand on patient's right buttock.

10. Lean patient forward and to left side while supporting the left side with your right arm, and pull patient's right buttock toward front of wheelchair (Fig. 2-55*C*).

11. Move your left hand from patient's right buttock to right scapula.

12. Move your right hand from patient's left scapula to left buttock.

13. Lean patient forward and to right side while supporting right side with your left arm, and pull patient's left buttock toward front of wheelchair.

14. Continue steps 9 through 13 until patient is sitting on front half to two-thirds of wheelchair cushion.

Buttock may come forward only a small amount. This usually indicates a need to lean patient forward and to the side more.

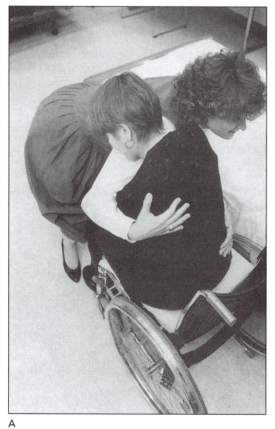

A

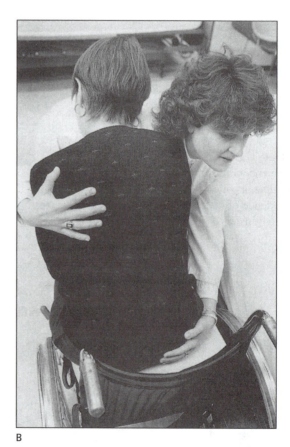

B

Figure 2-55   Moving the Patient Forward in a Wheelchair (Technique 1).

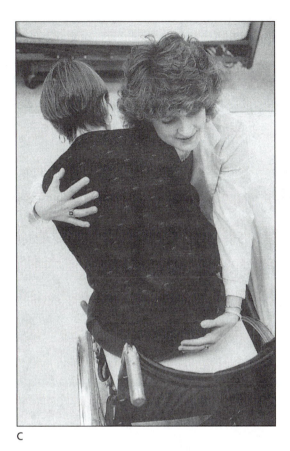

C

Figure 2-55 (continued)

Moving Backward

TECHNIQUE 1

 Steps

 Additional Information

1. Remove footrests.

2. Lock brakes.

3. Remove safety strap.

4. Have patient assist as much as possible.

5. Lean patient forward over either of your hips (Fig. 2-56A).

6. Encircle patient's trunk with your arms, grasping your wrists under patient's breasts (Fig. 2-56A).

7. Rock patient forward.

8. When patient's weight is over his or her legs, push against patient's shins or knees to move patient backward in chair (Fig. 2-56B).

9. Allow patient to come in contact with seat of wheelchair.

10. Continue steps 7 through 9 until patient is in appropriate sitting position.

Patient's feet should be securely on floor with wide base of support and toes quite a bit behind knees. If patient's feet do not touch floor, use technique 2.

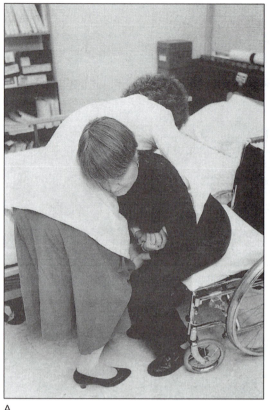 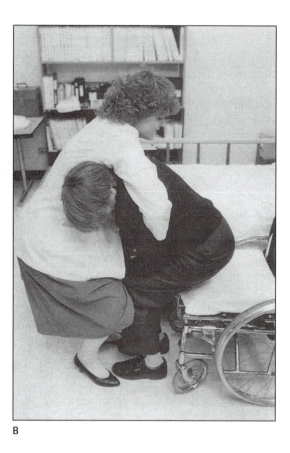

A   B

Figure 2-56   Moving the Patient Backward in a Wheelchair (Technique 1).

Moving Forward or Backward

TECHNIQUE 2

 Steps

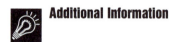 **Additional Information**

1. Get another person to assist you.
2. Stand behind patient, facing same way as patient.
3. Second person stands in front of patient, facing patient.
4. Second person places right shoulder to patient's right shoulder.
5. Second person leans patient forward and holds him or her there by cupping his or her scapulae.
6. First person encircles patient's chest under axillae, and with left hand grasps patient's right wrist and with right hand grasps patient's left wrist (Fig. 2-57A).
7. Second person lets patient rest back against first person, moves to face patient, and places a hand under each thigh above knee (Fig. 2-57B).
8. On count of three, lift up patient's trunk by lifting patient with your forearms against patient's ribs. Second person lifts patient's thighs and buttocks back or forward in wheelchair (Fig. 2-57C).
9. Continue with transfer techniques or complete appropriate patient positioning in wheelchair.

Second person should hold patient's thighs close to his or her own chest, bend knees, and have wide base of support.

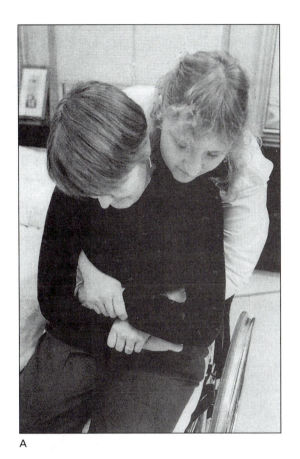

A

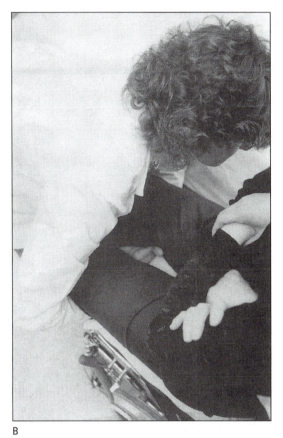

B

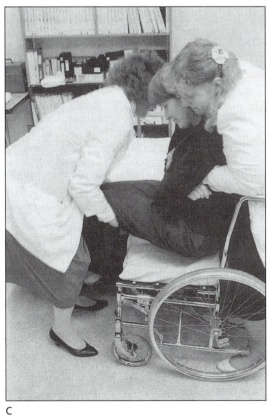

C

Figure 2-57   Moving the Patient Forward or Backward in a Wheelchair (Technique 2).

DOCUMENTATION

1. Note the effectiveness of patient and family teaching.
2. Document any unusual occurrences.
3. Note any change in the amount of assistance needed.
4. Note the amount and kind of assistance needed.
5. Note any special precautions, needs, or equipment.

Squat Pivot Transfer

PURPOSE

To transfer a patient safely from one surface to another

STAFF RESPONSIBLE

EQUIPMENT

1. Wheelchair
2. Bed or mat
3. Shower chair

GENERAL CONSIDERATIONS

1. This type of transfer is ideal for patients who have quadriplegia with increased tone, but it can be used with any patient who can bear weight on his or her legs (involuntarily or voluntarily). The patient need only be able to cooperate minimally but at least should not resist the procedure.

2. The use of a sliding board may facilitate the procedure, particularly with heavy or tall patients, or when there is a significant difference in height between the two surfaces or when going into the car, where the wheelchair cannot get close to the car seat.

3. The transferer must use good body mechanics to perform this procedure safely (i.e., keep the back straight and knees bent, have a wide base of support, pivot rather than twist, and carry weight at the center of the body).

4. Contraindications to using this transfer include:
   - Patients with leg or body casts
   - Patients with spinal orthoses (CTO, CTLSO, TLSO, or LSO)
   - Patients with trunk extension contractures
   - Patients with labile orthostatic hypotension or chronic obstructive pulmonary disease
   - Patients with arthritis or other diseases that prohibit flexion of hip and knee joints while weight bearing

PATIENT AND FAMILY EDUCATION

Teach this technique to the family. This method is recommended particularly for car transfers.

Procedure

Squat Pivot Transfer

 Steps

 Additional Information

1. Explain procedure to patient.

2. Position wheelchair 90 degrees to bed, shower chair, car seat, or other surface. Remove footrests and lock brakes. Remove armrest closest to location patient is going to.

3. Move patient forward in wheelchair or to side of bed so that feet are flat on floor and toes are behind knees with wide base of support (Fig. 2-58A).

Face patient, use wide base of support, and bend your knees, not your back.

See procedures for moving patient forward or backward in wheelchair. Ensure that patient is in anterior pelvic tilt, that trunk is symmetric, and that head is in midline.

4. Lean patient forward so that patient's shoulder rests against your hip opposite to surface to which patient is being transferred (Fig. 2-58*B*).

5. Reach under patient's breasts and clasp your wrists while leaning patient forward and placing your chest against patient's upper posterior trunk (Fig. 2-58*C*).

6. Rock patient's body forward a little and toward bed or chair, set patient down for a moment, then rock patient forward and over again until he or she is firmly on bed or chair (Fig. 2-58*C*).

7. Position patient appropriately in wheelchair or bed.

Place patient's arms in patient's lap.

Bend your legs and lean slightly backward. If patient feels heavy, try bending your knees more and leaning patient forward. Patient will be unable to resist transfer procedure.

If patient is heavy or too tall for transfer, a sliding board may be used to assist. A spotter may assist by positioning himself or herself behind patient's back and chair and helping lean and rock patient forward as needed. If you can't get your arms around the patient's trunk, you can lean them over your shoulder and hold onto the gait belt.

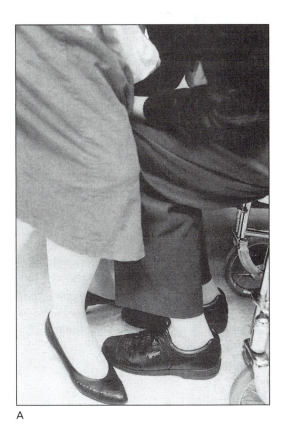

A

Figure 2-58   Dependent or Sitting Pivot Transfer

 DOCUMENTATION

1. Note the effectiveness of patient and family teaching.

2. Note the type of transfer.

3. Document the amount and kind of assistance required.

4. Note any special precautions, needs, or equipment.

5. Note any difficulty in completing the transfer.

6. Document any unusual occurrences.

7. Note any change in the amount of assistance needed.

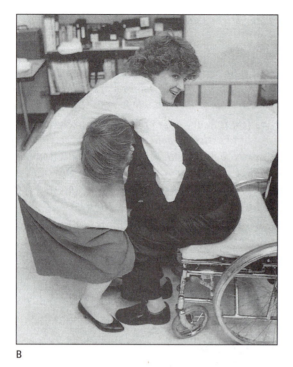

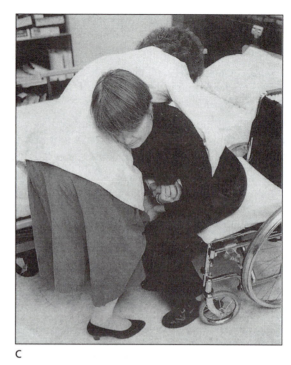

B

C

Figure 2-58 Dependent or Sitting Pivot Transfer (continued).

Stand Pivot Transfer

PURPOSE

To perform a safe stand pivot transfer to any surface

STAFF RESPONSIBLE

EQUIPMENT

1. Wheelchair
2. Shower chair
3. Toilet
4. Bed
5. Car

 GENERAL CONSIDERATIONS

1. In most cases, if the patient can voluntarily bear weight on one or both legs, a standing pivot transfer can be performed.

2. The patient with hemiplegia or brain damage may have any or all of the following problems:

- Partial or complete loss of function on one side of the body
- Partial or total lack of sensation
- Increased or decreased tone in the involved side
- Aphasia
- Perceptual problems
- Neglect of one side of the body
- Confusion
- Emotional lability
- Intellectual impairment
- Impaired vision

3. The person with hemiplegia has a sound arm and leg that should be utilized to their fullest extent when performing a transfer.

4. The less variance there is in the physical environment, the easier it is for the patient to transfer. Repetition in the same situation is valuable.

5. The armrest may or may not be removed, depending on the patient's level of ability. Removable legrests are desirable.

6. Familiarize yourself with body mechanics and transfer techniques so that you can perform the transfer properly.

7. Complete the following activities before doing the transfer:

- Assess the patient's strengths and weaknesses

- Observe the patient's activity and determine his or her ability to assist
- Observe the patient's posture and balance
- Evaluate the patient's comprehension and ability to follow instructions

PATIENT AND FAMILY EDUCATION

Teach this technique to the patient and family. After repetition of the technique, the patient may be able to perform the transfer with less assistance and/or fewer cues.

Procedures

Stand Pivot Transfer

PREPARATION FOR TRANSFER

 Steps

1. Review procedure with patient.

2. Position wheelchair at 90-degree angle to surface from which you are transferring patient.

3. Lock brakes on wheelchair.

4. Remove armrest closest to patient (if not needed) and move legrests out of way.

5. Adjust height of bed.

6. Place proper, nonslip shoes on patient.

7. Lower side rail closest to wheelchair and remove safety strap.

 Additional Information

Keep instructions to one- or two-step commands if patient has comprehension problems.

If hemiplegia exists, initially position wheelchair so that patient is able to lead with his or her strongest side until transfers are perfected. Ideally, a patient with hemiplegia should be able to transfer from both sides for optimal community reentry.

Patients needing minimal assistance may use armrest to push to standing.

Adjust bed so that patient's legs will be flat on floor when sitting on edge of bed.

BED, CHAIR TO WHEELCHAIR, SHOWER CHAIR, OR BACK TO BED: MAXIMAL ASSISTANCE

 Steps

1. Assist patient to sitting position.

2. Stand in front of patient.

3. Place patient's feet on floor with wide base of support and heels behind knees.

4. Place your legs on either side of patient's weak leg and bend your knees (Fig. 2-59*A*).

5. Put your hands on both sides of patient's chest, and place your right shoulder to patient's right shoulder (or your left shoulder to patient's left shoulder) (Fig. 2-59*B*).

 Additional Information

Do this by cradling trunk below shoulders while grasping lower extremities under knees. Simultaneously raise patient's head and slide legs off side of bed, pivoting trunk.

Place a gait belt around patient's waist to give you something firm to grasp. Depending on your size and patient's size, it may be helpful to place your hands under patient's buttocks. Do not allow patient to put arms around your neck. Instead, instruct patient to use arms to push off bed or to clasp hands and extend arms in front of himself or herself to weaker side. A rocking motion helps.

6. Have patient lean as far forward as possible and, on count of three, come to standing position (Fig. 2-59C).

Rock patient forward rhythmically three times and, on third time, stand. If patient is able, have him or her extend both arms straight out in front; otherwise keep patient's arms in his or her lap. Leaning forward will prevent patient from falling backward into wheelchair.

7. Pivot patient toward chair, stop when patient is in front of it.
8. Bend at knees to lower patient to chair.

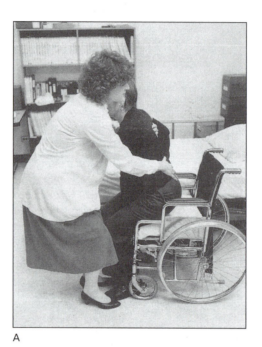

A

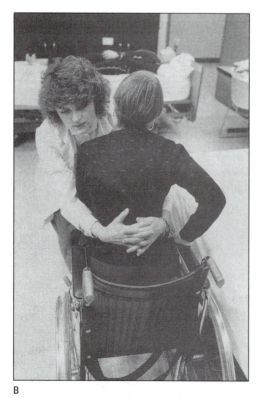

B

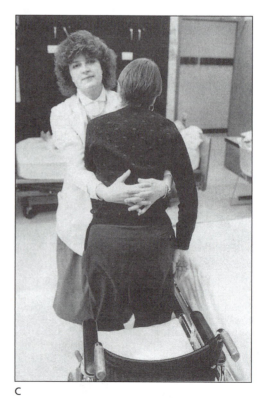

C

Figure 2-59 Standing Pivot Transfer, Maximal Assistance.

BED, CHAIR TO WHEELCHAIR, SHOWER CHAIR, OR BACK TO BED: MINIMAL ASSISTANCE

 Steps

1. Have patient come to sitting position with feet flat on floor (toes under knees).

2. Have patient place his or her strong hand on armrest of chair or side of bed.

3. Have patient lean forward, push against chair, and come to standing position.

4. Have patient pivot toward chair.

5. Have patient bend at waist and lean forward.

6. Have patient sit down.

 Additional Information

Assistance may be needed to maintain balance (put your hands on either side of patient's chest or give step-by-step directions).

Have patient look up when standing and look toward direction in which he or she is moving. Allow patient to get balance before pivoting.

You may want to have patient reach back to touch surface before sitting down.

 DOCUMENTATION

1. Document the type of transfer.

2. Note the amount and kind of assistance needed.

3. Note any special precautions, needs, or equipment.

4. Note any difficulty in completing the transfer.

5. Document any unusual occurrences.

6. Note any change in the amount of assistance needed.

7. Note the effectiveness of patient and family teaching.

Slide Board Transfer

PURPOSE

To transfer a patient safely from one surface to another

STAFF RESPONSIBLE

EQUIPMENT

1. Wheelchair

2. Shower chair

3. Transfer board/sliding board

4. Car

 GENERAL CONSIDERATIONS

1. This type of transfer may be used with a wide range of patients, from those requiring no assistance to those who are totally dependent. The patient need only cooperate minimally but at least should not resist the procedure. This transfer technique is especially helpful with car transfers.

2. The transferer must use good body mechanics to perform this procedure safely (i.e., keep the back straight and knees bent, have a wide base of support, pivot rather than twist, and carry weight at the center of the body). A helper may be used for very large or complicated patients. The helper should be positioned behind the patient and use the gait belt to help patient lean forward or slide.

3. Contraindications to using this transfer include:
   • Patients with trunk extension contractions, and
   • Patients who are resistive to the technique or who are uncooperative.

4. This type of transfer is often the first step in developing an independent lateral transfer for patients with paraplegia or paresis. The amount of energy and upper extremity strength required is substantially less when the sliding board is used.

PATIENT AND FAMILY EDUCATION

Teach this technique to the patient and family. It is especially helpful in performing transfers across uneven surfaces, including car transfers.

Procedure

Slide Board Transfer

 Steps

 Additional Information

1. Explain procedure to patient.

2. Position wheelchair 90 degrees to bed or whatever surface you want to transfer to.

3. Remove footrests.

4. Lock brakes.

5. Remove armrest closest to bed or chair or car.

6. Remove safety strap.

7. Move patient forward in wheelchair or to side of bed so that feet are flat on floor and toes are behind knees with wide base of support and toes are slightly between the two surfaces.

   Patients with casts or who cannot bear weight may have legs on bed but must compensate by leaning forward.

8. Lean patient to side away from chair or bed or car.

   Optimally, patient should be moving from higher surface to lower one.

9. Holding board at 45 degrees to bed or chair, slide it under patient's upper thighs (not buttocks) (Fig. 2-60*A*).

10. Reposition patient upright.

11. Aim free end of board to distant rear corner of chair or middle of bed (Fig. 2-60*B*) or car seat.

12. If patient is dependent:
    • Lean patient forward over your hip opposite to surface to which patient is being transferred
    • Circle patient's chest under breasts with your arms, and clasp your wrists
    • Slide patient along board (Fig. 2-60*C*)

    Place patient's arms in his or her lap. Alternatively, lean patient over your shoulder and grasp gait belt.

13. If patient is able to assist, have patient lean forward and slide himself or herself by shifting weight.

    Guard patient by placing your arms around patient's chest or waist and your legs between patient's legs. If patient's legs give out, lean patient forward more and brace his or her shin with yours.

14. If patient is independent, have him or her perform as many steps as possible (Fig 2-61).

    Eventually, as upper extremity strength and endurance increase, the sliding board becomes unnecessary.

15. Position patient in wheelchair or bed or car as appropriate.

 DOCUMENTATION

1. Note the type of transfer.

2. Document the amount and kind of assistance needed.

3. Document any special precautions, needs, or equipment.

4. Note any difficulties in completing the transfer.

5. Note any unusual occurrences.

6. Note any change in amount of assistance needed.

7. Document the effectiveness of patient and family teaching.

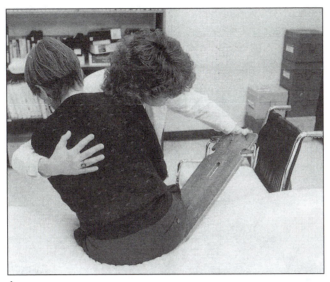

A

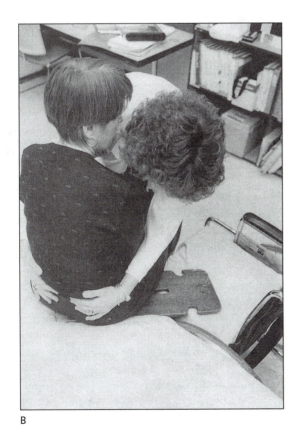

B

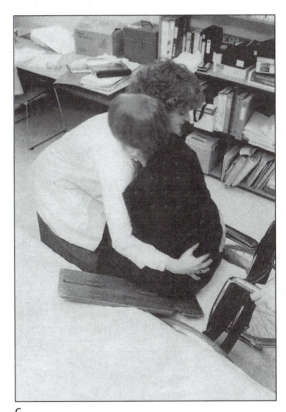

C

Figure 2-60   Sliding Board Transfer for Dependent Patient.

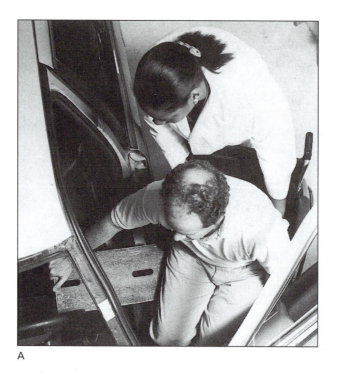

A

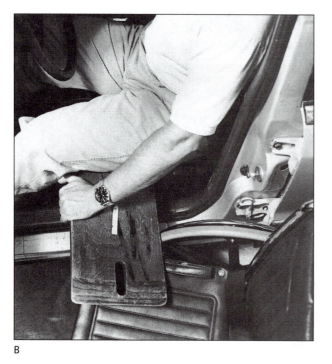

B

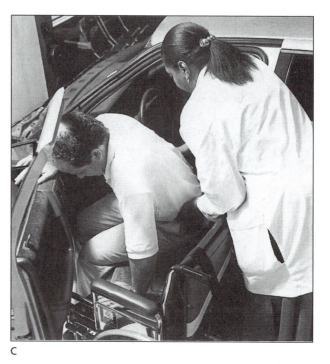

C

Figure 2-61 Sliding Board Transfer for Independent Patient.

Two-Person Lift

PURPOSE

To lift a patient safely from one surface to another

STAFF RESPONSIBLE

EQUIPMENT

1. Wheelchair with removable armrests and legrests
2. Shower chair
3. Toilet
4. Bed or mat

GENERAL CONSIDERATIONS

1. In most cases, any patient who sits at 60 degrees or higher can be transferred by the two-person lift technique.

2. Patients who consistently require a two-person lift should consider using a mechanical lifting device or transfer assistance device (sliding board). Such a patient may also be a candidate for a squat pivot transfer. The physical therapist should be consulted regarding this decision.

3. Patients requiring a two-person lift may have any or all of the following problems:
   - Paralyzed upper or lower extremities (or both)
   - Loss of sensation
   - Loss of position sense
   - Spasticity
   - Loss of trunk stability or balance in sitting
   - Contraindicated weight bearing in trunk or legs (i.e., fractures, contractures, or arthritis)

4. Familiarize yourself with body mechanics and transfer techniques so that you can perform the transfer properly.

5. Complete the following activities before performing the transfer:
   - Assess the patient's strengths and weaknesses
   - Observe the patient's activities and determine his or her ability to assist
   - Observe the patient's posture and balance
   - Evaluate the patient's comprehension and ability to follow instructions
   - Consider the patient's height and weight (patients weighing more than 150 lb should not be lifted, depending on your institution's lifting policy)

PATIENT AND FAMILY EDUCATION

1. The patient is not able to assist with this procedure.

2. The procedure requires two persons (not always available in the community setting), good body mechanics, and strength.

Procedure

Bed to Wheelchair or Shower Chair and Back

 Steps

1. Review procedure with patient.
2. Move patient to side of bed where transfer will take place, securing catheter, IV tubing, and so forth from harm.
3. Move wheelchair parallel to side of bed at hip level and facing foot of bed.
4. Lock wheels. Remove armrest closest to bed and both legrests if possible.
5. Raise bed so that it is at same level or slightly higher than seat cushion of wheelchair.
6. Bring patient to sitting position.

 Additional Information

Depending on environmental setup, this may be either right or left side.

Legrests can be moved out of the way; if not removable, raise them.

For those patients who experience orthostatic hypotension, head of bed should be raised 5 to 10 min before transfer. This may also help if patient has poor trunk balance or is obese.

7. Have patient cross arms on chest or cross them for him or her.

8. Stand behind patient with one knee on bed, slide arms under patient's axillae, and firmly grasp patient's forearms (Fig. 2-62*A*).

Put firm pressure with your forearms against patient's ribs rather than axillae. The humeral head can be forced into subacromial arch, causing pain on lifting.

9. The second person stands facing bed in front of wheelchair and places one arm under patient's thighs and one arm under knees (Fig. 2-62*B*).

This person should have wide base of support, bend at knees, and keep back as straight as possible.

10. On the count of three, patient is lifted into chair. Shift weight from knee on bed to leg behind chair; other person should step back (Fig. 2-62*C*).

Lift completely and slowly so as not to cause trauma to patient's skin or extremities. Be sure that patient is held close to your body (center of gravity), and do not bend your back.

11. Adjust patient's position as necessary.

12. Attach safety belt, replace armrests, and adjust legrests.

For patients with poor trunk stability, person at feet should stabilize patient until trunk supports are secured.

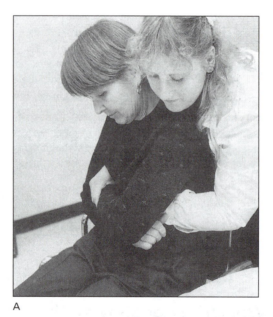

A

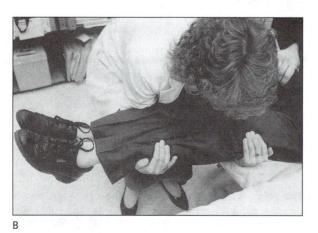

B

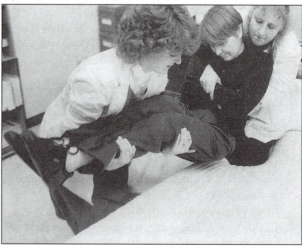

C

Figure 2-62   Two-Person Lift.

DOCUMENTATION

1. Note the type of transfer.
2. Document the amount and kind of assistance needed.
3. Note any special precautions (e.g., painful shoulders).

4. Note any difficulties in completing the transfer.
5. Note any unusual occurrences.
6. Document the effectiveness of patient and family teaching.

Showering Devices: Surgilift Transfer

PURPOSE

To transfer a patient safely by means of the Surgilift for bed or cart transfers or showers

STAFF RESPONSIBLE

EQUIPMENT

1. Surgilift
2. Surgilift netting
3. Restraint straps (optional, as needed)

GENERAL CONSIDERATIONS

1. Use of the Surgilift permits safe transfer of a patient by one staff member and minimizes strain on personnel and the patient.

2. The Surgilift should not be used on patients with unstable spines while braces are off unless specific prescriptions are written by the physician.
3. Some beds with casters removed do not permit Surgilift use because of low ground clearance.
4. The Surgilift safely carries 400 lb. Surgilift netting should be monitored for wear on the straps and replaced when this becomes evident.
5. The spring locks on the Surgilift frame are designed to lock tighter the more weight that is placed on the netting.
6. Surgilift netting is washed daily. Wash with warm water and disinfectant, rinse well, and air dry.
7. Surgilift netting is washed in the washer with hot water (140°F) and bleach after each use by patients who contaminate the netting with body secretions of any type during use (i.e., drainage that has soaked through dressing, incontinence of urine, and the like).
8. Patients can be showered while on the Surgilift. Netting allows for washing, rinsing, and drying of back and legs.

Procedure

 Steps

1. Place patient's bed in flat position.
2. Position patient to side of bed with head in position in which it will be on netting.

3. Fan-fold Surgilift netting and place it under patient.

4. Raise Surgilift frame to bed level by turning crank on side clockwise.
5. Lift frame to vertical position.
6. Slide wheels of Surgilift under bed while holding frame in vertical position.

 Additional Information

Try placing lifter over bed so that you can position patient such that lifter will fit around bed wheels and patient's head will be supported.

This can be done by rolling patient from side to side. Top of patient's head should be even with top end of netting.

7. Gently lower frame over patient, encircling him or her.

8. Lift up latches of spring locks, and thread netting straps through them.

9. Place restraining straps if needed over patient (e.g., if patient is agitated, impulsive, spastic, or mobile).

10. Raise Surgilift by turning knob so that patient's trunk is high enough to clear bed.

11. Take patient to desired location.

12. Reverse procedure to take patient off Surgilift.

Patients taller than 7 feet will be too long for frame. Their legs can be positioned so that they are supported with a pillow over top of frame, or they can be suspended in netting so that legs clear below frame.

Secure locks by pressing down on latches when straps are all in place.

Do not leave patient unattended on Surgilift.

Lower bed to lowest position to facilitate clearance.

DOCUMENTATION

1. Document the type of transfer.

2. Note any unusual occurrences during the Surgilift procedure.

3. Note any special precautions, needs, or equipment.

4. Note any difficulties in completing the transfer.

SHOWER CHAIRS (REGULAR AND RECLINING)

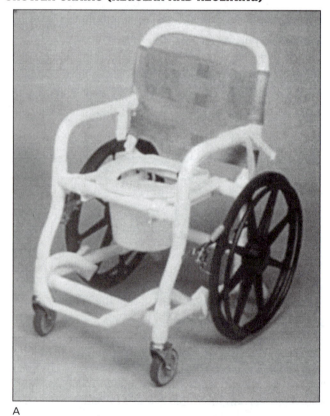

A

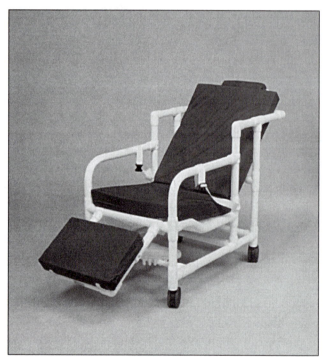

B

Figure 2-63   Reprinted with Permission from Duralife Inc., South Williamsport, PA.

SHOWER TROLLEY

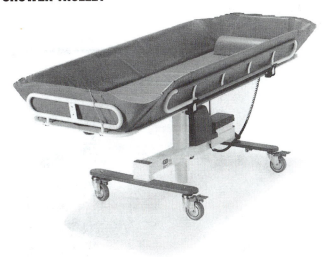

Figure 2-64   Reprinted with Permission from Arjo, Morton Grove, IL.

Floor to Chair Transfer

PURPOSE

To assist patient up from the floor

STAFF RESPONSIBLE

EQUIPMENT

No equipment necessary.

 GENERAL CONSIDERATIONS

1. This technique is for weak patients who find themselves on the floor. Patients with hip precautions or limitations in shoulder range of motion should not use this method.

Procedure

Floor to Chair Transfer

 Steps

1. Roll patient to one side.

2. Cue patient to come up on stronger arm (Fig. 2-65*A*).

3. Cue patient to come up on both arms (Fig. 2-65*B*).

4. Stabilize patient so (s)he gets on all fours (Fig. 2-65*C*).

5. Cue him or her to put first the strong arm, then the weaker arm, on the chair seat (Fig. 2-65*D*).

 Additional Information

Patient should do as much for himself or herself as possible. A gait belt is applied. If the patient has a stronger side, it should be on the bottom.

This will provide best use of patient's mobility skills.

Chair should be locked or stabilized.

6. Assist him or her to get the weaker foot and leg up and flexed with foot flat on floor; then the stronger foot and leg, up and flexed (Fig. 2-65E).

7. Have patient push down off their leg(s) and arms, lifting and twisting their hips into the seat (Fig. 2-65F).

8. Stabilize patient as (s)he straightens up and pivots into chair seat (Fig. 2-65G).

Patients with hemiplegia can often flex their weaker leg and foot but can't push down.

This will propel their weaker side into the chair first.

Use gait belt and good body mechanics.

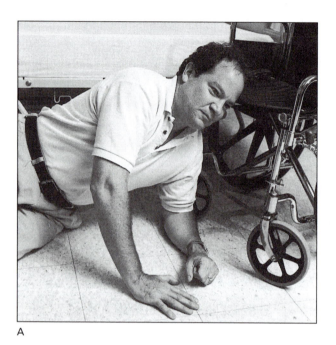

A

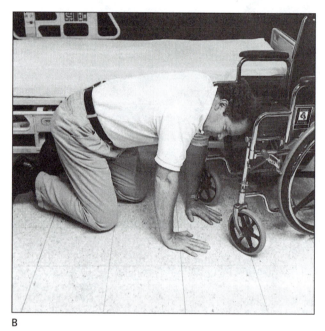

B

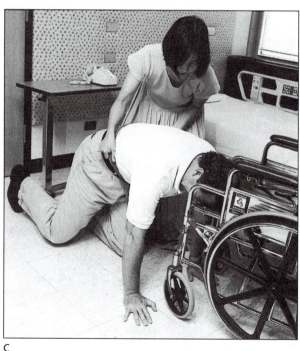

C

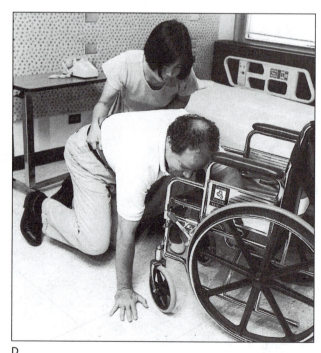

D

Figure 2-65   Floor to Chair Transfer.

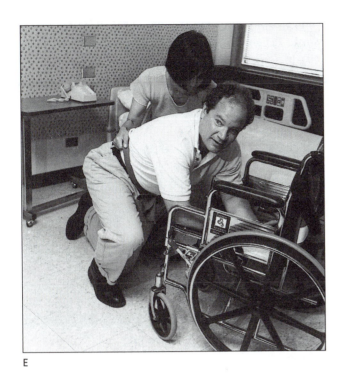

E

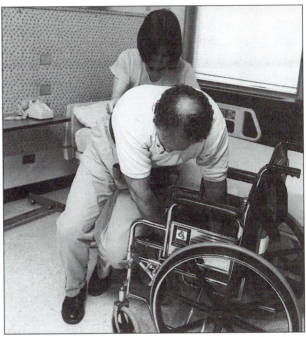

F

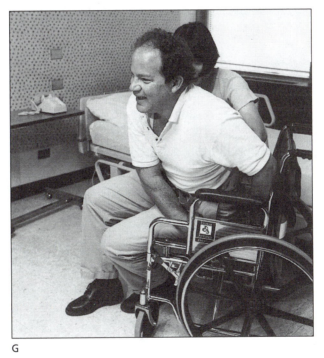

G

Figure 2-65 (continued)

REFERENCES

Carr, J. and Shepherd, R. (1983) *A Motor Relearning Program for Stroke* Rockville, MD: Aspen.

Crescimbeni, J.A. (1997) "From Bed to Chair: Transferring the Non-Weight-Bearing Patient" *Orthopaedic Nursing* 16(2):47–50.

DeGeorge, P. and Dunwoody, C. (1995) "Transfer Techniques of the Lower Extremity with an External Fixator" *Orthopaedic Nursing* 14(6):17–21.

Gee, Z.L. and Passarella, P.M. (1978) "Starting Right" *American Journal of Nursing* 87:802–808.

Gee, Z.L. and Passarella, P.M. (1985) *Nursing Care of the Stroke Patient* Pittsburgh, PA: AREN.

Johnstone, M. (1976) *The Stroke Patient: Principles of Rehabilitation* Edinburgh: Churchill-Livingstone.

Johnstone, M. (1978) *Restoration of Motor Function of the Stroke Patient* Edinburgh: Churchill-Livingstone.

O'Brien, M.T. and Pallett, P.J. (1978) *Total Care of the Stroke Patient* Boston: Little, Brown & Company.

Pallett, P.J. and O'Brien, M.T. (1985) *Textbook of Neurological Nursing* Boston: Little, Brown & Company.

CHAPTER 3

Procedures to Establish and Maintain Elimination

Introduction

Patients with physical disability, bowel and bladder incontinence, or complicated bladder management routines can experience major impediments to their ability to work and socialize or to reenter community life.

Management of the urinary tract may be one of the most significant factors in the patient's ability to function in his or her daily life and may profoundly affect his or her longevity. Urinary tract complications may lead to life-threatening situations in the patient with disability. An unmanaged bowel may cause the complications of constipation leading to impaction or incontinent bowel movements. With the help of skillful rehabilitation nurses, many of these problems can be prevented. The information in this chapter provides the nurse with current knowledge and techniques to avoid such problems. The following procedures should help establish simple, effective bladder programs and regular bowel habits.

The chapter is divided into two main sections: bowel elimination procedures and urinary elimination procedures. The bowel elimination procedures include establishing bowel programs, preventing complications, rectal digital stimulation techniques, and administration of suppositories. The urinary elimination procedures include establishing bladder programs, indwelling catheters, catheterizations, and home care procedures on preparation of solutions and disinfecting urinary equipment.

Aseptic technique is vital in the care of patients requiring bladder management. Effective hand-washing techniques before and after implementing each procedure are essential in prevention of iatrogenic complications. The goals of the elimination procedures are to:

1. Prevent complications of the bowel and urinary tracts by
   - Establishing programs for each patient that will minimize complications
   - Carefully adhering to established guidelines for avoidance of complications (e.g., principles of asepsis) when carrying out these procedures

2. Establish bowel and bladder programs that will maximize the patient's ability to function in his or her chosen lifestyle

3. Promote the patient and primary caregiver's ability to facilitate the maintenance of a healthy bowel and urinary tract

For further information on urinary incontinence in adults, an excellent resource is the Agency for Health Care Policy and Research's *Clinical Practice Guidelines: Urinary Incontinence in Adults* (U.S. Department of Health and Human Services, AHCPR Pub. No. 92-0039, Rockville, MD).

Other resources for incontinent patients include:

- National Association for Continence (formerly H.I.P.) P.O. Box 8310, Spartanburg, SC 29305-8310. (864) 579-7900 or (800) BLADDER.

- Simon Foundation for Continence P.O. Box 835, Wilmette, IL 60091. (800) 23-SIMON

Procedures for Bowel Elimination

Establishing and Revising a Bowel Program

PURPOSE

To establish a reliable, safe, inexpensive, and convenient method of managing bowel evacuation or fecal incontinence. The goals of any bowel program include:

1. Development of a method to establish regular bowel elimination and habit time
2. Management of fecal incontinence through establishment of fecal continence
3. Assistance in development of positive patient self-esteem

STAFF RESPONSIBLE

EQUIPMENT

No equipment necessary.

 GENERAL CONSIDERATIONS

1. A bowel program utilizes a method of rectal stimulation: chemical stimulation (suppository administration) or mechanical stimulation (digital stimulation). Other methods utilized include diet, fluid, medications, activity level, and establishing a habit time.

2. Review the patient's past bowel habits:
   - Frequency and pattern before disability
   - Use of laxatives and enemas
   - Fluid intake
   - Eating patterns and food preferences
   - Age and level of activity
   - Gastrointestinal history (diarrhea, constipation, hemorrhoids, or diverticulitis)

3. Further, consider any present factors that affect regular bowel evacuation:
   - Immobility or inactivity
   - Spinal precautions
   - Postural or tone abnormalities

   - Use of medications (stool softeners; laxatives; and medications causing sensitivity, diarrhea, or constipation; Table 3-1)
   - Tube feeding schedule
   - Diet (ability to chew and swallow and volume of fluid taken in)
   - Present program or use of suppositories

4. Assess the patient's ability to communicate the need to defecate. The level of sensory awareness and state of mental arousal must also be evaluated before a successful bowel program can be established.

5. The patient populations that can benefit from a regular bowel program include those with spinal cord injury, neuromuscular disease, traumatic brain injury, or cerebrovascular problems.

6. Precautions to be considered include the following:
   - Maintain spinal stability as appropriate for each individual patient, or work around postural tone abnormalities that prevent the patient from sitting upright at 90-degree angles
   - Observe for signs and symptoms of autonomic dysreflexia in persons with spinal cord injury above T6 and in those with traumatic brain injuries.

7. Bowel programs are developed in collaboration with the patient's attending physician as well as with the patient.

8. When initiating a program, start with a thorough assessment and the simplest, yet most effective, program for that patient. Patients with lower motor neuron lesions seem to respond best to a program with carbon dioxide suppository use or manual removal. Patients with upper motor neuron lesions may start with a daily bisacodyl suppository, advance to every other day use, and eventually substitute digital stimulation every other day. A glycerine suppository to provide local rectal irritation on a daily basis may be what is necessary for a patient with head injury or stroke.

9. Consider all aspects of the bowel program, including:
   - Medications
     - Softeners
     - Laxatives
     - Suppositories
   - Mechanical stimulation
     - Digital stimulation to relax rectal sphincter tone

- Suppositories (most effective after meals when peristalsis is increased)
- Diet and bulk intake
- Fluid intake
- Level of activity
- Timing (establish a consistent time)

10. Review or familiarize yourself with suppositories and medications available at your institution or facility.

11. Consider the patient's stage of growth and development.

12. Enlist the support of the patient, family, and staff through education.

13. When making changes, change only one aspect of a program at a time and evaluate the change through three or four administrations before making further changes. This approach allows for objective evaluation of the one component and of demonstrated consistency relating to the change.

14. Consistent time of suppository administration each day assists in establishing the pattern. Repeating the suppository if there are no results within a certain time frame is important.

15. Always provide privacy for bowel procedures.

PATIENT AND FAMILY EDUCATION

Teach the patient and family:

1. Basic gastrointestinal tract anatomy

2. Basic bowel physiology and pathophysiology as they relate to etiology or patient needs

3. Five basic aspects of good bowel function:
   - Diet
   - Fluids
   - Activity
   - Medication (see Table 3-1)
   - Habit time

Discuss the rationale for and choice of bowel program and explain the specifics. Discuss problem solving and provide practice in problem solving.

Table 3-1	Suppositories and Medications Used for Bowel Programs in Patients with Spinal Cord Injury		
Product	**Action**		**Considerations**
Laxatives			
Stimulant (contact laxative)			
Glycerine			
Bisacodyl	Acts on colonic mucosa to produce normal peristalsis through parasympathetic reflexes		Very effective for initial bowel regulation for upper motor neuron lesion (reflex bowel); can be irritating to persons with rectal sensation
Carbon dioxide evacuant	Acts by releasing carbon dioxide into rectum, stimulating peristalsis		Expensive; may cause autonomic dysreflexia, bowel distention
Medications			
Stool softeners	Wetting agents that promote absorption of water and emulsifying fats		Works well initially with Dulcolax suppository for patients with upper motor neuron lesion (reflex bowel)
Colace			
Surfax			
Peristaltic stimulators	Most are stool softeners and mild irritants that stimulate peristalsis		Indicated initially for those with delayed response to bowel program
Pericolace			
Doxidan			
Senecot (stimulator only)			
Bulk formers	Dietary fibers that aid in absorbing water from intestinal contents and provide bulk		Ensure adequate fluid intake; effective with patients who have recurring problem of loose or semiformed stools and who are unable to get bulk from foods (i.e., on tube feedings)
Metamucil			
Fibermed			
Lactinex	Assist in reinstating normal gastrointestinal flora		Indicated for persons with prolonged loose stools associated with antibiotic therapy.
Yogurt	Same as above		Same as above

SOURCE: From *Spinal Cord Injury. A Guide to Rehabilitation Nursing* (p. 113) by P.J. Matthews, C.E. Carlson, and N.B. Holt, 1987, Rockville, MD: Aspen Publishers, Inc. Copyright © 1987 by Aspen Publishers, Inc.

Procedure

Establishing a Bowel Program

 Steps

1. Complete nursing assessment.

2. Review factors influencing bowel program: diet, fluid, medications, and level of activity.

3. For patients with spinal cord injury, neuromuscular disease, or history of severe constipation or poor bowel results, begin with daily bisacodyl suppository, repeating application if there are no results in 30 to 60 min.

4. Record results and evaluate patient response for three to four administrations.

 Additional Information

Include rectal check to rule out impaction, check consistency of stool, and obtain hemoccult as ordered. For patients with sensation or autonomic dysreflexic problems, consider use of anesthetic ointment to minimize discomfort.

Identify problems, and implement appropriate action to correct as needed.

When evaluating results, look for any emerging patterns (i.e., inconsistencies or lack of results). Program can be reviewed or revised when a consistent pattern is identified.

 DOCUMENTATION

1. Document the results of the assessment.
2. Note all elements and the time of administration of the bowel program.
3. Note the patient and family education.
4. Document the results of the bowel program.
5. Note the patient's response to the program.

REFERENCES

Burkitt, D. P. and Meisner, P. (1979) "How to Manage Constipation with High Fiber Diet" *Geriatrics* 33:33–38.

Cannon, B. (1981) "Bowel Function" in Martin, N., Holt, N.B., and Hicks, D. (Eds.) *Comprehensive Rehabilitation Nursing.* New York: McGraw Hill, pp. 223–241.

Consortium for spinal cord medicine. (1998) *Clinical Practice Guidelines: Neurogenic Bowel Management in Adults with Spinal Cord Injury.* Paralyzed Veterans of America.

Harari, D., et al. (1997) "Constipation-Related Symptoms and Bowel Program Concerning Individuals with Spinal Cord Injury." *Spinal Cord* June 35(6):394–401.

Juckel-Regan, H. (1983) "Gastrointestinal System" in Benda, S. (Ed.) *Spinal Cord Injury Nursing Education— Suggested Content.* Chicago: American Spinal Injury Association, pp. 85–91.

King, R.B., Boyink, M., Keenan, M. (1977) *Rehabilitation Guide.* Chicago: Rehabilitation Institute of Chicago.

Kirshblum, S.C., et. al. (1998) "Bowel Care Practices in Chronic Spinal Cord Injury Patients" *Archives of Physical Medicine and Rehabilitation* 79(1):20–23.

Matthews, P.J. (1978) "Elimination" in Matthews, P.J. and Carlson, C. (Eds.) *Spinal Cord Injury: A Guide to Rehabilitation Nursing.* Rockville, MD: Aspen.

Munchiando, J.F. and Kendall, K. (1993) "Comparison of the Effectiveness of Two Bowel Programs for CVA Patients" *Rehabilitation Nursing* May: 18(3):168–172.

Stass, W. and Denault, P. (1973) "Bowel Control" *American Family Physician* 7:90–100.

Steins, S.A., Biener Bergman, S., Goetz, L.L. (1997) "Neurogenic Bowel Dysfunction after Spinal Cord Injury: Clinical Evaluation and Rehabilitative Management" [Review] *Archives of Physical Medicine and Rehabilitation* 78:s86–s102.

Procedure

Revising a Bowel Program

 Steps

1. Review bowel record and identify patterns and results.

2. Change only one aspect of bowel program at a time:
   - Suppository frequency
   - Number of suppositories
   - Suppository type
   - Diet (change to tube feeding, increase bulk, add prune juice or prunes as able)
   - Fluid volume
   - Activity
   - Medication

3. Upgrade program until:
   - Fecal continence is achieved
   - Management of fecal incontinence is achieved
   - Regular routine bowel elimination or habit time is established

 Additional Information

Allow 7 days or three to four administrations before making further changes.

 DOCUMENTATION

1. Note any changes or adaptations in the nursing care plan as indicated.

2. Document the results and patient response.

REFERENCES

Burkitt, D. P. and Meisner, P. (1979) "How to Manage Constipation with High Fiber Diet" *Geriatrics* 33:33–38.

Cannon, B. (1981) "Bowel Function" in Martin, N., Holt, N.B., and Hicks, D. (Eds.) *Comprehensive Rehabilitation Nursing* New York: McGraw-Hill, pp. 223–241.

Consortium for spinal cord medicine. (1998) *Clinical Practice Guidelines: Neurogenic Bowel Management in Adults with Spinal Cord Injury*. Paralyzed Veterans of America.

Harari, D., et al. (1997) "Constipation-Related Symptoms and Bowel Program Concerning Individuals with Spinal Cord Injury." *Spinal Cord* June 35(6):394–401.

Juckel-Regan, H. (1983) "Gastrointestinal System" in Benda, S. (Ed.) *Spinal Cord Injury Nursing Education—Suggested Content*. Chicago: American Spinal Injury Association, pp. 85–91.

King, R.B., Boyink, M., Keenan, M. (1977) *Rehabilitation Guide*. Chicago: Rehabilitation Institute of Chicago.

Kirshblum, S.C., et al. (1998) "Bowel Care Practices in Chronic Spinal Cord Injury Patients" *Archives of Physical Medicine and Rehabilitation* 79(1):20–23.

Matthews, P.J. (1978) "Elimination" in Matthews, P.J. and Carlson, C. (Eds.) *Spinal Cord Injury: A Guide to Rehabilitation Nursing*. Rockville, MD: Aspen.

Munchiando, J.F. and Kendall, K. (1993) "Comparison of the Effectiveness of Two Bowel Programs for CVA Patients" *Rehabilitation Nursing* May: 18(3):168–172.

Stass, W. and Denault, P. (1973) "Bowel Control" *American Family Physician* 7:90–100.

Steins, S.A., Biener Bergman, S., Goetz, L.L. (1997) "Neurogenic Bowel Dysfunction after Spinal Cord Injury: Clinical Evaluation and Rehabilitative Management" [Review] *Archives of Physical Medicine and Rehabilitation* 78:s86–s102.

Prevention and Control of Complications Related to Bowel Management

PURPOSE

To prevent, reduce, or eliminate complications related to bowel management. The complications to be addressed are constipation, impaction, diarrhea, hemorrhoids, delayed bowel program results, and autonomic dysreflexia.

STAFF RESPONSIBLE

EQUIPMENT

1. Bowel record, nursing admission, or health history form

GENERAL CONSIDERATIONS

1. Constipation is defined as the infrequent passage of hard stool. It is usually associated with straining or a feeling of fullness, distention, cramping, anorexia, and malaise. Occasional complaints of lower left quadrant tenderness may be present. If constipation is left untreated, it may result in impaction. Frequent problems with constipation may contribute to the development of hemorrhoids.

2. A decrease in activity level may promote constipation. Keeping the person as active as possible (i.e., allowing regular participation in all activities of daily living and allowing for a regular exercise program) helps alleviate problems with constipation.

3. Some foods may cause constipation. Patients should be encouraged to experiment with their diet and to avoid foods that cause problems. Adhering to a regular bowel program also assists in the prevention of constipation and other bowel complications.

4. Diarrhea is the frequent passage of watery stool (more than three loose, watery stools in 24 h). It may be accompanied by abdominal cramping. Infection, drug side effects, and dietary intake are a few of the causes of diarrhea. Adhering to a regular bowel program will assist in the prevention of these complications.

5. Adjust diet, fluid intake, medication, level of activity, and frequency of suppositories as needed for the individual patient.

6. Patient populations who may experience problems with bowel complications include elderly patients and those with spinal cord injuries, neuromuscular disease, and traumatic brain injury.

PATIENT AND FAMILY EDUCATION

Teach the patient and family:

1. The signs, causes, and corrective actions of: constipation, impaction, diarrhea, hemorrhoids, delayed results, and autonomic dysreflexia.

2. Prevention of bowel complications regarding choice of diet, fluid intake, and medication actions and side effects.

Procedure

Preventing Constipation

 Steps

 Additional Information

1. Complete nursing assessment to ascertain cause or causes of constipation. Investigate:
   - Diet
   - Fluid intake
   - Decreased activity
   - Medication
   - Problems adhering to bowel program
   - Availability of primary caregiver
   - Accessibility of bathroom

If there are no results from suppository program, repeat suppository in 30 to 60 min. If no results at that time or if results are small, repeat on next day. If stool is hard or if results take too long, add 4 to 6 oz of prune juice or four to six prunes to diet. Bran also may be added to diet.

2. Adjust present program.

3. Consult physician about need to increase or start stool softener or laxative.

Eliminating Fecal Impaction

 Steps

 Additional Information

1. Ascertain that problem being dealt with is indeed fecal impaction.

Remember that leakage of watery stool around impaction may be interpreted as diarrhea rather than impaction. A kidney-ureter-bladder (KUB) x-ray is the best way to differentiate between these two complications when impaction is high in bowel. A KUB is not needed for low impaction.

2. Attempt to remove low impaction with gloved and lubricated finger.

3. If impaction is high up in bowel, consult physician for oral medications (e.g., bisacodyl tabs or magnesium citrate).

Anesthetic ointment may be needed for decreasing noxious stimuli. Cardiac precautions may contraindicate this procedure.

4. Use oil retention enema in combination with above to loosen stool.

5. Use tap water enema if there are no results from oil retention. Repeat until clear.

6. When problem is alleviated, adjust program to remove cause.

Controlling Diarrhea

 Steps

 Additional Information

1. Assess patient to ascertain cause or causes.

Evaluate for factors that cause diarrhea, such as increased alcohol consumption, diet, or stool softeners. Perform rectal check to rule out impaction. Note fever because diarrhea may be caused by medical illness. Presence of diarrhea requires meticulous hygiene to prevent skin breakdown.

2. If diet is cause, remove offending foods or fluids.

3. If stool softeners are possible cause, request medication hold order from physician.

Consult physician regarding adjusting medications or stool softener to achieve desired stool firmness or to treat medical illness.

4. Resume program after diarrhea is no longer an issue.

Management of Hemorrhoids

 Steps

1. Assess patient for red, bulging areas inside and outside rectum, pain (if sensation is present), bleeding, and history or presence of constipation.
2. Consult with physician regarding treatment plan (may order such treatments as stool softeners, oil retention enema, sitz bath, ice, creams, and the like).
3. Correct and manage constipation if present.
4. Consult with physician regarding administration of mild laxative for short period of time.
5. Discourage straining and use of digital stimulation.
6. Return to previous program when flare-up is decreased. Include methods in program to manage or eliminate hard stool or constipation.

Methods to Correct Delayed Bowel Program Results

 Steps

1. Any one or a combination of the following methods may correct delayed results:
   - Give suppository close to mealtime or in conjunction with hot or cold drink (mealtimes produce increased peristalsis; hot or cold drinks stimulate gastrocolic reflex to aid in evacuation).
   - Repeat digital stimulation frequently to relax rectal sphincter.
   - Repeat suppository to increase chemical stimulation of bowel.
   - Assist patient with abdominal massage (right to left) to increase peristalsis.
   - Assist patient to assume upright or squatting position (position patient on commode or in shower chair or place patient's feet on stool and lean trunk forward).
   - Try using two suppositories as part of program.

Managing Autonomic Dysreflexia

 Steps

1. See Chap. 6, "Procedures for Prevention of Autonomic Dysreflexia Episodes and Identification and Treatment of an Acute Episode of Dysreflexia."

DOCUMENTATION

1. Note the assessment and changes in the program. Note and describe the complication (type, frequency, and results) and document the patient's response.

2. Document notification of the physician.

REFERENCES

Burkitt, D. P. and Meisner, P. (1979) "How to Manage Constipation with High Fiber Diet" *Geriatrics* 33:33–38.

Cannon, B. (1981) "Bowel Function" in Martin, N., Holt, N.B., and Hicks, D. (Eds.) *Comprehensive Rehabilitation Nursing* New York: McGraw Hill, pp. 223–241.

Consortium for spinal cord medicine. (1998) *Clinical Practice Guidelines: Neurogenic Bowel Management in Adults with Spinal Cord Injury*. Paralyzed Veterans of America.

Harari, D., et al. (1997) "Constipation-Related Symptoms and Bowel Program Concerning Individuals with Spinal Cord Injury." *Spinal Cord* June 35(6):394–401.

Juckel-Regan, H. (1983) "Gastrointestinal System" in Benda, S. (Ed.) *Spinal Cord Injury Nursing Education—Suggested Content*. Chicago: American Spinal Injury Association, pp. 85–91.

King, R.B., Boyink, M., Keenan, M. (1977) *Rehabilitation Guide*. Chicago: Rehabilitation Institute of Chicago.

Kirshblum, S.C., et. al. (1998) "Bowel Care Practices in Chronic Spinal Cord Injury Patients" *Archives of Physical Medicine and Rehabilitation* 79(1):20–23.

Matthews, P.J. (1978) "Elimination" in Matthews, P.J. and Carlson, C. (Eds.) *Spinal Cord Injury: A Guide to Rehabilitation Nursing*. Rockville, MD: Aspen.

Munchiando, J.F. and Kendall, K. (1993) "Comparison of the effectiveness of two bowel programs for CVA patients" *Rehabilitation Nursing* May: 18(3):168–172.

Stass, W. and Denault, P. (1973) "Bowel Control" *American Family Physician* 7:90–100.

Steins, S.A., Biener Bergman, S., Goetz, L.L. (1997) "Neurogenic Bowel Dysfunction after Spinal Cord Injury: Clinical Evaluation and Rehabilitative Management" [Review] *Archives of Physical Medicine and Rehabilitation* 78:s86–s102.

Rectal Digital Stimulation

PURPOSE

To produce bowel evacuation through relaxation of the anal sphincter to produce reflex defecation.

STAFF RESPONSIBLE

EQUIPMENT

1. Water-soluble lubricant
2. Incontinence pads
3. Gloves, soap, water, and washcloth
4. Medicinal lubricant as prescribed by physician (optional)

GENERAL CONSIDERATIONS

1. Digital stimulation of the anal sphincter produces mechanical relaxation of the sphincter, which may produce a bowel evacuation, speed up the effect of a suppository, or assist in complete bowel emptying. Digital stimulation also may precede suppository insertion to relax the anal sphincter and to aid in suppository administration.

2. If digital stimulation is used to facilitate the effect of a suppository, experience has shown that it is more effective to wait at least 15 min after suppository insertion to perform it. Digital stimulation may follow bowel evacuation to ensure complete emptying.

3. Digital stimulation is contraindicated in patients with a cardiac history and in whom there is indication of nausea and vomiting, abdominal pain, rectal bleeding, or increased sphincter spasticity.

4. Patients with sensation may find the procedure painful.

5. As with all bowel-related procedures, adhere to infection control practices and indications.

6. Additional complications are present with spinal cord injury above T6. If the patient is prone to autonomic dysreflexia, he or she should be observed for symptoms (e.g., sudden pounding headache, unexplained sweating, flushing, chills, or sudden increased blood pressure) during digital stimulation.

7. An anesthetic ointment can be used with patients who experience autonomic dysreflexia during digital stimulation or if hemorrhoids or pain are a problem. Deep breathing and relaxation techniques may help relieve discomfort.

8. Digital stimulation is also contraindicated in patients with a flaccid sphincter secondary to a lower motor neuron lesion because it is usually not effective in producing bowel results.

9. Digital stimulation can be performed with the patient side lying in bed or positioned on a commode chair or toilet. It is most effective, however, when the patient is in a sitting position to defecate because the stool evacuation is then aided by gravity.

PATIENT AND FAMILY EDUCATION

1. Teach the patient and family the general considerations.
2. Demonstrate the procedure and then encourage a return demonstration.
3. Discuss the role of digital stimulation in the present bowel program.
4. Discuss the need to evaluate effectiveness and problem solve. Provide practice situations.

Procedure

Rectal Digital Stimulation

 Steps

 Additional Information

1. Wash hands.
2. Assist patient with transfer to toilet or commode chair, or place incontinence pads under side-lying patient in bed.
3. Glove dominant hand and lubricate index or middle finger.
4. Locate anal opening and insert index or middle finger to check for stool.
5. If stool is present, gently remove it.
6. Reapply lubricant if needed, and reinsert finger approximately ½ to 1 in. into anal opening.
7. Gently rotate finger in circular motion against wall of anal sphincter for 30 s. May need to continue for 30 to 60 s and up to 2 min until sphincter relaxes.

Digital stimulation should be done until anal sphincter relaxes or up to 2 min or until defecation is achieved.

8. Wait about 15 to 20 min for reflex peristalsis to produce bowel movement.
9. If no bowel movement occurs, repeat digital stimulation or use suppository if these are the only elements in bowel program.

 DOCUMENTATION

1. Note the date, time, and method utilized; the time of evacuation; and the characteristics of the results.
2. Note the effectiveness and frequency of digital stimulation.
3. Note any complications or difficulties encountered during the procedure.
4. Document patient and caregiver education.

REFERENCES

Burkitt, D. P. and Meisner, P. (1979) "How to Manage Constipation with High Fiber Diet" *Geriatrics* 33:33–38.

Cannon, B. (1981) "Bowel Function" in Martin, N., Holt, N.B., and Hicks, D. (Eds.) *Comprehensive Rehabilitation Nursing* New York: McGraw Hill, pp. 223–241.

Consortium for spinal cord medicine. (1998) *Clinical Practice Guidelines: Neurogenic Bowel Management in Adults with Spinal Cord Injury.* Paralyzed Veterans of America.

Harari, D., et al. (1997) "Constipation-Related Symptoms and Bowel Program Concerning Individuals with Spinal Cord Injury" *Spinal Cord* June 35(6):394–401.

Juckel-Regan, H. (1983) "Gastrointestinal System" in Benda, S. (Ed.) *Spinal Cord Injury Nursing Education— Suggested Content*. Chicago: American Spinal Injury Association, pp. 85–91.

King, R.B., Boyink, M., Keenan, M. (1977) *Rehabilitation Guide*. Chicago: Rehabilitation Institute of Chicago.

Kirshblum, S.C., et. al. (1998) "Bowel Care Practices in Chronic Spinal Cord Injury Patients" *Archives of Physical Medicine and Rehabilitation* 79(1):20–23.

Matthews, P.J. (1978) "Elimination" in Matthews, P.J. and Carlson, C. (Eds.) *Spinal Cord Injury: A Guide to Rehabilitation Nursing*. Rockville, MD: Aspen.

Munchiando, J.F. and Kendall, K. (1993) "Comparison of the Effectiveness of Two Bowel Programs for CVA Patients" *Rehabilitation Nursing* May: 18(3):168–172.

Stass, W. and Denault, P. (1973) "Bowel Control" *American Family Physician* 7:90–100.

Steins, S.A., Biener Bergman, S., Goetz, L.L. (1997) "Neurogenic Bowel Dysfunction after Spinal Cord Injury: Clinical Evaluation and Rehabilitative Management" [Review] *Archives of Physical Medicine and Rehabilitation* 78:s86–s102.

Rectal Suppository Administration

PURPOSE

To achieve proper insertion and placement of rectal suppository

STAFF RESPONSIBLE

EQUIPMENT

1. Incontinence pads
2. Commode chair or shower chair
3. Gloves
4. Water-soluble lubricant
5. Glycerine suppository
6. Bisacodyl suppository
7. Other suppository
8. Anesthetic ointment

 ## GENERAL CONSIDERATIONS

1. Administering the suppository with the patient positioned on the left side is ideal because anatomically it eases suppository insertion and maintains the suppository position in the bowel.

2. A lubricant is not necessary, unless the patient experiences autonomic dysreflexia during administration. An anesthetic ointment may be prescribed in these cases or when the patient finds suppository insertion painful.

3. Generally, glycerine suppositories act mechanically to stimulate rectal mucosa, and bisacodyl suppositories act chemically to stimulate bowel movements. Familiarize yourself with the actions and uses of suppositories available in your facility. Obtain a medical order for suppository use.

4. Before administering any suppository, the nurse should assess the patient as outlined in the procedure for establishing a bowel program.

5. Use proper infection control guidelines: Wash hands before and after the procedure and dispose of all wastes according to infection control policy.

6. Observe patients who are prone to autonomic dysreflexia for symptoms of sudden onset of flushing, chills, unexplained diaphoresis, or increase of blood pressure.

7. If patient complains of nausea, vomiting, severe abdominal pain, or other symptoms of bowel impactions or obstruction, or if rectal bleeding is noted, report to the physician and make appropriate changes in the bowel program as needed.

PATIENT AND FAMILY EDUCATION

Teach the patient and family:

1. The general considerations

2. The role of the suppository in the bowel program and any side effects if the suppository is medicated

3. The basic procedure

4. Obtain a return demonstration, and evaluate effectiveness and problem-solving.

Procedure

Rectal Suppository Administration

 Steps

 Additional Information

1. Wash hands.

2. Prepare bed with incontinence pads. Place patient on *left* side with *right* top knee flexed.

   This is to aid access to intestine.

3. Apply gloves. Unwrap suppository if necessary.

4. Lubricate index or middle finger of dominant hand.

5. Locate anal opening and gently insert finger.

6. If stool is present, remove only stool blocking anal opening.

7. Use anesthetic ointment or other lubricant if needed.

   Do not lubricate suppository itself because this decreases its effectiveness. The carbon dioxide suppository should be activated by inserting the suppository in a cup of water until it starts to fizz.

   The carbon dioxide suppository does not need to be placed against intestinal wall.

8. Insert narrowest end of suppository into rectum. Turn suppository and place it along rectal wall as far up as possible, making certain that it is placed against wall of colon above sphincter and not embedded in stool.

9. Allow 15 to 20 min to pass before performing digital stimulation or transferring patient to toilet.

   Most suppositories work within 15 to 60 min of insertion; see product information.

10. Cleanse patient.

11. Dispose of all materials.

    Use infection control procedures.

 DOCUMENTATION

1. Note the time, date, and type of suppository insertion; the time at which evacuation occurred; and the characteristics of the results (amount and consistency).

2. Note the effectiveness, time, and frequency of digital stimulation if used.

3. Document any complications or difficulties encountered during the procedure.

REFERENCES

Burkitt, D. P. and Meisner, P. (1979) "How to Manage Constipation with High Fiber Diet" *Geriatrics* 33:33–38.

Cannon, B. (1981) "Bowel Function" in Martin, N., Holt, N.B., and Hicks, D. (Eds.) *Comprehensive Rehabilitation Nursing* New York: McGraw Hill, pp. 223–241.

Consortium for spinal cord medicine. (1998) *Clinical Practice Guidelines: Neurogenic Bowel Management in Adults with Spinal Cord Injury*. Paralyzed Veterans of America.

Harari, D., et al. (1997) "Constipation-Related Symptoms and Bowel Program Concerning Individuals with Spinal Cord Injury." *Spinal Cord* June 35(6):394–401.

Juckel-Regan, H. (1983) "Gastrointestinal System" in Benda, S. (Ed.) *Spinal Cord Injury Nursing Education—Suggested Content*. Chicago: American Spinal Injury Association, pp. 85–91.

King, R.B., Boyink, M., Keenan, M. (1977) *Rehabilitation Guide*. Chicago: Rehabilitation Institute of Chicago.

Kirshblum, S.C., et. al. (1998) "Bowel Care Practices in Chronic Spinal Cord Injury Patients" *Archives of Physical Medicine and Rehabilitation* 79(1):20–23.

Matthews, P.J. (1978) "Elimination" in Matthews, P.J. and Carlson, C. (Eds.) *Spinal Cord Injury: A Guide to Rehabilitation Nursing*. Rockville, MD: Aspen.

Munchiando, J.F. and Kendall, K. (1993) "Comparison of the Effectiveness of Two Bowel Programs for CVA Patients" *Rehabilitation Nursing* May: 18(3):168–172.

Stass, W. and Denault, P. (1973) "Bowel Control" *American Family Physician* 7:90–100.

Steins, S.A., Biener Bergman, S., Goetz, L.L. (1997) "Neurogenic Bowel Dysfunction after Spinal Cord Injury: Clinical Evaluation and Rehabilitative Management" [Review] *Archives of Physical Medicine and Rehabilitation* 78:s86–s102.

Enema Administration

PURPOSE

To introduce a solution into the colon to aid in stimulating peristalsis to promote bowel evacuation or soften stool.

STAFF RESPONSIBLE

EQUIPMENT

1. Enema or enema kit
2. Bedpan or commode
3. Incontinence pads
4. Toilet tissue
5. Linen
6. Lubricant (water-soluble)

 GENERAL CONSIDERATIONS

1. A physician's order is generally needed to administer an enema and should include the type and amount of solution to instill.
2. Caution should be exercised if the patient has complained of nausea, vomiting, or abdominal pain or if the temperature or white blood cell count is elevated. The patient should be evaluated for signs and symptoms of impaction.
3. Before enema administration, thorough assessment of the patient's physical status, cardiac concerns, and bowel history is essential. Approximate recommended volume amounts that may be instilled are as follows:
   - Adult, 500 to 1000 mL
   - Child, 250 to 400 mL
   - Infant, 15 to 60 mL
4. Large quantities of hypotonic solutions such as tap water can be absorbed through the bowel and cause water intoxication. Observe the patient for symptoms of weakness, pallor, vomiting, coughing, or dizziness.
5. Autonomic dysreflexia can be triggered by distention created by the enema solution.
6. Some patients with spinal cord injury may be unable to retain or expel the enema solution.

PATIENT AND FAMILY EDUCATION

1. Teach the patient and family the general considerations and precautions.
2. Demonstrate the procedure, and obtain a return demonstration.
3. Discuss the role of the enema to treat constipation or impaction.
4. Evaluate effectiveness and problem solving skills.

Procedure

Enema Administration

 Steps

 Additional Information

1. Asess patient and need for enema.
2. Check or obtain physician order.
3. Wash hands.
4. Gather equipment. Prepare solutions as prescribed.
5. Explain procedure and reason for enema administration to patient. Provide privacy.
6. Position patient on left side with knees flexed, and prepare bed with incontinence pads and linens.
7. Locate rectal opening (anus) and gently insert lubricated tip.

This is to aid access to intestine.

8. Encourage patient to take slow, deep breaths while liquid is being instilled.

9. Remove tip from rectum when all liquid is instilled and encourage patient to hold solution as long as possible (at least 10 to 15 min).

If patient is not able to hold it, gently apply pressure to rectum with a pad of toilet paper.

10. Assist patient into safe and comfortable position to expel enema (toilet, commode, or bedpan).

11. Observe amount, consistency, color, or unusual odor of returned enema.

Oil retention enema solution is absorbed into hard stool, so volume returned may be significantly less.

12. Clean patient and reposition him or her in clean, safe, and comfortable environment.

13. Dispose of all materials according to infection control guidelines.

DOCUMENTATION

1. Note the date and time of enema administration, the time of evacuation, and the characteristics of the results.

2. Note the volume of contents expelled.

3. Document any complications or difficulties encountered during the procedure.

Removal of Fecal Impaction

PURPOSE

To remove stool manually from the bowel to promote evacuation, to treat or relieve impaction, or to clear the rectum before suppository insertion.

STAFF RESPONSIBLE

EQUIPMENT

1. Gloves
2. Lubricant
3. Incontinence pads
4. Soap, water, washcloth, and towel

GENERAL CONSIDERATIONS

1. The procedure must be performed gently to avoid injury to the bowel wall or to hemorrhoids, if present.

2. If the stool is high up in the intestine, a small oil retention enema may be used to help soften hard stool.

3. Prevention of constipation and impaction is the key to management.

PATIENT AND FAMILY EDUCATION

1. Teach the patient and family the general considerations as they apply.

2. Demonstrate and obtain a return demonstration.

3. Discuss problem solving and follow-up.

4. Discuss changes in the program to alleviate constipation or impaction.

Procedure

Removal of Fecal Impaction

 Steps

1. Explain procedure.
2. Place incontinence pads beneath patient.
3. Position patient on left side.
4. Apply gloves.
5. Lubricate index or middle finger.
6. Insert gloved finger into patient's rectum.
7. Remove any hardened stool gently and dispose of properly.
8. Cleanse patient and dry his or her skin.

 Additional Information

This is to aid access to intestine.

Dispose of all materials according to infection control guidelines.

 DOCUMENTATION

1. Note the date and time of the procedure, the amount of stool removed, and the characteristics of the results.
2. Document any complications or difficulties encountered during the procedure.

REFERENCES

Burkitt, D. P. and Meisner, P. (1979) "How to Manage Constipation with High Fiber Diet" *Geriatrics* 33:33–38.

Cannon, B. (1981) "Bowel Function" in Martin, N., Holt, N.B., and Hicks, D. (Eds.) *Comprehensive Rehabilitation Nursing* New York: McGraw Hill, pp. 223–241.

Consortium for spinal cord medicine. (1998) *Clinical Practice Guidelines: Neurogenic Bowel Management in Adults with Spinal Cord Injury*. Paralyzed Veterans of America.

Harari, D., et al. (1997) "Constipation-Related Symptoms and Bowel Program Concerning Individuals with Spinal Cord Injury." *Spinal Cord* June 35(6):394–401.

Juckel-Regan, H. (1983) "Gastrointestinal System" in Benda, S. (Ed.) *Spinal Cord Injury Nursing Education—Suggested Content*. Chicago: American Spinal Injury Association, pp. 85–91.

King, R.B., Boyink, M., Keenan, M. (1977) *Rehabilitation Guide*. Chicago: Rehabilitation Institute of Chicago.

Kirshblum, S.C., et. al. (1998) "Bowel Care Practices in Chronic Spinal Cord Injury Patients" *Archives of Physical Medicine and Rehabilitation* 79(1):20–23.

Matthews, P.J. (1978) "Elimination" in Matthews, P.J. and Carlson, C. (Eds.) *Spinal Cord Injury: A Guide to Rehabilitation Nursing*. Rockville, MD: Aspen.

Munchiando, J.F. and Kendall, K. (1993) "Comparison of the Effectiveness of Two Bowel Programs for CVA Patients" *Rehabilitation Nursing* May: 18(3):168–172.

Stass, W. and Denault, P. (1973) "Bowel Control" *American Family Physician* 7:90–100.

Steins, S.A., Biener Bergman, S., Goetz, L.L. (1997) "Neurogenic Bowel Dysfunction after Spinal Cord Injury: Clinical Evaluation and Rehabilitative Management" [Review] *Archives of Physical Medicine and Rehabilitation* 78:s86–s102.

Procedures for Urinary Elimination: Establishing Bladder Programs

Intermittent Catheterization

PURPOSE

To provide complete and regular bladder drainage, either permanently or until reflex voiding is well established; to decrease trauma to the bladder and urethra associated with the use of an indwelling catheter; to prevent incontinence by combining intermittent catheterization with regulated fluid intake; to minimize the occurrence of urinary tract infections

STAFF RESPONSIBLE

EQUIPMENT

1. Clean catheter or catheterization pack
2. External catheter (optional)
3. Incontinence pads or panties (optional)
4. Measurement device to measure urine volume (if not in pack)
5. Disposable nonsterile gloves
6. Syringe to deflate balloon of indwelling catheter (when appropriate)

 ### GENERAL CONSIDERATIONS

1. The return of adequate reflex bladder activity is favorably influenced by the avoidance of overdistention and chronic infection, which can damage the neural and muscular elements of the bladder wall. Maintenance of a good blood supply to the bladder by avoiding increased pressures caused by bladder overdistention is thought to be a key factor in the prevention of urinary tract infection.

2. It is possible to significantly decrease the incidence of urinary infection by using intermittent catheterization rather than an indwelling catheter. An indwelling catheter can provoke sepsis if it becomes obstructed and allows the bladder to overdistend markedly. Bladder overdistention is also thought to contribute to the development of

vesicoureteral reflux. Infection also occurs if bacteria enter the bladder during catheterization and multiply because of prolonged intervals between catheterizations/bladder emptying.

3. Clean intermittent catheterization is used if catheterizations occur every 6 h or more often. If done less frequently, perform sterile technique (King et al., 1992).

4. Sterile urine can be maintained if catheterizations are performed often enough to prevent bladder distention and multiplication of bacteria.

5. Catheter size and type will vary according to the patient's age and special needs. A #14 French catheter is used by older adolescents and adults. Younger patients will use a smaller size catheter and very small children may need to use a feeding tube since it is possible to obtain sizes smaller than #8 French in feeding tubes but not catheters. Insert catheter or feeding tube only as far as necessary to obtain urine flow and use urinary catheters whenever possible to avoid looping or knotting of tube (Carlson & Mowery, 1997).

6. High residual urine volumes are thought to interfere with the antibacterial action of the bladder wall. Incomplete emptying of the bladder allows bacteria present to increase rapidly, whereas complete emptying of the bladder can help to eliminate bacteria and result in a sterile urine.

7. A physician's prescription is required when initiating or changing any individual's intermittent catheterization program, though the patient or caregiver may elect to catheterize more often if deemed necessary.

8. Complications and related problems include the following:
   • Bladder-sphincter dyssynergia (intravesical pressure not adequate to overcome resistance at bladder neck): signs of bladder overdistention secondary to bladder-sphincter dyssynergia may indicate a need for immediate catheterization. Medication may be ordered to relax the bladder neck. The patient may need to continue on lifelong intermittent catheterizations, undergo surgical intervention, or have an indwelling catheter inserted.
   • Perineal or genital dermatitis: excoriation and rash experienced by some patients are primarily a result of the procedure used to apply and maintain the external

catheter and indicate the need for more frequent changing of incontinence devices, or poor hygiene. Prevention of incontinence in patients on long-term or permanent intermittent catheterization may require drug therapy to decrease incontinence.

- Hydronephrosis: may develop with sterile urine and no overt symptoms and has been seen in patients who are catheter free. Obstruction, infection, reflux, and neurogenic factors can contribute to hydronephrosis (Shields, 1981). The threat of this complication is reduced when patients thoroughly understand and follow the bladder program. Close postdischarge follow-up is indicated to prevent this condition. If hydronephrosis is detected, an alternate method of bladder drainage may be initiated (i.e., indwelling catheter or surgical intervention).

- Autonomic dysreflexia (hyperreflexia): the symptoms may be caused by bladder distention or infection and may be seen for the first time when intermittent catheterization is started. This is a medical emergency and demands prompt evaluation and treatment (see Chap. 6, "Procedures for Prevention of Autonomic Dysreflexia Episodes and Identification and Treatment of an Acute Episode of Dysreflexia"). Frequent episodes of dysreflexia may be severe enough to warrant discontinuing an intermittent catheterization program.

- Other reasons for unsuccessful intermittent catheterization programs include previously acquired urinary tract complications (periurethral abscess, penoscrotal fistula, strictures, and the like). Meticulous attention to indwelling catheter care from the start of the disability and early placement on intermittent catheterization programs may be keys to preventing these problems. A failure to develop spontaneous voiding, high residual urine volumes, lack of patient problem-solving abilities, and poor cooperation may also interfere with attempts to become catheter free.

- Decreased manual dexterity in people with progressive disabilities and the inability to adjust to procedural routines may be contraindications to home catheterization programs. For patients who are dependent in self-catheterizations, postdischarge intermittent catheterization may be impractical if the caregiver's assistance is inadequate.

9. If incontinence between catheterizations interferes with activities, an external condom collecting device should be applied (usually used for men). An external device is not necessary for the individual who has not started to void. External condom collecting devices applied with fixatives on the penis itself (Crixiline strips, Freedom, Skin Bond, Urosan, and so forth) are considered only when postvoiding residual is done no more frequently than daily. When obtaining a postvoiding residual, a padded urinal can be propped for male patients to void into before catheterization. Triggering techniques such as tapping or anal stretch may be used. For female patients, sanitary pads, external

catheters, or incontinence pants with liners may be used. When the goal is dryness, incontinence must be recorded and reported to the attending physician to maintain effective management of the pharmacologic regimen.

10. The program is started as early as possible to avoid complications associated with an indwelling catheter. The physician writes specific orders regarding catheterization schedule.

11. When voiding is completely absent, catheterizations are initially performed every 4 h, day and night, and more often if bladder overdistention is observed. Ideally, catheterized urine volumes should not exceed bladder capacity (which may be as little as 100 to 200 mL). In the absence of data on bladder capacity, it is generally recommended that volumes not exceed 400 mL.

12. Some individuals may experience bladder overdistention at night and in the early morning. Individuals with lower-extremity paralysis may develop dependent edema during the day and then diurese when supine. If they do not void, bladder overdistention could occur. This may be minimized by doing one or more of the following:
    - Elevating the lower extremities periodically during the day
    - Wearing support stockings
    - Increasing the frequency of catheterizations during the night
    - Limiting or eliminating fluids early in the evening and throughout the night

13. Tests for assessing urinary function (Table 3-2) may be recommended for some patients with neurogenic bladders. Intravenous pyelography (IVP) and measurements of serum creatinine and blood urea nitrogen are used to evaluate kidney function. After baseline IVP, renal ultrasonography may be used for follow-up. Voiding cystourethrography (VCG) is used to assess bladder capacity, reflux, reflex voiding, and sensation for distention. Urodynamics procedures assess the bladder-urethral pressure profile; findings are used to diagnose detrusor-sphincter dyssynergy. The physician determines the appropriateness of diagnostic tests. There is some controversy surrounding the criteria and timing of performing VCG and measuring urodynamics.

14. When monitoring the patient for spontaneous voiding, it is sometimes found that patients with normally flaccid bladders may urinate a small amount. If the patient is catheterized after a small void and if the volume of the catheterization is high, it is likely that the patient did not have a true void. This is considered overflow incontinence.

15. Initially it may be helpful to structure the program by instructing the patient to drink a specific amount every hour or two. At the start of the program, fluids may be restricted after 8 or 9 P.M. (except small amounts) to avoid bladder overdistention. After a patient begins to void

Table 3-2 Common Tests for Assessing Urinary Tract Function

Test	Purpose	Procedure
Intravenous Pyelogram (IVP)	To demonstrate kidney function and rule out stones, obstructions, stenosis; recommended every year (every 6 mos. for high risk)	Contrast dye administered IV followed by serial x-rays as dye is excreted; requires bowel prep prior to procedure
Renal Ultrasound	As above; may be used in place of follow-up IVP; ideally, patient should have a baseline IVP initially	Noninvasive; requires bowel prep prior to procedure
Cystourethrogram	To assess bladder capacity, reflux, reflex voiding, and sensation for distention	Indwelling catheter is placed; dye is instilled into bladder; x-ray is taken and catheter is removed and patient tries to void
Urodynamics	To assess bladder-urethral pressure profile and diagnose detrusor-sphincter dyssynergy	Indwelling catheter is placed; fluid is instilled into bladder and sensor placed to detect detrusor pressure and sphincter contraction
Serum Creatinine	Normal value: 0.5–1.0	Blood drawn
Blood Urea Nitrogen	Normal value: 10–20	Blood drawn
Urinalysis	To determine presence and amount of bacteria, glucose, blood, protein in urine	Random sample of urine; does not have to be sterile
Culture and Sensitivity	To determine type of bacteria and its sensitivity to antibiotics	Requires sterile specimen either through aspiration from indwelling catheter, sterile catheterization, or midstream void

SOURCE: From *Spinal Cord Injury: A Guide to Rehabilitation Nursing* (p. 103) by P.J. Matthews, C.E. Carlson, and N.B. Holt, 1987, Rockville, MD: Aspen Publishers, Inc. Copyright © 1987 by Aspen Publishers, Inc.

spontaneously, fluid restrictions can be liberalized or eliminated if bladder distention does not occur. If the patient does not have spontaneous voids and is to be on long-term intermittent catheterization, experimentation with fluid intake and catheterization schedule to provide flexibility is advised.

16. The parasympathetic nervous system is primarily responsible for bladder emptying, and drugs that stimulate or inhibit this system can be used either to aid weak bladder contractions or to decrease overactivity of bladder contractions. Urecholine (bethanechol chloride) has probably been the most widely used cholinergic drug to increase bladder contraction. *Caution is necessary because reflux of urine can occur if dyssynergia is present.* Anticholinergic drugs, such as Pro-Banthine and Ditropan, have been used for patients with uncontrolled bladder contractions and incontinence. They are particularly important in female patients who are incontinent. The sympathetic nervous system influences the bladder neck (internal sphincter region), and drugs that modify internal sphincter resistance can be used to decrease resistance to urine outflow, which can help combat urine retention. Therefore, sympatholytic drugs such as Dibenzyline may decrease resistance at the bladder neck and contribute to more complete emptying. Drugs affecting the autonomic nervous system can have serious side effects. Patient and family education and close monitoring of patient response are of primary import.

17. Bladder ultrasound may be performed to measure volume of urine in the bladder and to measure postvoid residual volumes. This may reduce the number of catheterizations needed, thus reducing risk of UTI and other complications.

18. For females, a mirror can be used to learn the anatomy and to identify the urethral meatus until location can be identified by tactile perception.

19. Certain positions will provide easier access to the meatus especially for females.
   • In the wheelchair it may be helpful to elevate one leg for access to the genitals which can be achieved by putting one foot on a low table, footstool, rung of chair; by raising the footrest; or by placing the leg over the side of the wheelchair.
   • In bed prop up in a sitting position with the knees flexed (Taylor position) and legs placed outward with the soles of the feet touching. This position may be maintained by placing a pillow under one knee or crossing the legs at the ankle.

20. The need for adaptive equipment (i.e., thigh abductor/spreader, splints, and/or clothing adaptations) to facilitate independent catheterization should be explored. Occupational therapy can be helpful in providing these adaptations.

21. Be alert for symptoms of latex allergy, as patients with chronic urologic conditions are at risk for developing latex allergies (Brown, 1994).

PATIENT AND FAMILY EDUCATION

1. For successful outcomes, the patient must participate fully in the program. Initiation of the program, fluid restrictions, action and side effects of medications, frequency of catheterization, progress, and termination of the program must be thoroughly explained to the patient and family. The attending physician and nurse are responsible for the initial explanation of the program and goal identification.

2. If injury to the spinal cord is above T6, the patient or caregiver is taught about the possibility of autonomic dysreflexia before beginning on an intermittent catheterization program.

3. Before discharge, the patient or caregiver must understand the importance of routine reevaluation.

4. A home health referral is usually indicated to assist with community adjustment to the program and to provide reinforcement.

5. The clean catheterization procedure is to be taught prior to discharge as a method of urinary management to be used in the home setting unless contraindicated. Contraindications include: catheterization less frequently than every 6 h, a resistant organism is present, or patient is performing catheterization to obtain postvoid residual. If any contraindications exist then sterile catheterization is to be done.

6. Consider age, growth and development stage, and learning ability when assessing a child's readiness to learn self-intermittent catheterization. Typically children are able to perform the procedure at 4 to 5 years of age.

Procedure

Intermittent Catheterization

 Steps

 Additional Information

1. Nursing assessment includes the following:
   - Type of neurogenic bladder (reflexic or areflexic)
   - Sensation for distention
   - Sensation for voiding
   - History of autonomic dysreflexia
   - Condition of urinary meatus and external genitalia (discharge, skin irritation, potential problems with fitting of external catheter)
   - Pattern and adequacy of fluid intake and pattern of output, with particular attention to patterns of sudden diuresis (see General Considerations 9)
   - Medication (urologic, other)
   - Concurrent medical conditions (e.g., infection, renal disease, hydration status, electrolyte imbalance)
   - Patient and caregiver problem-solving ability, motivation, cognitive status, and knowledge of urinary system and intermittent catheterization program

   A reflexic bladder results from lesions above the sacral spinal cord segments. Reflex voiding with varying degrees of residual urine occurs. An areflexic bladder results from lesions in the sacral reflex center or in the spinal roots. This type of bladder is characterized by retention of urine with bladder overdistention. Areflexic bladders can occur during spinal shock. If patient has frequent episodes of dysreflexia from bladder-related causes and if small volumes trigger voiding episodes, he or she may not be a good candidate for intermittent catheterization. Some patients are unable to restrict their fluids because of concurrent medical problems or excessive thirst. These patients may not be good candidates at this time. Patients and caregivers who are poorly motivated, unreliable, or poor problem-solvers may not be good candidates for this program.

2. Physician writes an order to begin program, including frequency of catheterizations and fluid restrictions.

   Physician's order is required to alter frequency of catheterizations and fluid restriction.

3. Instruct patient in purpose of program, frequency of catheterizations, and fluid restrictions. Also instruct patient to monitor for voids. Patient is to notify nurse if he or she voids or feels distended.

   Some patients may have normal sensation for distention and voids. Other patients may notice subtle sensations (i.e., flushing, tingling, goosebumps). Still others will not have any sensation. It is important that patient and caregiver begin to take responsibility for program well before discharge. Patient may need to decrease fluids or to increase frequency of catheterizations.

4. Catheterize patient at prescribed frequency. If patient has spontaneous void, use Bladder Volume Instrument immediately to estimate postvoid residual.

   Overdistention is thought to contribute to infections, vesicoureteral reflux and interferes with reflex activity.

5. Document all spontaneous voids and catheterization volumes. Note time of each event.

6. Encourage the patient to request fluids at appropriate intervals.

7. Monitor catheterization volumes and notify physician if:
   • Volumes are too high
   • Volumes are too low
   • Patient is having spontaneous voids with low postvoid residuals

8. If patient is having spontaneous voids:
   • Obtain and apply external catheter
   • Attempt to stimulate voids at regular intervals and before catheterizations

9. Well before discharge, assess appropriateness of program for home.

Patient may need to increase fluids or to decrease frequency of catheterizations. Patient will need adequate volume to trigger void if reflex activity is present.

If patient is voiding and if catheterization volumes never exceed 300 to 400 mL, he or she no longer needs fluid restriction. If postvoid residuals are consistently low, program may be discontinued with occasional checking of postvoid residuals. See procedure on external catheters.

See procedure on methods to stimulate voids. Adequate resources must exist for patients to be considered safe with an intermittent catheterization program at home (i.e., independent with procedure; adequate caregivers, supplies, problem-solving abilities). Sterile self-catheterization for home use is expensive. Clean intermittent catheterization is easier to perform and maintain in routines of daily living at home. Clean intermittent catheterization has been found to be safe in home environment.

10. If patient will be catheterized at least every 6 h, teach patient and caregiver clean catheterization technique for home use. Obtain physician order to begin this program.

 ## DOCUMENTATION

1. Record all urine measurements. It may be helpful to keep a flow sheet at the bedside for this purpose.

2. It is important that voiding between catheterizations be recorded. Note the time and amount.

3. Document all patient and caregiver education regarding the program.

4. Document when the program starts and when changes occur. Inability to comply with the program is significant and should be documented.

REFERENCES

Agency for Health Care Policy and Research (1992) *Clinical Practice Guidelines: Urinary Incontinence in Adults.* (AHCPR 92-0038) Rockville, MD: Department of Health and Human Services.

Broadwell, D. and Jackson, B. (1982) *Principles of Ostomy Care* St. Louis, MO: Mosby.

Brown, J.P. (1994) "Latex Allergy Requires Attention in Orthopaedic Nursing" *Orthopaedic Nursing* 13(1):7–11.

Carlson, D. and Mowery, B.D. (1997) "Standards to Prevent Complications of Urinary Catheterization in Children: Should and Should-Knots." *Journal of Pediatric Nursing* 2(1):37–41.

Johnson, J. (1980) "Rehabilitative Aspects of Neurologic Bladder Dysfunction: Symposium on Rehabilitation Nursing" *Nursing Clinics of North America* 15:293–308.

King, R.B., Carlson, C.E., Mervine, J., et al. (1992) "Clean and Sterile Intermittent Catheterization Methods in Hospitalized Patients with Spinal Cord Injury" *Archives of Physical Medicine & Rehabilitation* 73:798–802.

Matthews, P.J. (1987) In Matthews, P.J., Carlson, C., and Holt, N. (Eds.) *Spinal Cord Injury: A Guide to Rehabilitation Nursing.* Rockville, MD: Aspen.

Shields, L. (1981) "Urinary Function" In Martin, N., Holt, N., and Hicks, D. (Eds.) *Comprehensive Rehabilitation Nursing* New York: McGraw-Hill; pp. 186–222.

Wu, Y., (1983) "Total Bladder Care for the Spinal Cord Injured Patient" *Annals of the Academy of Medicine (Singapore)* 12:391.

Establishing Bladder Programs for Patients with Brain Damage

PURPOSE

To eliminate the use of indwelling catheters; to avoid catheter-related complications; to achieve urinary continence through scheduled voidings and fluid restrictions if needed; to promote the individual's self-esteem

STAFF RESPONSIBLE

EQUIPMENT

If needed:

1. Commode chair, bedpan, toilet, or raised toilet seat

2. Incontinence pads or briefs or external catheters

3. Adaptive clothing and equipment

 GENERAL CONSIDERATIONS

1. Voluntary inhibition of the micturition (voiding) reflex is mediated through the influence of the midbrain and other centers of the brain. These centers inhibit bladder contractions and facilitate relaxation of the external urinary sphincter and pelvic floor to allow bladder emptying. Since bladder function in the cerebral cortex is bilateral, patients with unilateral injury generally have successful bladder retraining (O'Brien and Pallett, 1978).

2. A brain lesion that disrupts the inhibitory centers can result in frequent, uninhibited bladder contractions (uninhibited bladder). Urinary frequency, urgency, and incontinence are symptoms of this condition. Bilateral brain damage may result in loss of voluntary micturition.

3. Most patients with brain damage from a stroke can be continent of urine because bladder emptying is possible: the sacral reflex arc remains intact, and there is at least partial sensation of bladder filling along with partial voluntary control of bladder emptying.

4. Other factors contributing to incontinence after brain damage include:
   - Impaired sensory feedback
   - Impaired motor ability
   - Impaired cognition, especially disorientation to time, memory deficits, and problem-solving difficulties (Owen et al., 1995)
   - Impaired communication

   - Organic problems such as urinary tract infection, changes due to aging, disease, or trauma

   Gelber et al. (1993) found three major mechanisms responsible for poststroke urinary incontinence: (1) disruption of the neuromicturition pathways, resulting in bladder hyperreflexia and urgency incontinence; (2) incontinence due to stroke-related cognitive and language deficits, with normal bladder function; and (3) concurrent neuropathy or medication use, resulting in bladder hyporeflexia and overflow incontinence. Urodynamic studies are of benefit in establishing the cause of incontinence. Gross (1998) found incontinent stroke patients took longer to be transferred to rehabilitation poststroke, had more episodes of incontinence on their first rehabilitation day, had lower FIM (functional independence measures) scores on admission, and smaller gains in these scores when compared to continent stroke patients at discharge.

5. Before implementing bladder programs, the nurse assesses the patient to determine the etiology of the bladder incontinence. Assessment of present voiding patterns, factors contributing to incontinence, appropriateness of toileting schedule, and appropriateness of present bladder program are important in identifying any limiting factors. Evaluation of the home environment, especially location of toileting facilities, is also useful. Bladder toileting programs are based on the etiology of incontinence, the data base obtained through assessment, and the goals of patient care.

6. Once the program is established, communication to the nursing staff (by means of the nursing care plan and incontinence flow sheet), physician, patient, family, and interdisciplinary team is essential for its success.

7. The incontinence flow sheet is a worksheet for assessing the pattern of incontinence and fluid intake, factors contributing to incontinence, and for monitoring the effectiveness of a toileting program.

8. Initial goals of bladder programs are usually very modest (i.e., daytime continence). External catheters or incontinence briefs or pads may be utilized through the night.

9. It is important to provide privacy for urinary elimination. Consideration of the patient's self-esteem and dignity is essential to a successful program, along with consideration of the toileting facility to be utilized and the position of the patient for voiding.

10. Continence programs require a team approach and involve the nurse, physician, physical therapist, occupational therapist, and others as needed.

11. Consultation with the occupational therapy department may be needed to assist with the fabrication of adaptive clothing. Velcro closures, zipper pulls, or clothing hooks may be useful.

12. Generally speaking, if an indwelling catheter has been in place for several months, a urinary system evaluation may be ordered by the physician prior to catheter removal.

13. If pharmacologic management is necessary to improve bladder tone, the patient should be observed for medication effect on the program and for side effects.

14. Meticulous skin care is needed to prevent perineal skin irritation related to incontinence.

15. Constipation can contribute to urinary incontinence. Assess and treat constipation.

16. Bladder ultrasound may be performed as needed to evaluate volume of urine in bladder and to measure postvoid residual volumes.

PATIENT AND FAMILY EDUCATION

1. Teach the patient and family the general considerations as they apply to the patient, inclusive of basic anatomy and physiology.

2. Teach the goals of the bladder program.

3. Explain the present program, responsibilities for the program, and the use of the incontinence flow sheet.

4. Evaluate the program's effectiveness and the patient's problem-solving skills.

5. Note the use and care of equipment if used.

Procedure

Establishing Bladder Programs for Patients with Brain Damage

 Steps

 Additional Information

1. Obtain history of incontinence from patient or family members. Assess:
   - Ability to communicate bladder fullness
   - Awareness of sensation of fullness
   - Frequency of incontinence
   - Sensation of urgency

2. Initiate recording of intake and output.

Initial assessment of present bladder function is important to any retraining program. A 24-h record of fluid intake and output provides baseline data.

3. Place call light within reach, and instruct patient in use.

If patient is aphasic, develop system to communicate need to toilet. Place commode near bed if urgency is severe.

4. Initiate incontinence flow sheet (Exhibit 3-1) and indicate bladder program, goals, and fluid and toileting directions.

Flow sheet can be used to assess pattern of incontinence if patient is not on a bladder program or effectiveness of current bladder program. Notify patient, family, and appropriate interdisciplinary staff.

5. To use flow sheet:
   - Chart fluid and toileting amounts in measured volumes in proper cells and columns. Estimate volume of incontinence on basis of the following amounts: small, 50 to 100 mL; medium, 100 to 175 mL; large, more than 200 mL.

Knowledge of relationship between amount of fluid taken in and voiding intervals will assist when developing bladder program. If there is no void when patient is toileted, toilet patient 1 h later. Toilet time or prompt is specified time from the last void. For example, patient may drink small amount of fluids and be incontinent in 30 to 40 min, or patient may drink 400 mL with incontinence 2 h later. Toileting needs will vary in these situations.

   - Use comments section or mentation column to indicate patient's mental status, location of patient, or other circumstances under which incontinence occurred.

Knowledge of patient's mental status or level of awareness and location at time of incontinence will assist in progressing or developing plan.

Knowledge of patient position may be helpful; for example, in supine position it is difficult to relax perineal muscles completely. This may result in incomplete emptying. Privacy is important for many patients for complete bladder emptying.

	DATE: 12/13/85				DATE:				DATE:				DATE:				DATE:			
	FLUID INTAKE	TOILETED AMOUNT	INCONTINENT AMOUNT	MENTATION	FLUID INTAKE	TOILETED AMOUNT	INCONTINENT AMOUNT	MENTATION	FLUID INTAKE	TOILETED AMOUNT	INCONTINENT AMOUNT	MENTATION	FLUID INTAKE	TOILETED AMOUNT	INCONTINENT AMOUNT	MENTATION	FLUID INTAKE	TOILETED AMOUNT	INCONTINENT AMOUNT	MENTATION
8-9a	250																			
9-10a		100																		
10-11a	100																			
11-12a		0																		
12-1p	300																			
1-2p		300																		
2-3p	150																			
3-4p		0																		
4-5p	250																			
5-6p		100																		
6-7p	100																			
7-8p		300																		
8-9p	150																			
9-10p		0																		
10-11p																				
12-1a																				
1-2a	50	200		0																
2-3a																				
3-4a																				
4-5a			approx 100	S/A																
5-6a																				
6-7a																				
7-8a	50	0																		

JOHN DOE
DR. P. BROWN
Rehabilitation Institute of Chicago
Division of Nursing

INCONTINENCE FLOW SHEET

PRESENT PROGRAM (include MD's order for caths if no void in a specific time):

Toilet every 2 hours during day
Toilet every 4 hours during night
No fluid restrictions
Push Fluids!!

KEY

Fluid Intake = amount in cc's
Toileted Amount = amount in cc's, indicate 0 if no void

Mentation = C - Confused
            S - Sleeping
            O - Oriented
            A - Aware Wet

COMMENTS:
Include cath time and amts.
coffee in a.m. & at dinner
does not drink a lot of fluids
requested toileting at 1 a.m.
incontinent at 4:30 a.m.

COMMENTS:
Include cath time and amts.

COMMENTS:
Include cath time and amts.

COMMENTS:
Include cath time and amts.

COMMENTS:
Include cath time and amts.

Source: Courtesy of Division of Nursing, Rehabilitation Institute of Chicago.

Exhibit 3-1   Incontinence Flow Sheet

- Indicate in comments section if incontinence occurred off nursing unit, in bed, on the way to toilet, and so on.
- Indicate in comments section any unusual occurrences (i.e., frequency, urgency, burning).

6. Assess baseline data on incontinence flow sheet for patterns.

7. Revise toileting frequency on basis of patterns of incontinence observed.

8. Review findings with physician.

9. Review total fluid intake for adequacy and evaluate need for restriction of fluids.

10. Consider use of behavioral intervention program if timed fluids, toileting, and medication are ineffective.

Patients may be incontinent when in unfamiliar environments.

Urinary infection contributes to urgency and frequency.

Pattern is usually noted in 2 to 3 days but may take longer. Toileting schedule must be consistent. If pattern is obscure, offer toileting every 2 h (or prompt patient). If patient has frequent periods of dryness, increase intervals between toileting and evaluate. Decrease intervals to 1 h if incontinence has not improved. Advance to establishing voiding pattern by offering toileting at key times: in early morning, before and after meals, before scheduled therapies, before rest periods, or at bedtime. Nighttime toileting with restricted fluids may be scheduled for every 3 to 4 h.

If medications are ordered to treat urinary tract infection, urgency, or frequency, evaluate effectiveness and for side effects. Continue use of flow sheet for evaluation.

Establish fluid schedule every 2 h if there is no clear incontinence pattern or if patient intake is poor. If incontinence occurs through night and if medical condition allows, restrict amount of fluids after 8 P.M. Limiting fluids at night is not indicated if patient is dehydrated or if other medical condition contraindicates. Eventually, most patients do not need strict fluid schedule.

Behavioral programs are individualized and somewhat complex. Refer to McCormick, Scheve, and Leahy (1988) for extensive references.

 ## DOCUMENTATION

1. Document the amount, frequency, and circumstances related to incontinence, intake, and output.
2. Document emerging patterns of incontinence and of progress toward goals.
3. Document the patient and family response to the program.
4. Document the elements of the plan to control incontinence and to achieve continence: goals, fluids (type, amount, and frequency), toileting frequency, prompts (cueing, if used), and protective devices or clothing used.

REFERENCES

Agency for Health Care Policy and Research (1992) *Clinical Practice Guidelines: Urinary Incontinence in Adults* (AHCPR 92-0038) Rockville, MD: Department of Health and Human Services.

Gelber, D.A., Good, D.C., Laren, L.J., Verhuest, S. J. (1993) "Causes of Urinary Incontinence after Acute Hemispheric Stroke" *Stroke* 24(3), 378–82.

Gross, J.C. (1998) "A Comparison of the Characteristics of Incontinent and Continent Stroke Patients in a Rehabilitation Program" *Rehabilitation Nursing* 23(3):132–40.

McCormick, K.A., Scheve, A. S., and Leahy, E. (1988) "Nursing Management of Urinary Incontinence in Geriatric Inpatients" *Nursing Clinics of North America* 23:231–363.

O'Brien, M.T., and Pallett, P.J. (1978) *Total Care of the Stroke Patient.* Boston: Little, Brown.

Owen, D. C., Getz, P. A., Bulla, S. (1995) "A Comparison of Characteristics of Patients with Completed Stroke: Those Who Completed Continence and Those Who Did Not" *Rehabilitation Nursing* 20(4):197–203.

Pallett, P.J., and O'Brien, M.T. (1985) *Textbook of Neurosurgical Nursing.* Boston: Little, Brown.

Methods to Stimulate Voiding and to Empty the Bladder in Patients with Spinal Cord Injuries

PURPOSE

To initiate voiding or to empty the bladder in the patient with spinal cord injury

STAFF RESPONSIBLE

EQUIPMENT

1. Nonsterile gloves
2. Water-soluble lubricant (for anal stretch)

 GENERAL CONSIDERATIONS

1. Methods of stimulation should *not* be used if the patient has detrusor-sphincter dyssynergia because it could cause reflux of urine into the ureters and kidney.
2. Urodynamic studies should be performed to evaluate the effects of Credé and Valsalva maneuvers, abdominal tapping, and anal stretch techniques.

3. Anal stretch is used with patients with complete spinal cord lesions above the sacral segments or with a reflex neurogenic bladder.
4. Anal stretch requires a physician's orders.
5. When using anal stretch, the patient may also need to do Credé or Valsalva maneuvers to empty the bladder because anal stretch inhibits detrusor and urethral sphincter contractions (Matthews, 1987).
6. Credé and Valsalva maneuvers may be effective for patients with lower motor neuron lesions that have resulted in an areflexic bladder. To avoid vesicoureteral reflux, detrusor-sphincter dyssynergia should be ruled out or voiding should be initiated before using Credé maneuver.
7. Credé maneuver requires a physician's order.
8. For more information about types of bladder dysfunction, see Matthews (1987).

PATIENT AND FAMILY EDUCATION

1. Education should include the purpose of the procedure, the proper technique to stimulate voiding, measuring the effectiveness of the technique, and any possible complications.
2. Whenever possible, involve the patient and family in the procedure.

Procedures

Anal Stretch

 Steps

1. Obtain physician's order.

2. Explain purpose and procedure to patient. Provide privacy.
3. Position patient comfortably on side or on toilet.
4. Don glove and lubricate index and middle fingers.
5. Insert first one then two fingers gently into rectum (Fig. 3-1*A*).
6. Spread fingers apart (Fig. 3-1*B*).

 Additional Information

This procedure may cause vesicoureteral reflux in patients with detrusor-sphincter dyssynergia.

Go only as far as necessary to stretch anal sphincter (usually about 3 cm).

Observe for signs and symptoms of autonomic dysreflexia. Assess for bowel movement.

7. Withdraw fingers gently once voiding is complete.

If patient begins to void, have him or her perform Valsalva or Credé maneuver to increase intraabdominal pressure to facilitate emptying.

8. Clean patient and make him or her comfortable.

Dispose of soiled materials according to infection control procedures.

9. Catheterize for residual urine as ordered by physician.
10. Document according to guidelines.

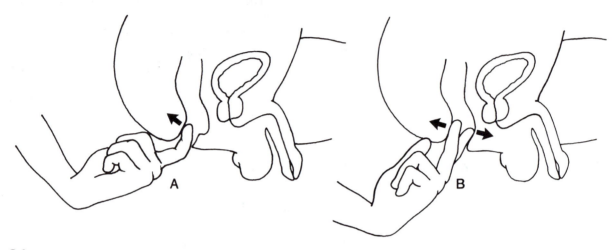

Figure 3-1

Credé Maneuver

 Steps

1. Obtain physician's order.

2. Explain purpose and procedure to patient. Provide privacy.

3. Place hands flat against patient's abdomen lateral to and below umbilicus.

4. With hands, use firm downward and medial stroke toward bladder, then press with both hands directly over bladder.

5. Repeat several times.

6. Catheterize for residual urine if ordered by physician.

7. Return patient to comfortable position and appropriate dress.

8. Document according to guidelines.

 Additional Information

This procedure may cause vesicoureteral reflux in patients with detrusor-sphincter dyssynergia.

Patient may be positioned in Fowler's position in bed or seated on toilet or commode.

This will manually express urine from bladder.

Valsalva Maneuver

 Steps

1. Explain purpose and procedure to patient. Provide privacy.
2. Instruct patient to hold breath while straining to urinate and move bowels.
3. Repeat several times.
4. Catheterize for residual urine if ordered by physician.
5. Document according to guidelines.

 Additional Information

This procedure is contraindicated for some cardiac patients. Consult physician.

Patient may be positioned in Fowler's position in bed or seated on toilet or commode.

Monitor for syncope and cardiac changes.

Other Techniques for Patients with Reflexic Neurogenic Bladders

 Steps

1. Explain purpose and procedure to patient. Provide privacy.

2. Tap with fingers over patient's suprapubic region for 2 to 3 min (about 50 taps). If ineffective, stop and wait 1 min.
3. Try stroking medial thigh in area along adductor magnus for 2 to 3 min. If ineffective, stop and wait 1 min.
4. Try pinching abdomen above inguinal ligaments for 2 to 3 min. If ineffective, stop and wait 1 min.
5. Try pulling patient's pubic hair for 2 to 3 min. If ineffective, stop and wait 1 min.
6. Try massaging the male patient's penoscrotal area. If ineffective, stop and wait 1 min.
7. Try pinching posterior aspect of male patient's glans penis for 2 to 3 min. If ineffective, stop.
8. Catheterize for residual urine if ordered by physician.
9. Document according to guidelines.

 Additional Information

See Shields (1981) for further information about other techniques.

These techniques may seem unusually harsh. Patients should be fully informed of specific procedures and desired results.

 DOCUMENTATION

1. Document the procedure, the effectiveness of the techniques, the most successful methods to stimulate voiding or to empty the bladder, the amount voided, and the type of catheterization.
2. Document any complications or unusual observations.
3. Document patient and primary caregiver education and involvement in the procedure.

REFERENCES

Agency for Health Care Policy and Research (1992) *Clinical Practice Guidelines: Urinary Incontinence in Adults.* (AHCPR 92-0038) Rockville, MD: Department of Health and Human Services.

Cardenas, D. D., Kelly, E., and Mayo, M.E. (1985) "Manual Stimulation of Reflex Voiding after Spinal Cord Injury" *Archives of Physical Medicine and Rehabilitation* 66:459–462.

Kivat, Zimmerman and Donovan (1975) "Sphincter Stretch: New Technique Resulting in Continence and Complete Voiding in Paraplegics" *Journal of Urology* 114:895–897.

Matthews, P.J. (1987) In Matthews, P.J., Carlson, C., and Holt, N. (Eds.) *Spinal Cord Injury: A Guide to Rehabilitation Nursing*. Rockville, MD: Aspen.

Shields, L. (1981) "Urinary Function" In Martin, N., Holt, N., and Hicks, D. (Eds.) *Comprehensive Rehabilitation Nursing* New York: McGraw-Hill; pp. 186–222.

Wu, Y. (1983) "Total Bladder Care for the Spinal Cord Injured Patient" *Annals of the Academy of Medicine (Singapore)* 12:391.

Wu, Y., Nanninga, J.B., and Hamilton, B.B. (1986) "Inhibition of the External Urethral Sphincter and Sacral Reflex by Anal Stretch in Spinal Cord Injured Patients" *Archives of Physical Medicine and Rehabilitation* 67: 135–136.

Procedures for Urinary Elimination: External Catheters

Male External Catheter Application and Removal

PURPOSE

To apply an external catheter to a male patient for urine collection; to remove the catheter without injury to the patient

STAFF RESPONSIBLE

EQUIPMENT

Choice of external appliance and fixative: See local/national manufacturers for available appliances and fixatives.

For all appliances:

1. Soap, water, and towel
2. Leg bag
3. Extension tubing
4. Nonsterile gloves

 GENERAL CONSIDERATIONS

1. It is recommended that an external catheter is changed at least once every 24 h until patient tolerance has developed. With proper supervision, some external catheters have been worn safely for longer periods of time. The catheter should be left off to allow the skin to air for an hour or so between changes.

2. External catheters can be removed at night for patients who are prone to skin problems. A urinal may be positioned in place with the rim padded. The care plan should indicate this intervention and include frequent skin checks. If urinal positioning is not possible because of increased tone, incontinence briefs or pads can be used instead.

3. A check on patients who are dependent in application or require supervision at least once a shift ensures that the external catheter is not applied too tightly or becomes too tight over time. Patients who are independent are taught to perform self-checks.

4. External catheters are *not* to be applied over red or broken skin areas. If possible, the catheter is to be applied distal to the open area. A Crixiline strip may be applied over the open area to provide a waterproof barrier and to assist in healing, and the external catheter can be applied over this strip. If neither option is available, the external catheter is not worn. A pad or incontinence briefs with proper skin care can be used to manage the incontinence until area heals.

5. If applied to an erect penis, external catheters should not be applied tightly. Clipping the ring that forms at the base of the condom will prevent a tourniquet effect if the patient experiences frequent or prolonged erections.

6. A foreskin that is not pulled forward over the glans penis may act as a tourniquet when the patient has an erection.

7. Decisions regarding the type of external catheter and fixative are to be made by the nurse, and directions must be written in the nursing care plan. Sample options are shown in Tables 3-3 and 3-4. The following assessments are to be made before this decision:
   - Cost of the external catheter and fixative, considering reusability
   - Frequency of removal (i.e., for intermittent catheterizations)
   - Ease of application and construction for the person who usually applies the device
   - Penis size (flaccid and erect)
   - Reaction to a skin patch test with fixatives before routine use to rule out sensitivity
   - Degree of sensation
   - Patient's cognitive status
   - Frequency and duration of erections
   - Activity level, including positions assumed throughout the day
   - Previous use, success, and problems
   - Availability of the external catheter when the patient is outside the hospital
   - Type of drainage tubing and bag to be used

8. Different fixatives may be combined. Try fixatives, one at a time, starting with the simplest and least expensive first. The patient should be monitored at least every shift each time the type of external catheter or fixative is altered until tolerance and appropriateness are determined. No

Table 3-3	**Sample Product Options for Male External Catheters**	
Type of External Catheter	**Sizes**	**Considerations**
Bardic Urosheath	Small, medium, large and X-large	Rigid; no expansion; reusable; very durable; firm base that prevents twisting. Clean by washing with soap and water and rinsing thoroughly.
Condom with latex tubing	One size	Disposable; parts can be reused with a new condom. Tubing can be cut to custom length for drainage. Be sure that a drainage hole is made in condom. (See Fig. 3-2.)
Condom with Texas or similar adaptor	One size	Disposable; parts can be reused with a new condom. Be sure that a drainage hole is made in condom.
Gizmo	Standard and small	Reusable with Crixiline tape or Posey strap. Bulb at base prevents twisting.
Hollister self-adhesive catheter	Standard, medium, pediatric, geriatric	Disposable; design prevents kinking and twisting; sheath contains nonirritating adhesive inside; long wear time. Retracted penis pouch and reusable external device are available.
Mentor Freedom	Medium and standard	No adhesive required because fixative is already applied to sheath. Recommended for use with retractable penis. A protective skin dressing can be used for application provided that it is allowed to dry completely. Not recommended if external catheter needs to be changed more than twice a day.
Texas prepackaged	One size	Disposable; parts should be saved and reused with a new condom to reduce cost.
Uri-Drain	Standard, pediatric, and geriatric	Reusable if used with Crixiline strips or Posey strap. Firm base prevents twisting.
Urosan	Standard and small	Disposable; one-time use only. Do not use if external catheter is removed more than once a day. Use only with Urosan adhesive tape and skin protectant.

NOTE: These are sample products that are now available. New products are continually being developed.

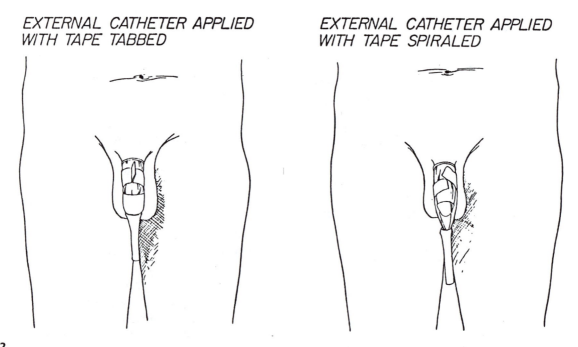

EXTERNAL CATHETER APPLIED WITH TAPE TABBED

EXTERNAL CATHETER APPLIED WITH TAPE SPIRALED

Figure 3-2

Table 3-4   Product Options for Fixatives

Fixative	Considerations
Nonadhesive sheath holder Posey sheath holder	Reusable; washable. If holder gets wet with urine or from washing, be sure that it dries completely before putting it back on. Monitor at frequent intervals for development of pressure areas on shaft of penis. Holder can also be adapted by occupational therapist for patients with limited hand function.
Latex sheath holder	Not recommended. Tendency to cause pressure areas.
Single-sided adhesives applied over sheath Elastic tape	Expands if applied with spiral or tab technique (Fig. 3-3). Use 1-in. tape. Use new external catheter with each change because tape will tear catheter when removing.
Double-sided adhesives applied between penile shaft and sheath	Same as above. All brands are applied to penis with spiral technique; external catheter is applied over adhesive. Difficult to apply with limited hand function. These double-sided adhesives should not be used on patients who need to remove catheter more than once or twice a day.
Uriliner, Urofoam, Crixiline strips, Uristrips	*Crixiline:* Available in 1- to 6-in. strips. Strips are not water soluble and turn to gel at body temperature. Allows for expansion and contraction. Can be placed over small pressure areas to aid healing. Wash off with soap and water. Must be removed and new strips applied every 24 h. *Unistrips:* Cannot be purchased separately; packaged with Urosan external catheter and a Skin Prep swab.
Liquid adhesives Tincture of benzoin	May be used alone or with one-sided adhesive or sheath holder.

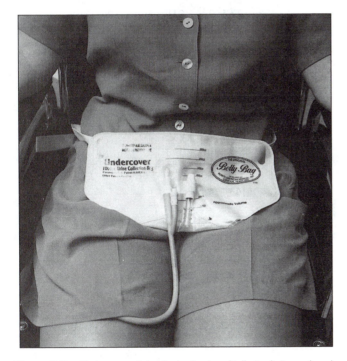

Figure 3-3 Undercover abdominal urine bag (Belly Bag). Reproduced with permission from North American Medical, Inc., Lubbock, TX.

additional fixatives should be used with strapless or self-adhesive external catheters such as Freedom.

9. Patients or primary caregivers are to be taught external catheter application and removal.

10. The nurse should periodically document progress or tolerance to the external catheter.

11. Follow any and all infection control guidelines, and always discard used equipment in the appropriate manner.

12. Durable external appliances are available. The patient is fitted for the appliance by the manufacturer's representative. Additional fixatives are not necessary.

PATIENT AND FAMILY EDUCATION

1. Education should include the purpose of male external catheter application, its removal, and the proper techniques involved.

2. The patient and caregiver should be included in decision making with regard to the type of external catheter and its method of application. Also instruct as to potential complications associated with these devices and how to observe for, prevent, and alleviate complications.

3. Whenever possible, involve the patient and family in the procedure.

Procedure

Applying and Removing an External Catheter with Adhesives or Skin Barrier

This method of application can be used for all types of external catheters except the Freedom Mentor catheter.

Application

 Steps

 Additional Information

1. Collect necessary equipment.
2. Wash hands with soap and water.
3. Provide for patient's privacy.

   Apply nonsterile gloves.

4. Perform groin care (if foreskin is present, clean beneath it and pull it forward and down to original position).
5. Check skin for any reddened or open areas.
6. Trim or shave any pubic hairs if they will become entangled in external catheter.
7. Apply the following if being used:
   - Skin barrier
   - Crixiline strip (in spiral fashion on shaft of penis)
   - Benzoin spray (to shaft of penis)
   - Skin Bond cement

   Apply to shaft of penis. When it becomes tacky, apply external catheter. A fenestrated, disposable washcloth may be used as a shield to keep from spraying pubic hairs.

   Put on external catheter before spray dries completely.

8. Position catheter 1 in. below head of penis.
9. Roll catheter up shaft of penis.
10. Connect to drainage equipment (either directly to drainage bag or to adaptor with extension tubing).

Removal

 Steps

Additional Information

1. Provide privacy.
2. Loosen tape or remove adhesive.

   Put on nonsterile gloves.

3. To remove adhesive:
   - Apply adhesive remover per product directions
   - Wash penis with soap and water, rinse, and dry thoroughly

   Caution: *Do not cut external catheter to remove. Always peel gently to roll off.*

4. Inspect skin on penis.
5. Clean reusable external catheter with soap and water; dry before reusing.

Procedure

Applying and Removing an External Catheter with Elastic Tape or Posey Sheath Holder

Caution: When frequent erections occur, the potential for pressure sore development exists. To test the tension of the Posey holder or tape, apply it to fingers held together of a size similar to that of the penis and place the fingers in a dependent position. Simulate the erection size with the fingers and check the circulation in the nailbeds.

Application

 Steps

 Additional Information

1. Follow steps 1 through 6, applying and removing an external catheter, above.

2. Cut a strip of Elastic tape equal to 1⅛ times circumference of penis shaft.

3. Position external catheter 1 in. below head of penis, and roll it up shaft of penis.

4. Secure Elastic tape or Posey sheath holder below penoscrotal junction:
   • If Elastic tape is applied (see Fig. 3-2).
   • If Posey sheath holder is applied, place blue surface against external catheter. Overlap fabric ends on anterior surface of penis. Put a finger under sheath holder while securing Velcro closure. Press Velcro in place with wrinkling (allowing for erection or voiding). Do not use Posey holder if it overlaps over half or more of circumference of penis. Check 2 h after application and once a shift.

Apply in spiral or tabbed manner. Spiral fashion allows for even pressure to be applied.

Removal

 Steps

 Additional Information

1. Loosen tape or Posey sheath. Gently peel and roll it off.

2. Inspect skin on penis.

3. Perform groin care.

4. Clean reusable external catheter and Posey sheath holder with soap and water.

Provide privacy.

Put on nonsterile gloves.

Caution: *Do not cut external catheter to remove.*

Procedure

Applying and Removing a Mentor Freedom External Catheter

Use of a skin barrier spray or pads is not necessary, but they can be used provided that the barrier dries completely before the external catheter is applied.

Application

 Steps

 Additional Information

1. Perform steps 1 through 6, applying and removing an external catheter, above.

2. Place cone end of rolled sheath next to head of penis.

3. Slowly unroll sheath all the way up length of penis.

If the penis recedes, grasp penis with one hand while rolling sheath on with other hand. Penis will retract again without sheath being pushed off.

4. Squeeze sheath all around penis to seal.

If there are many wrinkles in sheath, use a smaller external catheter. If patient has frequent erections, clip ring at top of external sheath to prevent tourniquet effect.

5. Connect to drainage equipment (either directly to drainage bag or to adaptor with extension tubing).

6. Report skin tolerance, success, or problems to nurse in charge.

Removal

 Steps

 Additional Information

1. Remove by grasping end of sheath at base of penis and gently rolling toward glans penis.

Apply nonsterile gloves

2. Inspect skin on penis, and perform groin care.

3. Clean reusable external catheter with soap and water.

 DOCUMENTATION

1. Document the type of appliance and fixative and the method of application, frequency of penile skin check, wearing times, and degree of assistance or supervision needed.

2. Document the patient's skin tolerance, degree of satisfaction, and any problems or complications.

3. Document patient and family teaching (success and problems).

REFERENCES

King, R.B., Boyink, M., Keenan, M. (1977) *Rehabilitation Guide* Chicago: Rehabilitation Institute of Chicago.

Newman, E., Price, M., Magney, J. (1986) *Care of the Disabled Urinary Tract* Springfield, IL: Thomas.

Procedures for Urinary Elimination: Indwelling Catheters

Overview: Selection and Care of the Indwelling Catheter

PURPOSE

To determine the most appropriate choice of an indwelling catheter; to prevent complications associated with indwelling catheterization

STAFF RESPONSIBLE

GENERAL CONSIDERATIONS

1. Although it is desirable to eliminate the use of an indwelling catheter, its use cannot be avoided in some situations. Other methods of urinary elimination that may be considered are intermittent catheterization, external catheters, timed voiding schedules, and methods to stimulate voiding.

2. The presence of a catheter carries numerous complications, the most serious of which is infection. Every effort must be made to avoid introduction of bacteria into the urinary system.

3. Other commonly occurring complications, such as peno-scrotal fistulas, urethritis, and urinary tract calculi, can be reduced with proper preventive care.

4. Provide for patient's privacy throughout any urinary procedures.

PATIENT AND FAMILY EDUCATION

1. Education should include the purpose and proper technique for the care of the indwelling catheter as well as how to prevent and observe for potential complications, such as urinary tract infection.

2. Whenever possible, involve the patient and family in the procedure.

3. Discuss patient's feeling regarding the indwelling catheters.

Procedure

Selection and Care of the Indwelling Catheter

 Steps

1. Choose catheter least likely to result in complications. Assess the following characteristics:
   - Size: the smallest possible size should be used to decrease urethral irritation. A # 16 catheter with a 5-mL balloon can be used by most adults.
   - Balloon size: the smallest amount necessary to keep catheter in bladder, usually 7 to 8 mL, is advised but may be increased to 10 mL if the catheter is easily dislodged (Kniep-Hardy et al., 1985; Moore, 1992). A small balloon allows more complete bladder emptying.
   - Catheter material: choices include latex, silicone, silicone-coated latex, and hydrogel-coated latex.

 Additional Information

Leaking around catheter is an indication to use a smaller catheter and/or balloon and is often due to constipation or bowel impaction (Ziemann et al., 1984).

Overfilling the balloon or using large balloons increases foreign body surface area in the bladder and may erode bladder mucosa (Moore, 1992) and may increase calculus formation. Large-size catheters and balloons can actually contribute to urine leakage (Kennedy et al., 1983).

Silicone and silicone-coated latex catheters may be less irritating and cause less encrustations; hydrogel-coated latex catheters may be less irritating and decrease infections by being more resistant to biofilm development (Nacey and Delahunt, 1991)

2. Maintain good urine flow in drainage system:
   - Monitor catheter for the following signs indicating catheter change needed:
     - Drainage is sluggish or absent
     - Significant grit has accumulated in the catheter
   - Check for plugging. Catheter should be changed if urine flow is obstructed. If plugging occurs frequently, the cause should be investigated. Irrigations are not used routinely.
   - Always keep drainage bag below level of bladder to prevent backflow of urine into bladder.
   - Empty drainage bag at least every 8 h or whenever large amount of urine is in bag.
   - Do not allow tubing to kink or to form dependent loop below level of the bag.

3. Tape catheter to thigh or abdomen to prevent trauma caused by tension on catheter.

4. Prevent contamination of urinary drainage system:
   - Always wash hands and wear gloves for any contact with urine or urinary equipment.
   - Minimize opening of drainage system as much as possible. Use leg bag only on patients who are upright and active.
   - If drainage device is found to be disconnected from catheter, replace with new, sterile device and tubing.
   - No special meatal care beyond routine cleaning is needed. Meatal care using special cleansing agents or ointments is ineffective in preventing urinary infections (Burke et al., 1983; Classen et al., 1991).
   - Never allow drainage bag or tubing to touch floor.
   - Try to separate patients with indwelling catheters as much as possible (i.e., place them in separate rooms), especially if a patient has urinary tract infection. Follow infection control guidelines, especially, for patients with multiple resistant organisms.

To test for grit, roll catheter between fingers and feel for any particles in catheter lumen.

Oral fluid intake that ensures urinary output of 2500 mL is best method of bladder irrigation. Prior to catheter change, check for kinks in tubing or other external obstruction.

Empty drainage bag before any transfer or turn during which bag may not stay well below level of bladder.

Be sure to empty bag before patient leaves unit for a significant length of time. See procedure on attaching drainage device.

See procedures on taping a catheter.

Try to time irrigations and other procedures with change of drainage device. Each opening of urinary drainage system significantly increases risk of urinary tract infection.

See procedures for Routine Urinary Meatal Hygiene for Patients with Indwelling Catheters. Always wash from urinary meatus down catheter.

Monitor patients for symptoms of urinary tract infections (i.e., cloudy urine, strong odor, complaint of burning or pain in area of catheter).

DOCUMENTATION

1. Document all urinary procedures and any problems or complications noted.

2. Document any signs or symptoms of urinary tract infection.

3. Document any participation in the procedure by the patient or primary caregiver.

4. Document patient and family education.

REFERENCES

Agency for Health Care Policy and Research (1992) *Clinical Practice Guidelines: Urinary Incontinence in Adults.* (AHCPR 92-0038) Rockville, MD: Department of Health and Human Services.

Brown, J.P. (1994) "Latex Allergy Requires Attention in Orthopaedic Nursing" *Orthopaedic Nursing* 13(1):7–11.

Brunner, L.S., and Suddarth, D.S. (1984) *Textbook of Medical Surgical Nursing.* Philadelphia: Lippincott.

Burke, J., Jacobson, J., Garibalki, R., et al. (1983) "Evaluation of Daily Meatal Care with Polyantibiotic

Ointment in Prevention of Urinary Catheter-Associated Bacteriuria." *Journal of Urology* 129:331–334.

Burkitt, D., and Randall, J. (1987) "Catheterization: Urethral Trauma" *Nursing Times* 83:43, 59–60, 63.

Classen, D.C., Larsen, R.A., Burke, J.B., et al. (1991) Daily Meatal Care for Prevention of Catheter-Associated Bacteriuria: Results Using Frequent Applications of Polyantibiotic Cream. *Infection Control and Hospital Epidemiology* 12(3):157–162.

Kennedy, A.P., Brocklehurst, J.C., and Lye, M.D.W. (1983) "Factors Related to the Problems of Long-Term Catheterization" *Journal of Advanced Nursing* 8:207–212.

Kniep-Hardy, M.J., Votava, K., and Stubbings, M.J. (1985) "Managing Indwelling Catheters at Home" *Geriatric Nursing* 6:280–285.

McConnell, E.A., and Zimmerman, M.F. (1983) *Care of Patients with Urologic Problems*. Philadelphia: Lippincott.

Moore, K.N. (1992) "Indwelling Catheters: Problems and Management" *The Canadian Nurse* 88(6):33–35.

Nacey, J.N. and Delahunt, B. (1991) "Toxicity Study of First and Second Generation Hydrogel-Coated Latex Urinary Catheters." *British Journal of Urology* 67:314–316.

Wilde, M. (1997) "Long-Term Indwelling Urinary Catheter Care: Conceptualizing the Research." *Journal of Advanced Nursing* 25:1252–1261.

Ziemann, L.K., Lastauskas, N.M., and Ambrosini, G. (1984) Incidence of Leakage from Indwelling Urinary Catheters in Home-Bound Patients. *Home Healthcare Nurse* 2(5):22–26.

Attaching a Drainage Device to an Indwelling or External Catheter

PURPOSE

To provide a sterile collecting device for patients with an indwelling or external catheter.

STAFF RESPONSIBLE

EQUIPMENT

1. Urinary drainage bag (bedside, leg, or abdominal/belly bag)
2. Extension tubing with 5-in. adaptors (if needed)
3. Adapted clamps (if needed)
4. Leg bag straps (adapted straps optional)
5. Tape (if needed)
6. Alcohol wipes
7. Plastic bags
8. Nonsterile gloves

 GENERAL CONSIDERATIONS

1. A closed, sterile urinary drainage system should be used for those patients with an indwelling catheter who remain in bed. For those who are up, dressed, and active, a leg bag or abdominal bag may be worn during the day. The leg bag may be worn day and night if it can be emptied often enough at night so that it is not overfilled. If so, be sure the bag is taken off the leg and laid on the bed at night to enhance drainage. The abdominal bag may also be worn day and night and may be laid on the bed or remain attached to the patient (see Fig. 3-3). Abdominal or belly bags are used with **indwelling catheters only**. Every effort should be made to maintain a closed system whenever possible.

2. If an open drainage system is used, be sure that the bedside drainage system is changed at least every 24 h or whenever contamination is suspected.

3. The bedside urinary drainage bag is to be used whenever a patient with an indwelling catheter will be supine for an extended length of time.

4. If a bladder irrigation is to be done, it should be performed when the drainage devices are changed. This minimizes the need to disconnect the catheter an additional time. Routine bladder irrigations are not recommended, however (AHCPR, 1992).

5. Whenever a catheter is disconnected, there is an opportunity for contamination of the urinary tract. Therefore, aseptic technique should be maintained throughout the procedure in regard to exposed ports and lumens.

6. Nonsterile gloves are used when handling urine or urinary equipment of any patient. Empty all urine from the existing drainage device before disconnection. Used drainage devices and tubing are discarded according to infection control procedures.

7. The following considerations refer to leg bag use:
   • The leg bag is used while the patient is up in the wheelchair.
   • Extension tubing is used for patients who prefer to wear the leg bag on the calf and for patients using external catheters.

- To facilitate independent management of drainage devices, the occupational therapist can adapt leg bag straps and provide special clamps.
- The leg bag should be applied to the right and left legs on alternating days. Straps should be loose so as not to compromise circulation or to cause pressure.
- Location of the leg bag on the leg is based on patient preference.

PATIENT AND FAMILY EDUCATION

1. Education should include the purpose and proper technique for attaching a drainage device and how to prevent and observe for potential complications such as infection or obstructed drainage.
2. Whenever possible, involve the patient and family in the procedure.

Procedure

Attaching a Drainage Device to an Indwelling or External Catheter

 Steps

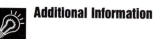 **Additional Information**

1. Wash hands.
2. Explain procedure and provide for privacy.
3. Check drainage bag.

Ensure that cover is on at end of tubing. Ensure that clamp is closed at bottom of drainage bag. If cap is not in place, discard unit and obtain a new one.

 Steps

 Additional Information

At Bedside

1. Open plastic bag for disposal of used equipment.
2. Loosen cover from catheter adaptor of drainage bag; do not remove cap yet.
3. Don nonsterile gloves.
4. Clean area of connection between indwelling catheter and existing drainage device with alcohol wipe.

Allow alcohol to dry before proceeding.

5. Pinch indwelling catheter tubing and separate catheter from present drainage device. If external catheter, allow all urine to drain into drainage device before disconnecting.

Ensure that tubing port of indwelling catheter remains sterile. Pinch is performed to prevent urine flow.

6. Remove cap of drainage bag with one hand, and connect (new) drainage bag to indwelling or external catheter.
7. Push together, then pull back slightly to ensure that connection is secure.

Prevent contamination of connection site during removal or once cap has been removed.

8. Tape indwelling catheter to thigh or abdomen of patient.

Refer to procedure on taping an indwelling catheter. This is to prevent kinking or formation of dependent loops that would hinder flow of urine. All tubing should be below level of bladder.

9. Coil extra tubing length on bed. Tape excess tubing to itself.
10. Suspend bag below level of bladder on bedframe with hanger provided.

Unnecessary with abdominal bag. Drainage bag should never be in contact with floor.

11. Dispose of used drainage bag.
12. Remove gloves; wash hands.

Disposal is according to infection control procedures.

DOCUMENTATION

1. Document the procedure, outcome, and any significant observations.

2. Document patient and primary caregiver education and involvement in the procedure.

REFERENCES

Agency for Health Care Policy and Research (1992) *Clinical Practice Guidelines: Urinary Incontinence in Adults.* (AHCPR 92-0038) Rockville, MD: Department of Health and Human Services.

King, R.B., Boyink, M., and Keenan, M. (1977) *Rehabilitation Guide* Chicago: Rehabilitation Institute of Chicago.

Undercover Abdominal Urine Bag (Belly Bag) developed by North American Medical, Inc. Lubbock, TX.

Taping an Indwelling Catheter: Male

PURPOSE

To secure an indwelling catheter to prevent urethral irritation and strictures, penoscrotal fistula, or tension on the catheter

STAFF RESPONSIBLE

EQUIPMENT

1. Tape, 1-in. width (select type of tape according to the patient's skin tolerance)

2. Nonsterile gloves

GENERAL CONSIDERATIONS

1. Securing the catheter to the patient's thigh reduces tension on the catheter and may reduce sphincter damage

(Burkitt & Randall, 1987) and trauma to the urethra and bladder (Edwards et al., 1983).

2. Rotate sites of taping to prevent skin irritation.

3. Place the tape over clean, intact skin. Apply skin protectant if skin is fragile.

4. If excessive hair is present, clip the hair with scissors.

5. Observe the catheter for kinking at the site of taping; adjust if kinking is present.

6. Tape the catheter to the abdomen at night and whenever the patient will be lying down for a long period of time. When the patient is sitting, the catheter should be taped laterally to the upper anterior thigh.

PATIENT AND FAMILY EDUCATION

1. Education should include the purpose and proper technique for taping an indwelling catheter and how to prevent and observe for potential complications such as local irritation or tension on the catheter.

2. Whenever possible, involve the patient and family in the procedure.

Procedure

Taping an Indwelling Catheter: Male

Steps	Additional Information

1. Gather equipment.

2. Provide privacy and explain procedure to patient.

3. Wash hands and don gloves.

4. Cut a 6-in. strip of 1-in. wide tape.

5. Wrap center of tape around catheter, approximately 2 to 3 in. from catheter's distal end and proximal to bifurcation.

6. Pinch tape to itself around catheter, allowing ends to remain free.

7. Secure both ends of tape to abdomen below navel, lifting penis off scrotum (Fig. 3-4), or to anterior thigh.

8. Retape as necessary after movement, position changes, catheter irrigations, or change of drainage bags.

Enough slack should be left in catheter to prevent tension and to allow for erections.

TAPING A CATHETER (MALE)

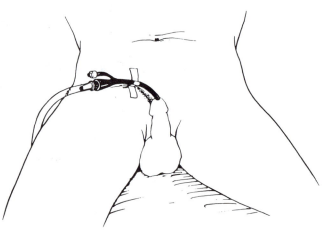

Figure 3-4

 DOCUMENTATION

1. Document the position of the tape and any problems or complications noted.

2. Document patient and primary caregiver education and involvement in the procedure.

REFERENCES

Agency for Health Care Policy and Research (1992) *Clinical Practice Guidelines: Urinary Incontinence in Adults* (AHCPR 92-0038) Rockville, MD: Department of Health and Human Services.

Burkitt, D. and Randall, J. (1987). "Catheterization: Urethral Trauma." *Nursing Times* 83(43):59–60,63.

Edwards, L.E., Lock, R. Powell, C. and Jones, P. (1983) "Post-Catheterisation Urethral Strictures: A Clinical and Experimental Study" *British Journal of Urology* 55:53–56.

King, R.B., Boyink, M., and Keenan, M. (1977) *Rehabilitation Guide* Chicago: Rehabilitation Institute of Chicago.

Taping an Indwelling Catheter: Female

PURPOSE

To secure an indwelling catheter to prevent tension on the catheter.

STAFF RESPONSIBLE

EQUIPMENT

1. Tape, 1-in. width (select type of tape according to the patient's skin tolerance)

2. Nonsterile gloves

 GENERAL CONSIDERATIONS

1. Rotate sites of taping to prevent skin irritation.

2. Place the tape over clean, intact skin. Use skin protectant if skin is fragile.

3. If excessive hair is present, trim the hair with scissors.

4. Observe the catheter for kinking at the site of taping; adjust if kinking is present.

PATIENT AND FAMILY EDUCATION

1. Education should include the purpose and proper technique for taping an indwelling catheter and how to prevent and observe for potential complications such as local irritation or tension on the catheter.

2. Whenever possible, involve the patient and family in the procedure.

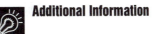

Taping an Indwelling Catheter: Female

 Steps

Additional Information

1. Gather equipment.

2. Provide privacy and explain procedure to patient.

3. Wash hands and don gloves.

4. Cut 6-in. strip of 1-in. wide tape.

5. Wrap center of tape around catheter, approximately 2 to 3 in. from catheter's distal end and proximal to bifurcation.

6. Pinch tape to itself around catheter, allowing ends to remain free.

7. Secure both ends of tape to inner thigh (Fig. 3-5).

Enough slack should be left in catheter to prevent tension.

8. Retape as necessary after movement, position changes, catheter irrigations, or change of drainage bags.

TAPING A CATHETER (FEMALE)

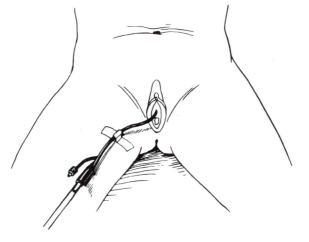

Figure 3-5

DOCUMENTATION

1. Document the position of the tape and any problems or complications noted.

2. Document patient and primary caregiver education and involvement in the procedure.

REFERENCES

Agency for Health Care Policy and Research (1992) *Clinical Practice Guidelines: Urinary Incontinence in Adults.*

(AHCPR 92-0038) Rockville, MD: Department of Health and Human Services.

Burkitt, D. and Randall, J. (1987). "Catheterization: Urethral Trauma." *Nursing Times* 83(43):59–60,63.

Edwards, L.E., Lock, R. Powell, C. and Jones, P. (1983) "Post-Catheterisation Urethral Strictures: A Clinical and Experimental Study" *British Journal of Urology* 55:53–56.

King, R.B., Boyink, M., and Keenan, M. (1977) *Rehabilitation Guide* Chicago: Rehabilitation Institute of Chicago.

Catheter Irrigation

PURPOSE

To assess and/or maintain the patency of an indwelling catheter. *Note:* This procedure is no longer common practice as a routine procedure for clearing accumulation of debris in the catheter because of the risk of infection associated with a break in the closed drainage system. Ruwalt (1983) found that routine bladder irrigation to be ineffective in eradicating bacteriuria. Furthermore, it may disrupt bladder epithelium, predisposing the patient to further infection.

This is primarily a home care procedure.

STAFF RESPONSIBLE

EQUIPMENT

1. Prepackaged sterile irrigation set
2. Sterile normal saline or other irrigating solution as ordered by physician
3. Nonsterile gloves
4. Alcohol prep pad

GENERAL CONSIDERATIONS

1. Sterile ("no touch") technique is used for this procedure.

2. Attempt to coordinate this procedure with the change of the urinary drainage system to decrease the possibility of contamination. A new, sterile drainage device should be used whenever possible after opening the catheter system.

3. All irrigating solutions must be labeled and checked for loose cap, precipitate, or expiration before use.

4. Follow agency policy regarding conditions for which irrigation is indicated.

5. An oral fluid intake that ensures a daily urinary output of 2500 mL or more is the best method of bladder irrigation.

6. Hematuria, pain, or symptoms of autonomic dysreflexia noted during the procedure should be promptly reported to the physician.

7. Aspiration of irrigation solution is not performed routinely but only under specific conditions (if there is no return of solution or on a specific physician's order for removal of blood clots or sediment). When aspiration is necessary, force is never used, nor are large amounts of solution instilled into the bladder.

PATIENT AND FAMILY EDUCATION

1. Education of the patient and caregiver should include the purpose and proper technique for catheter irrigation and how to prevent and observe for potential complications such as infection or overdistended bladder.

2. Whenever possible, involve the patient and family in the procedure.

Procedure

Catheter Irrigation

 Steps

 Additional Information

1. Prepare patient: give explanations and provide privacy. Gather equipment.

2. Wash hands and don nonsterile gloves.

3. Perform groin care and catheter care if needed at this time. If performed, wash hands and don new pair of nonsterile gloves.

4. Open irrigation set and bottle of solution. Place waterproof pad, plastic side down, under catheter and tubing connection.

5. Open extra sterile alcohol pad and place it near catheter connection site.

6. Lift syringe from container and remove protective cap from tip.

7. Pour at least 100 mL of solution into irrigation solution container and replace syringe.

8. Swab catheter tubing junction with alcohol and allow to dry.

9. Disconnect catheter from drainage device; place catheter in notch of sterile drainage tray.

10. Discard drainage device.

11. Draw up 30 mL of irrigation solution.

12. Hold end of catheter upward.

13. Set tip of syringe in catheter opening, allowing solution to enter catheter under gentle pressure.

14. Pinch off catheter, maintaining squeeze on bulb of syringe.

15. Disconnect catheter and syringe. Replace catheter in notch of collection tray and syringe into solution container.

16. Observe for return of the solution; note amount and characteristics.

17. If there is no return of solution and if other methods have been tried:
    - Instill 30 mL more solution into bladder.
    - Applying gentle suction, withdraw only 30 mL of solution. If solution returns readily, continue with irrigation procedures.

18. Repeat instillation of 30 mL of solution twice more or until urine is clear.

Check solution to ensure that it is safe (sterile, without precipitate, and within date of expiration).

This can be used to help prevent contamination of drainage system if it is to be reattached.

Syringe and inside of solution container must remain sterile. If they come into contact with anything, they must be replaced.

Place so that open end of catheter does not touch anything.

If reusing drainage device, place tip of tubing carefully in extra opened alcohol prep pad container or in sterile cap if provided.

Do not allow open end of catheter to touch anything.

If resistance is met, refer to procedures for changing catheter (Male/Female Indwelling Catheterization).

This is to prevent injecting air in bladder or placing suction on bladder mucosa.

All solution should be returned before continuing. If not, be sure catheter is below level of bladder, gently press over bladder, and rotate patient's position.

Do not force solution into bladder. Do not instill more solution if patient exhibits symptoms of autonomic dysreflexia. Only 30 mL of the 60 mL of solution in bladder is withdrawn to prevent trauma to bladder mucosa during aspiration. If this is not successful, refer to procedures for changing catheter (Male/Female Indwelling Catheterization).

A total of 90 mL or more of irrigant is used.

19. Reconnect catheter to drainage.

No touch technique is used to preserve sterility; new sterile drainage system is preferred.

20. Restore patient to comfortable position and appropriate dress.

Retape catheter to thigh or abdomen as appropriate.

21. Remove gloves and discard used equipment in appropriate manner.

Disposal is according to infection control procedures.

22. Wash hands.

23. Document as below.

 ## DOCUMENTATION

1. Document the procedure, the characteristics and amount of returned solution, and any unusual circumstances during the irrigation.

2. Document patient and primary caregiver education and involvement in the procedure.

REFERENCES

Ruwalt, M.M. (1983) "Irrigation of Indwelling Catheters" *Urology* 21(2):127–129.

Procedures for Urinary Elimination: Catheterization Procedures

Male Straight Catheterization

PURPOSE

To empty the bladder of urine or to measure the amount of urine remaining in the bladder immediately after voiding (residual urine)

STAFF RESPONSIBLE

EQUIPMENT

1. Prepackaged sterile catheterization tray with straight catheter
2. Washcloth, towel, soap, and water
3. Nonsterile gloves
4. Bag for disposal
5. Additional lubricant (optional)
6. Urinal (if attempting to stimulate void)
7. Coudé tip catheter if needed
8. Benzalkonium chloride prepackaged sterile catheterization tray (if patient is allergic to Betadine)

 ### GENERAL CONSIDERATIONS

1. A physician's order is required for catheterization.
2. Maintain privacy for the patient throughout the procedure.
3. If the patient is allergic to Betadine, order benzalkonium chloride solution in a prepackaged sterile catheterization tray. Indicate "Allergy To" per agency protocol.

4. If the foreskin is present, retract it over the head of the penis during catheterization. During groin care, wash the penis with the foreskin down and then with it retracted. After catheterization, perform this procedure in reverse.
5. When introducing the catheter, sometimes resistance is met. If resistance is suspected to be due to sphincter tone, try one or more of the following techniques:
   - Have the patient take a deep breath or use the incentive spirometer. As the patient exhales, gently advance the catheter.
   - Perform ROM to the lower extremities before catheter insertion.
   - Position the patient with his hips externally rotated and knees flexed (frog-leg position).
   - Position the patient on his side with his hips and knees flexed.
   - Try anal stretch (see "Methods to Stimulate Voiding and to Empty the Bladder").
   - If continued resistance is met, notify the physician.
6. If resistance is thought to be due to a stricture, consult the physician about the possible use of a coudé tip catheter and document the decision.
7. For patients with spinal cord injury at T6 or above, autonomic dysreflexia may be experienced during catheter insertion. Anesthetic lubricant may help in these patients.

PATIENT AND FAMILY EDUCATION

1. Education should include the purpose and proper technique for catheterization. Also instruct on how to observe for and prevent potential complications such as infection, incomplete emptying of bladder, and difficulty in introduction of the catheter.
2. Whenever possible, involve the patient and family in the procedure.

Procedure

Male Straight Catheterization

 Steps

1. Prepare patient, give explanations, and provide privacy.
2. Wash hands; don nonsterile gloves.

3. Perform groin care.
4. Remove gloves and wash hands.
5. Open kit and establish sterile field.
6. Remove top drape and place under patient's penis.
7. Remove second fenestrated drape and place over patient's penis.
8. Apply sterile gloves.
9. Open and pour Betadine over cotton balls.
10. Open lubricant and lubricate catheter from tip to near distal end.
11. With nondominant hand, grasp penis and hold upward at 60- to 90-degree angle to body.
12. Using forceps, cleanse head of penis with cotton balls in circular motion, starting at urinary meatus and continuing downward on penis.
13. Place tray on drape. Pick up catheter with dominant hand and hold it about 4 in. from tip.
14. Gently insert well-lubricated catheter to 1 or 2 in. beyond point where urine begins to flow.

15. Holding catheter firmly in place, allow urine to drain completely. Then withdraw catheter a slight amount, and observe for any further urine return.

16. Remove catheter and perform groin care.
17. Dispose of used equipment in appropriate manner.
18. Wash hands.
19. Restore patient to comfortable position and appropriate dress.

 Additional Information

If residual urine is ordered, stimulate void as directed in care plan or physician's orders.

Establish clean, uncluttered area.

Additional lubricant may be necessary. Return catheter to tray.
If foreskin is present, keep retracted throughout procedure.

Cleanse once with each cotton ball and discard each cotton ball after use.

Be sure distal end of catheter remains in tray.

Continue holding penis at 60- to 90-degree angle. If resistance is met, apply relaxation techniques or consult physician about possible use of coudé tip catheter. Check for signs and symptoms of autonomic dysreflexia.

If more than 500 mL of urine is in bladder, pinch catheter for 5 to 10 min before allowing remaining urine to drain or remove catheter and repeat catheterization procedure from step 5 in 5 to 10 min.

Disposal is according to infection control procedures.

 DOCUMENTATION

1. Record the procedure, the amount of urine, any attempts to stimulate voiding and voided amounts of urine, and any complications or unusual observations.
2. Record any participation by the patient or primary caregiver in the procedure.

REFERENCES

Agency for Health Care Policy and Research (1992) *Clinical Practice Guidelines: Urinary Incontinence in Adults* (AHCPR 92-0038) Rockville, MD: Department of Health and Human Services.

Brown, J.P. (1994) "Latex Allergy Requires Attention in Orthopaedic Nursing" *Orthopaedic Nursing* 13(1):7–11.

Wu, Y. (1983) "Total Bladder Care for the Spinal Cord Injured Patient" *Annals of the Academy of Medicine* (*Singapore*) 12:391.

Female Straight Catheterization

PURPOSE

To empty the bladder of urine or to measure the amount of urine remaining immediately after voiding (residual urine)

STAFF RESPONSIBLE

EQUIPMENT

1. Prepackaged sterile catheterization tray with straight catheter
2. Washcloth, towel, soap, and water
3. Nonsterile gloves
4. Bag for disposal
5. Urine container (if attempting to stimulate void)
6. Flashlight (optional)
7. Sheet or bath blanket
8. Coudé tip catheter if needed
9. Benzalkonium chloride prepackaged sterile catheterization tray (if patient is allergic to Betadine)

 ## GENERAL CONSIDERATIONS

1. A physician's order is required for catheterization.
2. Assistance may be needed to carry out the procedure if the patient's lower extremities are severely spastic, if the patient is unable to cooperate, or if adequate lighting is only available by flashlight.
3. Maintain privacy for the patient throughout the procedure.
4. If the patient is allergic to Betadine, order benzalkonium chloride solution in a prepackaged sterile catheterization tray. Indicate "Allergy To" per agency protocol.
5. If a spasm occurs during insertion of the catheter, stop and wait for it to subside. If continued resistance is met, do not use force. Stop and notify the physician.
6. For patients with spinal cord injury at T6 or above, autonomic dysreflexia may be experienced during catheter insertion. Anesthetic lubricant may help these patients.

PATIENT AND FAMILY EDUCATION

1. Education should include the purpose and proper technique for catheterization. Also instruct on how to observe for and prevent potential complications such as infection and incomplete emptying of bladder.
2. Whenever possible, involve the patient and family in the procedure.

Procedure

Female Straight Catheterization

 Steps

1. Prepare patient in supine position with knees flexed and hips abducted. Drape with sheet or bath blanket to allow for exposure from suprapubic area to knees.

2. Explain procedure to patient and caregiver.
3. Ensure adequate lighting.
4. Wash hands; don nonsterile gloves.
5. Cleanse perineal area with soap and water.

 Additional Information

If patient has loss of motor control in lower extremities, position may be better maintained with ankles crossed. If residual urine is ordered, stimulate void as directed in care plan or physician's orders.

A flashlight may be necessary.

Cleanse from clitoris toward anus.

6. Remove gloves and wash hands.

7. Open kit and establish sterile field.

Have clean, uncluttered area.

8. Position moisture-proof drape under patient's buttocks.

Maintain sterility of exposed surface of drape.

9. Apply sterile gloves.

10. Open and pour Betadine over cotton balls.

11. Open lubricant and lubricate catheter.

Lubricate from tip to several inches down on catheter.

12. Move equipment to between patient's legs.

13. Separate labia minora with your nondominant hand so that urinary meatus is well visualized; maintain this separation until catheterization is completed.

This hand is now contaminated.

14. Pick up cotton balls with forceps and cleanse around urinary meatus.

Cleanse with one downward stroke from clitoris toward anus for each cotton ball and then discard cotton ball; use all cotton balls. Cleanse both sides of meatus before cleaning meatus itself.

15. Place tray on drape close to, but not touching, perineal area.

16. Pick up catheter with dominant hand, holding it about 4 in. from tip with open end in tray.

17. Insert lubricated catheter slowly to 1 to 2 in. beyond point where urine begins to flow.

Sterile catheter and gloved hand must not touch labia or pubic hair.

18. Holding catheter firmly in place, allow urine to drain completely. Then withdraw catheter a slight amount and observe for any further urine return.

Observe for signs and symptoms of autonomic dysreflexia. If urine does not immediately flow, exert gentle pressure over bladder or ask patient to cough or deep breathe. If more than 500 mL of urine is in the bladder, pinch catheter for 5 to 10 min before allowing remaining urine to drain or remove catheter and repeat procedure from step 7 in 5 to 10 min.

19. Remove catheter and cleanse perineal area.

20. Dispose of equipment in appropriate manner.

Disposal is according to infection control procedures.

21. Remove gloves.

22. Restore patient to comfortable position and appropriate dress.

23. Wash hands.

 DOCUMENTATION

1. Record the procedure, the amount of urine, any attempts to stimulate void and voided amount of urine, and any complications or unusual observations.

2. Record any participation by the patient or primary caregiver in the procedure.

REFERENCES

Agency for Health Care Policy and Research (1992) *Clinical Practice Guidelines: Urinary Incontinence in Adults.* (AHCPR 92-0038) Rockville, MD: Department of Health and Human Services.

Broadwell, D., and Jackson, B. (1982) *Principles of Ostomy Care* St. Louis, MO: Mosby.

Johnson, J. (1980) "Rehabilitative Aspects of Neurologic Bladder Dysfunction: Symposium on Rehabilitation Nursing" *Nursing Clinics of North America* 15:293–308.

King, R.B., Carlson, C.E., Mervine, J., et al. (1992) "Clean and Sterile Intermittent Catheterization Methods in Hospitalized Patients with Spinal Cord Injury" *Archives of Physical Medicine & Rehabilitation* 73:798–802.

Matthews, P.J. (1987) In Matthews, P.J., Carlson, C., and Holt, N. (Eds.) *Spinal Cord Injury: A Guide to Rehabilitation Nursing.* Rockville, MD: Aspen.

Shields, L. (1981) "Urinary Function" In Martin, N., Holt, N., and Hicks, D. (Eds.) *Comprehensive Rehabilitation Nursing* (186–222) New York: McGraw-Hill.

Wu, Y., (1983) "Total Bladder Care for the Spinal Cord Injured Patient" *Annals of the Academy of Medicine (Singapore)* 12:391.

Male Indwelling Catheterization

PURPOSE

To establish urinary drainage or to facilitate certain diagnostic procedures and assessments

STAFF RESPONSIBLE

EQUIPMENT

1. Prepackaged sterile catheterization tray with appropriate size and type of indwelling catheter
2. Washcloths, towels, soap, and water
3. Sterile leg bag or bedside drainage bag
4. 10-mL syringe (if removing indwelling catheter)
5. Nonsterile gloves and bag for disposal
6. Additional lubricant (if needed)
7. Additional equipment for high-risk patients:
   - Irrigation set
   - Bottle of sterile normal saline solution
   - Measuring tape
8. Special indwelling catheters if needed (coudé tip, balloons with greater than 10-mL capacity)
9. Benzalkonium chloride prepackaged sterile catheterization trays (for patients who are allergic to Betadine solution)

GENERAL CONSIDERATIONS

1. A physician's order is required for catheterization.
2. Before the initial insertion or change of an indwelling catheter of a male patient, assessment of the patient's risk of developing urinary complications during catheterization (Exhibit 3-2) must be determined and documented in the progress notes or admission form.
3. Maintain privacy for the patient throughout the procedure.
4. If the patient is allergic to Betadine solution, order benzalkonium chloride solution in a prepackaged sterile catheterization tray. Indicate "Allergy To" per agency protocol.
5. If the foreskin is present, retract it over the head of the penis. If this is not possible or if the foreskin will not remain in position, notify the physician. While performing groin care, wash the penis with the foreskin down and then with the foreskin retracted. Be sure to repeat this procedure in reverse when performing groin care after indwelling catheterization.

Before inserting or changing an indwelling catheter in a male for the first time, ask the patient or primary caregiver the following questions (check the medical record if the patient or primary caregiver is unreliable or unavailable).

1. Have you ever had an indwelling catheter, one that stays in your body?
   YES ☐ (continue with rest of questions)
   NO ☐ (skip question 2)
2. Have you ever had bleeding from your penis during or after an indwelling catheter has been put in?
   YES ☐   NO ☐
   If YES, describe _____
3. Have you or anyone else ever had problems putting a catheter in you?
   YES ☐   NO ☐
   If YES, describe _____
4. Have you ever been told how to perform, or noticed others performing, an anal stretch or using a coudé tip catheter when putting a catheter in you?
   YES ☐   NO ☐
   If YES, describe _____
5. Have you ever had surgery on your bladder, such as a sphincterotomy, cystoscopy, transurethral resection, or urethral dilation?
   YES ☐   NO ☐
   If YES, describe _____
6. Have you ever had any injury or trauma to your bladder, penis, or urethra?
   YES ☐   NO ☐
   If YES, describe _____
7. Have you ever been told that you have a urethral stricture, enlarged prostate, or spastic bladder?
   YES ☐   NO ☐
   If YES, describe _____

Rating: If the answer was "no" to questions 2 through 7, consider the patient a normal risk. If the answer was "yes" to any question 2 through 7, consider the patient at high risk for urinary complications.

Exhibit 3-2   Risk assessment of indwelling catheter use for males.

---

6. When introducing the catheter, sometimes resistance is met. If resistance is suspected to be due to sphincter tone, try one or more of the following techniques:
   - Have the patient take a deep breath or use the incentive spirometer. When the patient exhales, gently advance the catheter.
   - Perform ROM to the lower extremities before catheter insertion.
   - Position the patient's legs in external rotation of the hips with flexed knees (frog-leg position).
   - Position the patient on his side with his hips and knees flexed.
   - Try anal stretch (see "Methods to Stimulate Voiding and to Empty the Bladder").

If none of these techniques work, stop and notify the physician.

7. If resistance is thought to be the result of stricture, the nurse should consult the physician with regard to the use of a coudé tip catheter. This should be noted in the progress notes.

8. The standard balloon size is 5 mL. Balloons should be inflated to 8 to 10 mL. Otherwise, the balloon may be expelled through the sphincter and into the urethra. Larger balloon sizes are not recommended for use in males unless ordered by the physician.

9. Follow these steps to assess for proper placement of the catheter:
   - Pressure exerted to inflate the balloon during testing should be equal to the pressure exerted to inflate the balloon after insertion. If pressure is greater after insertion, the balloon may be in the urethra.
   - After balloon insertion, if gentle withdrawal of the catheter does not produce movement, the balloon may be in the urethra.
   - Nonresolving symptoms of autonomic dysreflexia in patients with spinal cord injury above the level of T6 may indicate that the balloon is in the urethra.
   - Irrigate the catheter with 30 mL of normal saline solution. If the irrigation instills with ease and if all the solution returns through the lumen of the catheter, the balloon can be considered in the bladder. If there is resistance to instillation or if the solution returns from around the catheter, consider the balloon in the urethra.

10. If at any time an incident of tautness or pulling on the catheter occurs, placement should be reevaluated by any of the measures above.

11. If the balloon is considered in the urethra, deflate immediately. The catheter should be repositioned and assessed, or removed and a new catheter inserted. If the patient has had a sphincterotomy and if an indwelling catheter is needed, monitor for signs of balloon placement in the urethra. This is not an uncommon occurrence.

12. If there is no urine return after ensuring proper balloon placement, perform Credé maneuver on the patient's bladder, push fluids, and continue to observe for urine return.

13. If hemorrhage occurs during or after the catheterization, institute emergency measures and contact the physician immediately.

14. For patients with spinal cord injury at T6 or above, autonomic dysreflexia may occur during insertion.

15. An anesthetic lubricant may be used for chronic autonomic dysreflexia or for discomfort associated with catheterizations (allergies should be considered).

PATIENT AND FAMILY EDUCATION

1. Education should include the purpose and proper technique for catheterization. Also instruct on how to observe for potential complications such as infection, incomplete emptying of the bladder, difficulty in introduction of the catheter, or inflation of the balloon in the urethra.

2. Whenever possible, involve the patient and family in the procedure.

Procedure

Male Indwelling Catheterization

 Steps

 Additional Information

1. Check current catheter size, type, and measured length exposed.

   Measured length is attained by measuring distance from tip of penis to end of catheter.

2. Prepare patient: Explain procedure and provide privacy. Gather equipment and wash hands.

   If high-risk patient, have additional equipment on hand and conveniently placed (see Equipment, 7).

3. Don nonsterile gloves.

4. Completely deflate balloon of current catheter.

   Use 10-mL syringe or one of appropriate size (see "Deflating a Defective Indwelling Catheter Balloon" procedure if balloon does not deflate).

5. Gently remove catheter.

   Observe and feel tip for stones or grit.

6. Perform groin care. Remove gloves. Wash hands.

7. Determine optimum position of both patient and yourself. Open catheter tray and establish sterile field.

   Establish clean, uncluttered area. Provide bag for disposal.

8. Remove top drape and place under patient's penis.

   Place shiny side down against bed and touch only edges.

9. Remove second fenestrated drape and place over patient's penis.

10. Apply sterile gloves.

11. To test balloon, attach sterile water-filled syringe to balloon lumen and slowly inflate and deflate balloon completely.

Note amount of pressure required to inflate balloon. Discard catheter if it does not inflate and deflate easily.

12. Leave syringe attached to balloon lumen.

This will facilitate easy inflation of balloon later.

13. Open and pour Betadine over cotton balls.

14. Open lubricant and lubricate catheter to bifurcation near end.

Additional lubricant may be necessary.

15. Place equipment to between patient's legs or, if patient is side lying, next to upper thighs or lower abdomen.

16. Use nondominant hand to grasp penis firmly and hold upward at 60- to 90-degree angle to body.

This hand is now contaminated.

17. Cleanse head of penis with cotton balls (held in forceps) in circular motion, starting at urinary meatus.

18. Pick up catheter with dominant hand, holding it about 4 in. from tip with open end in collecting device.

19. Slowly insert well-lubricated catheter, noting when urine begins to flow.

If more than 500 mL of urine is in bladder, pinch catheter for 5 to 10 min before allowing remaining urine to drain.

20. Insert catheter 2 in. beyond point where flow of urine starts or up to bifurcation of catheter.

Evaluate to determine whether catheter is in bladder. If patient has erection, wait for it to resolve. If erection does not readily resolve, consult physician.

21. Inflate balloon with 8 to 10 mL of sterile water. Amount of pressure should be same as when testing balloon. Hold catheter firmly in place until balloon is inflated.

If amount of pressure is increased, evaluate placement; balloon may be in urethra. Evaluate and monitor patient for complications.

22. Gently withdraw catheter until balloon rests against bladder neck.

If patient has had a sphincterotomy, do not pull back on catheter.

23. Measure length of catheter exposed.

Length should be the same as or less than measured length at beginning of procedure.

24. Attach catheter to sterile drainage system.

25. Tape catheter to abdomen or upper anterior thigh.

26. Perform groin care.

27. Discard used equipment in appropriate manner.

Disposal is according to infection control procedures.

28. Remove gloves and wash hands.

29. Restore patient to comfortable position and appropriate dress.

DOCUMENTATION

1. Document your assessment of risk factors in the progress notes (see Exhibit 3-2).

2. Document in the care plan and patient record the size and type of catheter, size of the balloon, length of catheter exposed, the date of change, any special instructions, and the level of staff to perform the procedure.

3. Document any complications or significant observations and notify the physician.

4. Record any participation by the patient or the primary caregiver in the procedure.

REFERENCES

Agency for Health Care Policy and Research (1992) *Clinical Practice Guidelines: Urinary Incontinence in Adults* (AHCPR 92-0038) Rockville, MD: Department of Health and Human Services.

Brown, J.P. (1994) "Latex Allergy Requires Attention in Orthopaedic Nursing" *Orthopaedic Nursing* 13(1):7–11.

Brunner, L.S., and Suddarth, D.S. (1984) *Textbook of Medical Surgical Nursing* Philadelphia: Lippincott.

Burke, J., Jacobson, J., Garibalki, R., et al. (1983) "Evaluation of Daily Meatal Care with Polyantibiotic Ointment in Prevention of Urinary Catheter-Associated Bacteriuria." *Journal of Urology* 129: 331–334.

Burkitt, D., and Randall, J. (1987) "Catheterization: Urethral Trauma" *Nursing Times* 83:43, 59–60, 63.

Kennedy, A.P., Brocklehurst, J.C., and Lye, M.D.W. (1983) "Factors Related to the Problems of Long-Term Catheterization" *Journal of Advanced Nursing* 8:207–212.

Kniep-Hardy, M.J., Votava, K., and Stubbings, M.J. (1985) "Managing Indwelling Catheters at Home" *Geriatric Nursing* 6:280–285.

McConnell, E.A., and Zimmerman, M.F. (1983) *Care of Patients with Urologic Problems* Philadelphia: Lippincott.

Moore, K.N. (1992) "Indwelling Catheters: Problems and Management" *The Canadian Nurse* 88(6):33–35.

Nacey, J.N. and Delahunt, B. (1991) "Toxicity Study of First and Second Generation Hydrogel-Coated Latex Urinary Catheters." *British Journal of Urology* 67:314–316.

Wilde, M. (1997) "Long-Term Indwelling Urinary Catheter Care: Conceptualizing the Research." *Journal of Advanced Nursing* 25:1252–1261.

Female Indwelling Catheterization

PURPOSE

To establish urinary drainage or to facilitate certain diagnostic procedures and assessments

STAFF RESPONSIBLE

EQUIPMENT

1. Prepackaged sterile catheterization tray with appropriate size and type of indwelling catheter
2. Nonsterile gloves
3. Bag for disposal
4. Washcloths, towels, soap, and water
5. Sterile leg bag or bedside drainage bag
6. 10-mL syringe (if removing catheter)
7. Sheet or bath blanket
8. Optional: flashlight, irrigation set, and normal saline solution
9. Special indwelling catheters if needed (coudé tip, special size catheter or balloon)
10. Benzalkonium chloride prepackaged sterile catheterization tray (for patients who are allergic to Betadine)

GENERAL CONSIDERATIONS

1. A physician's order is required for catheterization.
2. Assistance may be needed to perform this procedure if the patient's lower extremities are severely spastic, if the patient is unable to cooperate, or if adequate lighting is available only by flashlight.
3. Maintain privacy for the patient throughout the procedure.
4. If the patient is allergic to Betadine solution, order benzalkonium chloride. Indicate "Allergy To" per agency protocol.
5. The standard balloon size is 5 mL. Balloons are to be inflated to a volume of 8 to 10 mL. Otherwise, the balloon may be expelled through the sphincter into the urethra.
6. If a spasm occurs during insertion of the catheter, stop and wait until it subsides. If continued resistance is met, do not use force. Stop and notify the physician.
7. Follow these steps to assess for proper placement of the catheter:
   - Pressure exerted to inflate the balloon during testing should be approximately equal to the pressure exerted to inflate the balloon after insertion. If the pressure is greater after insertion, the balloon may be in the urethra.
   - After balloon insertion, if gentle withdrawal of the catheter does not produce movement, the balloon may be in the urethra.
   - Nonresolving symptoms of autonomic dysreflexia in patients with spinal cord injury may indicate that the balloon is in the urethra.
   - Irrigate the catheter with 30 mL of normal saline solution. If the irrigation instills with ease and if all the solution returns through the lumen of the catheter, the balloon can be considered in the bladder. If there is resistance to instillation or if the solution returns from around the catheter, consider the balloon in the urethra.
8. If at any time an incident of tautness or pulling on the catheter occurs, placement should be reevaluated by means of any of the measures above.

9. If the balloon is considered in the urethra, it should immediately be deflated. The catheter should be repositioned and reassessment made, or the catheter should be removed and a new catheter inserted.

10. If there is no urine return after ensuring proper placement, perform Credé maneuver on the patient's bladder, push fluids, and observe for urine return.

11. If hemorrhage occurs during or after the catheterization, institute emergency measures and contact the physician immediately.

12. For patients with spinal cord injury at T6 or above, autonomic dysreflexia may occur during catheter insertion.

13. An anesthetic lubricant may be used for chronic autonomic dysreflexia or for severe discomfort associated with catheterizations (allergies should be considered).

PATIENT AND FAMILY EDUCATION

1. Education should include the purpose and proper technique for catheterization. Also instruct on how to observe for and prevent potential complications such as infection, incomplete emptying of the bladder, and inflation of the balloon in the urethra.

2. Whenever possible, involve the patient and/or family in the procedure.

Procedure

Female Indwelling Catheterization

 Steps

 Additional Information

1. Prepare patient in supine position with knees flexed and hips abducted. Drape with sheet or bath blanket to allow for exposure from suprapubic area to knees. Explain procedure to patient or caregiver.

If patient has loss of motor control in lower extremities, position may be better maintained with ankles crossed and legs supported with pillows.

2. Ensure adequate lighting.

A flashlight may be necessary.

3. Wash hands and don nonsterile gloves.

4. Completely deflate balloon of current catheter.

Use 10-mL syringe or one of appropriate size (see "Deflating a Defective Indwelling Catheter Balloon" procedure if balloon does not deflate).

5. Gently remove catheter and dispose of appropriately.

Observe and feel tip for stones or grit.

6. Cleanse perineal area with soap and water. Remove gloves and wash hands.

Cleanse from clitoris toward anus.

7. Open catheterization tray and establish sterile field.

Have clean, uncluttered area.

8. Position moisture-proof drape under patient's buttocks.

Maintain sterility of exposed surface of drape.

9. Apply sterile gloves.

10. To test balloon, attach sterile water-filled syringe to balloon lumen and slowly inflate and deflate balloon.

Discard catheter if it does not inflate and deflate easily. Note amount of pressure required to inflate balloon. Leave syringe attached to balloon lumen.

11. Open and pour Betadine over cotton balls.

Use benzalkonium chloride if patient is allergic to Betadine.

12. Open lubricant and lubricate catheter from tip to several inches down.

13. Move equipment to between patient's legs.

14. Separate labia minora with your nondominant hand so that meatus is well visualized; maintain this separation until catheterization is completed.

This hand is now contaminated.

15. With forceps holding cotton ball, cleanse meatus and urethral opening.

Cleanse with one downward stroke from clitoris toward anus for each cotton ball and then discard cotton ball; use all cotton balls. Cleanse along both sides of meatus before cleansing meatus itself.

16. Place tray on drape close to but not touching perineal area.

17. Pick up catheter with dominant hand, holding it about 4 in. from tip with open end in collecting device.

Sterile catheter or gloved hand must not touch labia or pubic hair.

18. Insert lubricated catheter slowly, noting when urine begins to flow.

19. Insert catheter 2 in. beyond point where flow of urine starts. Hold catheter firmly in place until balloon is inflated.

If more than 500 mL of urine is in bladder, pinch catheter for 5 to 10 min before allowing remaining urine to drain. Evaluate to determine whether catheter is placed in bladder.

20. If urine does not immediately flow, exert gentle pressure over bladder or ask patient to cough or deep breathe.

Catheter may need to be reinserted slightly in case it has been expelled a bit before inflation of balloon.

21. Inflate balloon with 8 to 10 mL of sterile water. Amount of pressure should be same as when testing balloon.

If amount of pressure is increased, evaluate placement; balloon may be in urethra. Evaluate and monitor patient for complications.

22. Gently withdraw catheter until balloon rests against bladder neck.

If patient has had a sphincterotomy, do not pull back on catheter.

23. Attach catheter to sterile drainage system.

24. Tape catheter to upper inner thigh.

25. Perform perineal care.

26. Discard used equipment in appropriate manner.

Disposal is according to infection control guidelines.

27. Remove gloves and wash hands.

28. Restore patient to comfortable position and appropriate dress.

 DOCUMENTATION

1. Document in the care plan and patient record the size and type of catheter, the size of the balloon, the date of change, any special instructions, and the level of staff to perform the procedure.

2. Document any complications or significant observations and notify the physician.

3. Record any participation by the patient or primary caregiver in the procedure.

REFERENCES

Agency for Health Care Policy and Research (1992) *Clinical Practice Guidelines: Urinary Incontinence in Adults* (AHCPR 92-0038) Rockville, MD: Department of Health and Human Services.

Brown, J.P. (1994) "Latex Allergy Requires Attention in Orthopaedic Nursing" *Orthopaedic Nursing* 13(1):7–11.

Brunner, L.S., and Suddarth, D.S. (1984) *Textbook of Medical Surgical Nursing* Philadelphia: Lippincott.

Burke, J., Jacobson, J., Garibalki, R., et al. (1983) "Evaluation of Daily Meatal Care with Polyantibiotic Ointment in Prevention of Urinary Catheter-Associated Bacteriuria." *Journal of Urology* 129: 331–334.

Burkitt, D., and Randall, J. (1987) "Catheterization: Urethral Trauma" *Nursing Times* 83:43, 59–60, 63.

Kennedy, A.P., Brocklehurst, J.C., and Lye, M.D.W. (1983) "Factors Related to the Problems of Long-Term Catheterization" *Journal of Advanced Nursing* 8:207–212.

Kniep-Hardy, M.J., Votava, K., and Stubbings, M.J. (1985) "Managing Indwelling Catheters at Home" *Geriatric Nursing* 6:280–285.

McConnell, E.A., and Zimmerman, M.F. (1983) *Care of Patients with Urologic Problems* Philadelphia: Lippincott.

Moore, K.N. (1992) "Indwelling Catheters: Problems and Management" *The Canadian Nurse* 88(6):33–35.

Nacey, J.N. and Delahunt, B. (1991) "Toxicity Study of First and Second Generation Hydrogel-Coated Latex Urinary Catheters." *British Journal of Urology* 67:314–316.

Wilde, M. (1997) "Long-Term Indwelling Urinary Catheter Care: Conceptualizing the Research." *Journal of Advanced Nursing* 25:1252–1261.

Suprapubic Cystostomy Catheterization

PURPOSE

To establish urinary drainage through a suprapubic cystostomy; to avoid the disadvantages and complications of a urethral indwelling catheter

STAFF RESPONSIBLE

EQUIPMENT

1. Prepackaged sterile catheterization tray (without catheter)
2. Indwelling catheter (size indicated by physician)
3. 30-mL syringe with approximately 22-gauge needle or needleless spike
4. Another 30-mL syringe (if changing catheter)
5. Sterile water vial
6. Nonsterile gloves
7. Washcloths, soap, and water
8. Plastic bags
9. Sheet or bath blanket
10. Sterile leg bag or bedside drainage bag
11. Tape
12. Two 4 × 4 fenestrated gauze pads

 GENERAL CONSIDERATIONS

1. The physician's order for catheterization must include the type and size of catheter and balloon and the amount of solution needed to inflate the balloon.
2. This procedure must be performed with sterile technique.
3. Assistance may be needed to carry out the procedure if the patient is severely spastic or unable to cooperate.
4. Maintain privacy throughout the procedure.
5. If the patient is allergic to Betadine, order benzalkonium chloride solution. Indicate "Allergy To" per agency protocol.

PATIENT AND FAMILY EDUCATION

1. Education should include the purpose and proper technique for catheterization as well as how to observe for and prevent complications such as infection.
2. Whenever possible, involve the patient and family in the procedure.

Procedure

Suprapubic Cystostomy Catheterization

 Steps

 Additional Information

1. Prepare patient for procedure: explain procedure and provide privacy. Gather equipment and adjust lighting.
2. Place patient in supine position with legs extended.

   If patient is severely spastic, you may need assistance to perform catheterization.

3. Wash hands and don nonsterile gloves.
4. Remove dressing from stoma site.

   Note any redness, drainage, and the like.

5. Pull existing catheter gently until resistance is met. Note catheter size and type and balloon size; measure length exposed.

   Measure with measuring tape or ruler from stoma site to end of catheter.

6. Aspirate fluid from balloon with 30-mL syringe and remove catheter.

   See "Deflating a Defective Indwelling Catheter Balloon" procedure if balloon does not deflate.

7. Gently remove catheter.

   Observe catheter for calculi, grit, or clots. Roll tip of catheter between fingers to note grit.

8. Dispose of catheter and draining bag appropriately.

   Disposal is according to infection control procedures.

9. Cleanse suprapubic stoma site with soap and water. Remove gloves, and wash hands.

10. Fill sterile 30-mL syringe with prescribed amount of sterile water.

Place filled syringe next to sterile field.

11. Open catheterization tray and establish sterile field. Open catheter package and place on sterile field.

12. Place top drape on or next to patient's abdomen or symphysis pubis.

13. Place second drape over suprapubic stoma site.

14. Put on sterile gloves.

15. Pour Betadine over cotton balls and lubricate catheter.

Lubricate from tip to approximate length as measured before.

16. To test balloon, hold sterile water-filled syringe with nondominant hand, attach to balloon lumen, and slowly inflate and deflate.

Discard catheter if balloon does not inflate or deflate easily.

17. Position nondominant hand lightly over stoma.

This acts as anchor during cleansing and catheter insertion. Nondominant hand is now contaminated.

18. Cleanse stoma with Betadine-soaked cotton balls held in forceps.

Cleansing motion should start at center of stoma and continue in spiral motion away from center. Discard each cotton ball after one use.

19. Pick up catheter with dominant hand, holding it about 4 in. from tip with open end in sterile collecting tray.

20. Gently insert well-lubricated catheter into stoma 1 to 2 in. beyond previously estimated length.

If resistance is felt, direct tip of catheter toward symphysis pubis. Notify physician if resistance continues.

21. If urine does not immediately flow, exert gentle pressure over bladder or ask patient to deep breathe.

If more than 500 mL of urine is in bladder, pinch catheter for 5 to 10 min before allowing remaining urine to drain.

22. Using prefilled syringe, inflate balloon with prescribed amount of sterile water.

23. Gently withdraw catheter until resistance is met.

24. Connect catheter to sterile drainage system.

25. Dress stoma with fenestrated 4 × 4 gauze pads. Tape securely.

Preserves skin integrity around stoma.

26. Discard used equipment in appropriate manner.

Disposal is according to infection control procedures.

27. Remove gloves.

28. Tape catheter to abdomen.

This prevents pulling or pressure on catheter.

29. Restore patient to comfortable position and appropriate dress.

30. Wash hands.

DOCUMENTATION

1. Document in the care plan and patient record the size and type of catheter, the size of the balloon, the length of catheter exposed, the date of change, any special instructions, and the level of staff to perform the procedure.

2. Document any complications or significant observations and notify the physician.

3. Record any participation by the patient or primary caregiver in the procedure.

REFERENCES

Agency for Health Care Policy and Research (1992) *Clinical Practice Guidelines: Urinary Incontinence in Adults* (AHCPR 92-0038) Rockville, MD: Department of Health and Human Services.

Brown, J.P. (1994) "Latex Allergy Requires Attention in Orthopaedic Nursing" *Orthopaedic Nursing* 13(1):7–11.

Brunner, L.S., and Suddarth, D.S. (1984) *Textbook of Medical Surgical Nursing* Philadelphia: Lippincott.

Burke, J., Jacobson, J., Garibalki, R., et al. (1983) "Evaluation of Daily Meatal Care with Polyantibiotic Ointment in Prevention of Urinary Catheter-Associated Bacteriuria." *Journal of Urology* 129: 331–334.

Burkitt, D., and Randall, J. (1987) "Catheterization: Urethral Trauma" *Nursing Times* 83:43, 59–60, 63.

Kennedy, A.P., Brocklehurst, J.C., and Lye, M.D.W. (1983) "Factors Related to the Problems of Long-Term Catheterization" *Journal of Advanced Nursing* 8:207–212.

Kniep-Hardy, M.J., Votava, K., and Stubbings, M.J. (1985) "Managing Indwelling Catheters at Home" *Geriatric Nursing* 6:280–285.

McConnell, E.A., and Zimmerman, M.F. (1983) *Care of Patients with Urologic Problems* Philadelphia: Lippincott.

Moore, K.N. (1992) "Indwelling Catheters: Problems and Management" *The Canadian Nurse* 88(6):33–35.

Nacey, J.N. and Delahunt, B. (1991) "Toxicity Study of First and Second Generation Hydrogel-Coated Latex Urinary Catheters." *British Journal of Urology* 67:314–316.

Wilde, M. (1997) "Long-Term Indwelling Urinary Catheter Care: Conceptualizing the Research." *Journal of Advanced Nursing* 25:1252–1261.

Male Sterile Intermittent Catheterization: Touchless

PURPOSE

To provide periodic drainage of urine from the bladder

STAFF RESPONSIBLE

EQUIPMENT

1. Touchless sterile catheter kit
2. Nonsterile gloves (2 pairs)
3. Washcloth, soap, and water

GENERAL CONSIDERATIONS

1. A physician's order is required for catheterization.
2. Assistance may be needed to carry out the procedure if the patient's legs are severely spastic or if he is unable to cooperate.
3. Sterile technique must be used with this procedure.
4. Maintain privacy for the patient throughout the procedure.
5. If the foreskin is present, retract it over the head of the penis. If this is not possible or if the foreskin will not remain in position, notify the physician. While performing groin care, wash the penis with the foreskin down and then with the foreskin retracted.

6. When introducing the catheter, sometimes resistance is met. If resistance is suspected to be due to sphincter tone, try one or more of the following techniques:
   • Have the patient take a deep breath or use the incentive spirometer. When the patient exhales, gently advance the catheter.
   • Perform ROM to the lower extremities before catheter insertion.
   • Position the patient's legs with his hips externally rotated and his knees flexed (frog-leg position).
   • Position the patient on his side with his hips and knees flexed.
   • Try anal stretch (see "Methods to Stimulate Voiding and to Empty the Bladder").
   If none of these techniques work, stop and notify the physician.
7. If resistance is thought to be the result of stricture, consult the physician regarding the use of a coudé tip catheter.
8. For patients with spinal cord injury at T6 or above, autonomic dysreflexia may occur during catheter insertion. Anesthetic lubricant may be used if this is a chronic problem.

PATIENT AND FAMILY EDUCATION

1. Education should include the purpose and proper technique for catheterization. Also instruct on how to observe for and prevent potential complications such as infection, incomplete emptying of the bladder, and difficulty in introduction of the catheter.
2. Whenever possible, involve the patient and family in the procedure.

Procedure

Male Sterile Intermittent Catheterization: Touchless

 Steps

 Additional Information

1. Prepare patient: Explain procedure and provide privacy. Gather equipment.

2. Wash hands and don nonsterile gloves.

3. Perform groin care. Remove gloves and wash hands.

4. Don nonsterile gloves.

5. Open catheterization kit and remove contents.

   Save outer package.

6. Open lubricant package and hold it between fingers.

7. Pick up catheter sheath and remove plastic cover at top. Do not let anything touch top of cuff.

   Top edge and inside of cuff must remain sterile.

8. Push on sides of cuff to form a round opening.

9. Squeeze lubricant into bottom of cuff chamber.

   Do not let lubricant package touch inside portion of cuff.

10. Push catheter up through clear plastic guide to lubricate it. Then slide catheter down below tip of catheter guide.

11. Place catheter sheath carefully across outer package.

    This will keep top edge of cuff from touching anything.

12. Open package of Betadine swabs.

    If patient is allergic to Betadine, benzalkonium chloride may be used.

13. Using nondominant hand, hold penis upward at 60- to 90-degree angle to body.

    If foreskin is present, it should be retracted and held in place during procedure.

14. Cleanse urinary meatus once with each swab. Cleanse in a circular motion, starting at meatus and working away from it.

    Cleanse entire head of penis and distal area of shaft.

15. Still holding penis at 60- to 90-degree angle, pick up catheter sheath near cuff.

    Do not touch top edge or inside of cuff.

16. Place cuff over head of penis and hold in place with non-dominant hand. Position so that urinary opening is against catheter guide.

    Use nondominant hand to hold penis and catheter guide and dominant hand to push catheter. Thumb and finger of non-dominant hand can pinch catheter through guide so that you can readjust fingers on catheter while advancing it.

17. Using dominant hand, push catheter up through catheter guide and gently insert catheter into urinary opening.

    If resistance is met, use suggested methods to overcome it. If resistance continues, stop and notify physician.

18. Insert catheter until you note a urine flow; advance catheter 1 in. beyond this point.

19. Holding catheter firmly in place, allow urine to flow until bladder is empty or bag is full.

    If more than 500 mL of urine is in bladder, pinch or remove catheter for 5 to 10 min and then continue draining bladder.

20. When flow stops, retract catheter slightly and observe for more urine flow.

    May need to perform gentle Credé maneuver to empty bladder completely.

21. Withdraw catheter. Note volume of urine collected and empty urine into toilet.

22. Perform groin care.

23. Dispose of used equipment appropriately.

    Disposal is according to infection control procedures.

24. Remove gloves, wash hands.

25. Restore patient to comfortable position and appropriate dress.

DOCUMENTATION

1. Document the amount of urine and the time of the procedure.

2. Document any complications or significant observations, and notify the physician.

3. Document patient and primary caregiver education and involvement in the procedure.

REFERENCES

Agency for Health Care Policy and Research (1992) *Clinical Practice Guidelines: Urinary Incontinence in Adults* (AHCPR 92-0038) Rockville, MD: Department of Health and Human Services.

Broadwell, D., and Jackson, B. (1982) *Principles of Ostomy Care* St. Louis, MO: Mosby.

Johnson, J. (1980) "Rehabilitative Aspects of Neurologic Bladder Dysfunction: Symposium on Rehabilitation Nursing" *Nursing Clinics of North America* 15:293–308.

King, R.B., Carlson, C.E., Mervine, J., et al. (1992) "Clean and Sterile Intermittent Catheterization Methods in Hospitalized Patients with Spinal Cord Injury" *Archives of Physical Medicine & Rehabilitation* 73:798–802.

Matthews, P.J. (1987) In Matthews, P.J., Carlson, C., and Holt, N. (Eds.) *Spinal Cord Injury: A Guide to Rehabilitation Nursing* Rockville, MD: Aspen.

Shields, L. (1981) "Urinary Function" In Martin, N., Holt, N., and Hicks, D. (Eds.) *Comprehensive Rehabilitation Nursing* New York: McGraw-Hill; pp. 186–222.

Wu, Y., (1983) "Total Bladder Care for the Spinal Cord Injured Patient" *Annals of the Academy of Medicine (Singapore)* 12:391.

Female Sterile Intermittent Catheterization: Touchless

PURPOSE

To perform periodic drainage of urine from the bladder

STAFF RESPONSIBLE

EQUIPMENT

1. Touchless sterile catheterization kit

2. Nonsterile gloves (2 pairs)

3. Washcloth, soap, and water

4. Flashlight (optional)

GENERAL CONSIDERATIONS

1. A physician's order is required for catheterization.

2. Assistance may be needed to carry out the procedure if the patient's legs are severely spastic, if she is unable to cooperate, or if lighting is poor.

3. Sterile technique must be used with this procedure.

4. Maintain privacy for the patient throughout the procedure.

5. For patients with spinal cord injury at T6 or above, autonomic dysreflexia may occur during catheter insertion. Anesthetic lubricant may be used if this is a chronic problem.

PATIENT AND FAMILY EDUCATION

1. Education should include the purpose and proper technique for catheterization as well as how to observe for and prevent complications such as infection or incomplete emptying of the bladder.

2. Whenever possible, involve the patient and family in the procedure.

Procedure

Female Sterile Intermittent Catheterization: Touchless

 Steps

 Additional Information

1. Prepare patient: Explain procedure and provide privacy. Gather equipment.

2. Wash hands. Don nonsterile gloves.

3. Perform perineal care. Remove gloves and wash hands.

4. Don nonsterile gloves.

5. Open catheter kit and remove contents.

   Save outer package.

6. Open lubricant package and hold it between fingers.

7. Pick up catheter sheath and remove plastic cover at top.

   Do not allow anything to touch catheter guide.

8. Squeeze lubricant into catheter guide.

   Do not touch lubricant package to catheter guide.

9. Advance catheter ½ to 1 in. above catheter guide to lubricate. Then slide catheter back below tip of catheter guide.

10. Open package of Betadine swabs.

    If patient is allergic to Betadine, benzalkonium chloride may be used.

11. Place catheter sheath across outer package so that catheter guide does not touch anything.

12. Using nondominant hand, hold labia minora apart so that urinary meatus is well visualized.

    Ensure adequate lighting.

13. Cleanse urinary meatus once with each swab.

    Cleanse downward once with each swab from clitoral area to vagina. Cleanse both sides of meatus before cleansing meatus itself.

14. Pick up catheter sheath with dominant hand, holding catheter through catheter guide. Advance tip of catheter slightly beyond tip of catheter guide.

    Continue holding labia open with nondominant hand.

15. Insert catheter tip into meatus.

    Be sure to maintain gentle pressure of catheter guide against meatus.

16. Hold soft, top end of catheter guide gently but firmly against meatus.

17. Move nondominant hand to catheter guide and dominant hand to bag, holding catheter 1 in. below guide.

18. Gently advance catheter with dominant hand.

    If resistance is met, ask patient to deep breathe and advance catheter on exhalation. If resistance continues, stop and notify physician.

19. Stabilize catheter through catheter guide with nondominant hand, and return dominant hand to below catheter guide.

20. Continue in this manner until urine starts to flow. Advance catheter slightly beyond this point.

    If more than 500 mL of urine is in bladder, pinch or remove catheter for 5 to 10 min and then continue draining bladder.

21. Holding catheter firmly in place, allow urine to flow until bladder is empty or bag is full.

    May perform gentle Credé maneuver to empty bladder completely.

22. When flow stops, retract catheter slightly and observe for more urine return.

23. Withdraw catheter. Note volume of urine collected and empty urine into toilet.

24. Perform perineal care.

25. Dispose of used equipment appropriately.

Disposal is according to infection control procedures.

26. Remove gloves. Wash hands.

27. Restore patient to comfortable position and appropriate dress.

 DOCUMENTATION

1. Document the amount of urine and the time of the procedure.

2. Document any complications or significant observations and notify the physician.

3. Document patient and primary caregiver education and involvement in the procedure.

REFERENCES

Agency for Health Care Policy and Research (1992) *Clinical Practice Guidelines: Urinary Incontinence in Adults* (AHCPR 92-0038) Rockville, MD: Department of Health and Human Services.

Broadwell, D., and Jackson, B. (1982) *Principles of Ostomy Care* St. Louis, MO: Mosby.

Johnson, J. (1980) "Rehabilitative Aspects of Neurologic Bladder Dysfunction: Symposium on Rehabilitation Nursing" *Nursing Clinics of North America* 15:293–308.

King, R.B., Carlson, C.E., Mervine, J., et al. (1992) "Clean and Sterile Intermittent Catheterization Methods in Hospitalized Patients with Spinal Cord Injury" *Archives of Physical Medicine & Rehabilitation* 73:798–802.

Matthews, P.J. (1987) In Matthews, P.J., Carlson, C., and Holt, N. (Eds.) *Spinal Cord Injury: A Guide to Rehabilitation Nursing* Rockville, MD: Aspen.

Shields, L. (1981) "Urinary Function" In Martin, N., Holt, N., and Hicks, D. (Eds.) *Comprehensive Rehabilitation Nursing* New York: McGraw-Hill; pp. 186–222.

Wu, Y., (1983) "Total Bladder Care for the Spinal Cord Injured Patient" *Annals of the Academy of Medicine (Singapore)* 12:391.

Preparation of Normal Saline Solution for Home Use

PURPOSE

To prepare sterile normal saline solution for home use

STAFF RESPONSIBLE

EQUIPMENT

1. Table salt, two level teaspoons
2. Distilled water, 1 qt
3. Deep pan or kettle with tight lid
4. Clean glass jar or wide-mouth bottle (1-qt size) with lid

 GENERAL CONSIDERATIONS

1. Two level teaspoons of table salt in one quart of distilled water is the formula commonly used to approximate normal saline solution.
2. The procedure should be taught to patients and families who will be performing procedures after discharge requiring normal saline solution and is not meant to be used as a routine in the hospital. It is much less costly than purchasing the solution at a pharmacy.
3. If distilled water is not available, boiled tap water may be used.
4. Allow the solution to cool or warm to room temperature before use.
5. The solution is good for 1 week (kept in the refrigerator) once the glass container has been opened.

Procedure

Preparation of Normal Saline Solution for Home Use

 Steps

1. Assemble supplies needed to prepare solution.
2. Pour two level teaspoons of table salt into glass quart-size jar or bottle.
3. Add distilled water to jar to make 1 qt of solution.

4. Tighten lid and mix well.
5. Loosen lid and place jar or bottle into deep pan or kettle.
6. Add water to pan or kettle to depth of 4 to 6 in.
7. Put lid on pan or kettle and boil for 20 min.
8. Allow to cool and tighten lid on glass container.
9. Label container with type of solution and date prepared.

 Additional Information

If distilled water is not available, boil needed amount of tap water for 5 min before use. Allow any sediment to settle to bottom before pouring into solution container.

A loosened lid allows for expansion during heating process.

DOCUMENTATION

1. Document the teaching done and patient and family outcomes of being able to prepare the solution.

Disinfecting Urinary Drainage Equipment for Home Use

PURPOSE

To disinfect urinary drainage equipment at home

STAFF RESPONSIBLE

EQUIPMENT

1. Leg bag or bedside drainage bag with tip covers
2. Tubing and cap
3. Bulb syringe or turkey baster
4. Bleach solution
5. Tap water, 2 qt (or more)
6. Cotton-tipped applicator (Q-Tips), toothpick, or small bottle brush
7. Soap and running water
8. Basin (dish pan or bath basin)

GENERAL CONSIDERATIONS

1. This procedure is utilized for patient education purposes and is not meant to be used as a routine in the hospital.
2. Patients with a resistant infection are not to clean their used equipment. Equipment is discarded after use for these patients.
3. As many leg bags as can be totally submerged in the bleach solution can be disinfected at the same time (an average basin holds three to five leg bags).

PATIENT AND FAMILY EDUCATION

Education should include the purpose and proper technique for disinfecting urinary drainage equipment as well as how to observe for and prevent potential complications such as infection and skin irritation from contact with bleach solution.

Procedure

Disinfecting Urinary Drainage Equipment for Home Use

 Steps

1. Disconnect rubber tubing from leg bag to be disinfected.
2. Wash bag and tubing in hot, soapy water.
3. Force soapy solution through top valve of bag with syringe. Clean out any material adherent to inside of leg bag with cotton-tipped applicator.
4. Turn leg bag upside-down when filled with soapy solution to test flutter valve at top.
5. Hold bag and tubing under faucet to rinse.
6. Mix bleach and water solution in basin.

 Additional Information

Wash cap if disinfecting night drainage bag.

If water runs out, throw bag away.

For leg bags, concentration of mixture should be 5 mL of bleach to 1 qt of water. Night drainage bags require 1 tbs of bleach to 1 gal of water.

7. Fill bag half full with bleach solution, then submerge bag and tubing in basin.

Use bulb syringe to fill. Solution should be in contact with entire inner surface of bag.

8. Soak bags for 1 h.

One hour is minimum time. They may also be left overnight; cover basin if left overnight.

9. To remove, drain enough solution from basin so that you can pick up bag and tubing without putting your hand in solution.

Allow solution to drain completely out of bag and tubing.

10. Attach hose to adaptors on top and bottom of bag without touching adaptors.

Use cap to cover adaptor or night drainage bag.

11. Store in clean, dry place until ready for use.

Recommended places include a cabinet or drawer.

DOCUMENTATION

1. Documentation should include patient and family education, any unusual circumstances or problems noted, and the ability of the patient and family to carry out the procedure safely.

Disinfecting Reusable Urinary Irrigation Syringe for Home Use

PURPOSE

To disinfect a reusable urinary irrigation syringe (Asepto bulb syringe) and jar at home

STAFF RESPONSIBLE

EQUIPMENT

1. Asepto glass or rubber bulb syringe
2. Small glass jar with metal lid (4 to 6 oz)
3. Soap and water
4. Pot with tight-fitting lid (2 to 4 qt)

GENERAL CONSIDERATIONS

1. This procedure is utilized for patient education purposes and is not meant to be used as a routine in the hospital.

2. A supply of Asepto syringes and jars may be made available in the hospital for patient education purposes. If a patient is to use this procedure in the hospital for reinforcement of learning, an Asepto bulb syringe for the individual patient must be ordered. In addition, this patient or family should bring a small jar from home for the irrigation solution.

3. Patients with resistant infection are not to disinfect used urinary equipment. Equipment is discarded after use for these patients.

PATIENT AND FAMILY EDUCATION

Education should include the purpose and proper technique for disinfection of the syringe as well as how to observe for and prevent potential complications such as infection.

Procedure

Disinfecting Reusable Urinary Irrigation Syringe for Home Use

 Steps

1. Wash bulb, glass syringe, jar, pan, and lid with soapy water and rinse.
2. Place glass syringe, rubber bulb, and jar with cover in pot and cover with water.
3. Boil 15 min (covered) at rolling boil.
4. Allow water and equipment to cool.
5. Pour off water (keep cover over pot while pouring).
6. Store equipment in pot (covered) until ready to use.
7. When ready to use, remove jar and then syringe and bulb (squirt water out of bulb).

 DOCUMENTATION

1. Documentation should include patient and family education, any unusual circumstances or problems noted, and the ability of the patient and family to carry out the procedure safely.

Procedure for Bladder Ultrasound: Bladder Volume Instrument (BVI 2500)

PURPOSE

To describe technique for use of Bladder Volume Instrument and cleaning/maintenance procedures

STAFF RESPONSIBLE

EQUIPMENT

1. Bladder Volume Instrument (2500)
2. Ultrasound Transmission Gel
3. Nonsterile gloves
4. Alcohol pad or Kwik-Wipe

GENERAL CONSIDERATIONS

1. Bladder ultrasound is a method for noninvasive measurement of bladder volume (Lewis, 1995). Studies have shown a reduction in urinary tract infections with bladder ultrasound instead of catheterization in rehabilitation patients (O'Malley and Mee, 1990, Salcido et al., 1991).

2. This procedure will describe the technique used with the Bladder Volume Instrument 2500 by Diagnostic Ultrasound Corp. and its recommended usage.

3. A physician order is required to use the Bladder Volume Instrument (BVI). The order should include when the instrument is to be used and parameters for action or physician notification.

4. Only individuals trained in use of the equipment may perform the procedure.

5. Equipment is stored near the nursing station at all times and should be returned immediately after use to allow for recharging.

6. The BVI may be used on all patients except pregnant women. However, it may be difficult to get a clear image on patients with certain conditions: obesity, s/p major abdominal surgery with reconstruction, and prolapsed bladders.

Procedure

Bladder Ultrasound

 Steps

 Additional Information

1. Explain procedure to the patient.
2. Assemble equipment.
3. Wash hands and don gloves.
4. Place patient in supine position.
5. Disconnect machine from charger.

   DO NOT OPERATE EQUIPMENT WHILE BATTERY IS BEING CHARGED.

6. Expose bladder area.

   Provide privacy for patient. Expose lower abdomen to symphysis pubis, genitals need not be exposed

7. Apply a generous amount of the ultrasound gel directly over the scan head.

8. Place the transducer with gel on it at a point midline on the pelvis directly above the symphysis pubis with a light touch.

   The transducer should be held in a sagittal (head-toe) plane. The figure on the transducer should match the patient's position.

9. Depress on/off switch on the front panel. An internal self-test will be performed. Press front panel switch indicating male or female patient.

10. Press scan button. Hold the scan head in place.

The scan head needs 4 s to perform a scan.

11. The screen will display a volume and a diagram of the scan.

The picture of the scan should be centered in the crosshairs.

12. If diagram is not centered, move the scan head slightly to get a centered reading. Press the scan button for a repeat scan.

When doing multiple scans, the machine will display the largest volume. The current scan volume will be displayed.

13. Clean gel from the patient with a washcloth and clean the scan head with a clean cloth and Kwik-wipe.

14. Place scan head back in storage system and return BVI to nursing station to be recharged.

15. Notify nurse of results obtained.

16. Record volume obtained.

Make certain to indicate the measurement was obtained with the BVI.

DOCUMENTATION

1. Bladder volume amount obtained by BVI in timed urine pathway.

3. Nurses document any supporting or unusual observations in patient progress notes in medical record as well as any further actions taken in response to the procedure.

REFERENCES

Diagnostic ultrasound bladderscan™ non-invasive bladder volume instrument, Diagnostic Ultrasound Corp. Redmond, WA.

Lewis, N.A. (1995) "Implementing a Bladder Ultrasound Program" *Rehabilitation Nursing* 20(4):215–217.

Massagli, T., Cardenas, D. and Kelly, E. (1989) "Experience with Portable Ultrasound Equipment and Measurement of Urine Volume—Inter-user Reliability and Factors of Patient Position" *The Journal of Urology* 142:969–971.

Murrey, M. (1990) "Pediatric application of the bladder volume instruments" *Journal of Pediatric Nursing* 5(4):290–291.

O'Malley, L.A. and Mee, R. (1990) "Noninvasive Bladder Volume Management: BVI" *Archives of Physical Medicine and Rehabilitation* 71:785.

Salcido, R., Fisher, S., Homes G. (1991) "Diagnostic Effectiveness of Bladder Ultrasound in a Large Population of Stroke Patients" *Archives of Physical Medicine and Rehabilitation* 72:787.

CHAPTER 4

Procedures to Maintain and Restore Tissue Integrity

Introduction

The emphasis of this chapter is prevention and management of pressure ulcers. Pressure ulcers are a source of morbidity and mortality for individuals with chronic illness and disability and can create tremendous financial, personal, and social costs. Pressure ulcers are a particular risk in conditions resulting in motor or sensory deficits or debilitation and among elderly persons with acute or chronic illness. It has been estimated that 5 to 10 percent (50,000 to 100,000) of patients hospitalized in the United States each year develop pressure ulcers (Shanon, 1982). The incidence of pressure ulcers varies widely according to the population studied, but several studies have demonstrated a high incidence in elderly patients (Norton, McLaren, and Exton-Smith, 1962; Barbenel et al., 1977) and persons with neurologic disorders.

A pressure ulcer is an area of soft tissue necrosis, generally found over bony prominences, that results from interruption of blood supply to the tissue. Although pressure is considered the primary factor in the development of pressure ulcers, the amount and duration required to produce tissue necrosis appear to vary. Multiple intrinsic factors, such as body temperature and metabolic status, and extrinsic factors, such as friction and shear, contribute to tissue necrosis. Therefore, assessment of factors that increase risk for pressure ulcers and interfere with wound healing is a critical nursing function. In recent years, nurse authors have suggested that the incidence of pressure ulcers can be decreased through improved assessment of risk and rigorous application of preventive measures for those at risk (King, 1981; Braden and Bergstrom, 1987; Gosnell, 1987). Several scales that systemize risk assessment have been developed (Norton et al., 1962; Bergstrom et al., 1987; Gosnell, 1973). Nurses are encouraged to evaluate these instruments for clinical application in a specific setting. Most scales employ the criteria of mobility, continence, nutrition, and mental alertness.

Over the years, a large variety of treatments have been proposed to aid healing of pressure ulcers. Until recent years, few treatments were based on controlled studies of wound healing. The nurse, in collaboration with the physician, should evaluate the merit of a potential treatment and should assess its effectiveness for an individual patient. Interventions to promote healing should be based on the classification of severity of breakdown and on the presence or absence of exudate and eschar. To assist in decision making in the choice of dressing, a procedure describes options for dressings on the basis of stage and characteristics of the pressure ulcer. A specific dressing procedure representing each option category is included. Additional information and research on dressing selection is also available in the AHCPR guidelines: Treatment of Pressure Ulcers.

Claims are made frequently for the pressure relief effectiveness of numerous support devices, but again, many claims are not based on research. Before selecting a support surface for institution-wide or individual patient use, it is wise to seek evidence of effectiveness in laboratory or clinical settings. Interest in the evaluation of support systems has resulted in the publication of a number of studies that provide a basis for decision making about special mattresses, beds, and cushions (Lilla et al., 1975; Wells and Geden, 1984; Krouskop et al., 1985; Maklebust et al., 1986).

Patient and family education is a primary consideration in prevention and management of pressure ulcers for individuals with chronic risk factors. Specific skin procedures for home care are available elsewhere and are not included in this manual (King et al., 1977). The clinical discipline responsible for some aspects of patient education related to skin care varies from agency to agency. For example, an occupational therapist, physical therapist, or nurse may select wheelchair cushions and teach pressure relief behavior. Nevertheless, nursing generally has primary responsibility for skin care education and is always responsible for reinforcing all aspects of skin care and for ensuring the correct use of equipment.

Decisions regarding preventive measures, as well as procedures to manage existing ulcers, are based on thorough assessment of the patient, environment, and activities. Socioemotional factors also influence patient and family education about skin care and decisions affecting postdischarge care and are a consideration for assessment.

An attempt has been made to be objective in describing wound care options and support surfaces. Inclusion of a product does not represent endorsement or recommendation for use.

Further information on prevention and treatment of pressure ulcers may be found in the following publications:

U.S. Department of Health and Human Services (1992) *Pressure Ulcers in Adults: Prediction and Prevention Clinical Practice Guideline No.3*. AHCPR Publication No. 92-0047. Rockville, MD: Agency for Health Care Policy and Research.

U.S. Department of Health and Human Services (1994) *Treatment of Pressure Ulcers. Clinical Practice Guideline No. 15*. AHCPR Publication No. 95-0652. Rockville, MD: Agency for Health Care Policy and Research.

Assessment

Assessment and Management of Pressure Ulcer Risk Factors

PURPOSE

To prevent pressure ulcers; to minimize risk factors; to prevent further damage; to promote healing

STAFF RESPONSIBLE

GENERAL CONSIDERATIONS

1. A patient's individual skin care plan should reflect the following considerations:

   - Risk factors
   - Economics
   - Feasibility
   - Compatibility with activities of daily living (ADLs)
   - Patient goals

2. Intrinsic (person-related) risk factors that appear to be most predictive of risk for pressure ulcers are:

   - Mental status
   - Mobility
   - Nutrition
   - Decreased sensation
   - Elevated temperature
   - Low diastolic blood pressure

3. Extrinsic factors that contribute to the development of pressure ulcers are:

   - Pressure in excess of capillary pressure that is sustained for long periods
   - Shear forces
   - Friction
   - Local moisture (incontinence, perspiration, or humidity)
   - Local temperature (elevated local temperature from contact with a surface)

4. The literature on pressure ulcers indicates that elderly patients (Norton et al., 1962; Lowthian, 1979) and individuals with spinal cord injuries (Young and Burns, 1981) have a high incidence of pressure ulcers.

5. Involve the patient and primary caregiver in planning the skin care program as soon as possible.

6. Assess the patient's and primary caregiver's knowledge of prevention and management of skin breakdown.

7. Avoid the use of agents that can dry the skin (alcohol and excess or harsh soap), especially for older persons. Avoid low humidity and cold temperatures.

8. For dry skin problems, use emollients.

9. Do not massage over a red area as it produces friction and increased pressure.

10. Routine pressure relief with a turning schedule is required for all persons at risk for pressure ulcers. Increased frequency of pressure relief or special support devices are advised for a patient who is at high risk (i.e., having several risk factors).

11. Inadequate nutrition contributes to the risk for pressure ulcer formation. Assess the patient's dietary intake and the presence of hypoproteinemia, anemia, or avitaminosis, and plan nutritional support as needed.

12. Cleanse patients after incontinence and apply emollient lotion, if needed. Change wet clothing and bed linens immediately. If needed, use quick absorbing incontinence pads or briefs and/or topical moisture barriers.

13. Mobilize patients and perform routine range of motion (ROM) to prevent contractures. Contractures and other body deformities alter pressure loading and can result in increased risk for pressure ulcers.

PATIENT AND FAMILY EDUCATION

1. Educate the patient and family about actual and potential risk factors and interventions to decrease risk when the risk for pressure ulcer development is chronic.

2. Teach and reinforce:

   - Assessment of risk factors and early signs of skin necrosis
   - Preventive skin care measures
   - Adaptation of the program to various community situations
   - Guidelines for safely upgrading skin tolerance
   - Methods to monitor skin problems
   - Management of skin redness or breakdown

Procedure

Assessment and Management of Pressure Sore Risk Factors

 Steps

 Additional Information

1. Assess patient's risk for pressure ulcers. Consider patient at high risk if he or she exhibits risk factors.
   - Attempt to minimize those risk factors that can be reduced through nursing interventions (marked with asterisk in right column).
   - Reassess patient routinely for changes in risk factors. Alter plan on basis of these factors. Frequency of assessment is based on acuity and severity of risk factors.

Consider use of Braden Scale (Fig. 4-1) (Bergstrom et al., 1987).
Risk factors include:
- *Advanced age (older than 60 years of age)*
- *Low diastolic blood pressure*
- *Decreased mobility**
- *Decreased sensation*
- *Fever or infection**
- *Moisture or diaphoresis**
- *Incontinence (bowel and bladder)**
- *Dry skin*
- *Edema**
- *Nutritional state (anemia, hypoproteinemia, or avitaminosis)**
- *Medication that can alter mental status**
- *Overweight or underweight**
- *Decreased muscle tone*
- *Decreased hydration**

2. Minimize duration of pressure:
   - Change patient's position frequently. Establish tissue tolerance time for patient when lying or sitting on basis of individual's ability to tolerate pressure and risk factors.
   - When patient is sitting, reinforce pressure relief every 15 to 30 min.
   - Upgrade skin tolerance time slowly (no more than 30 min at a time). Assess skin carefully when attempting new tolerance time.

See procedure on Turning and Positioning.
When patient is recumbent, attempt to incorporate as many different positions as possible (side, avoiding direct pressure on trochanter; back; and prone lying). Small shifts in position are also advised. Patients with multiple risk factors may not tolerate repositioning every 2 h. Turning hourly, making small shifts, and using supports that more evenly distribute pressure are options.

See procedures on Pressure Relief Activities.

Assess that established program is well tolerated (hyperemia resolves in 30 min or less) before continuing to upgrade tolerance.

3. Minimize intensity of pressure:
   - Use pressure relieving devices (special beds, mattress toppers, wheelchair cushions, and elbow and foot protectors).
   - Consider bridging bony prominences with pillows or foam blocks and using positioning techniques that distribute pressure more evenly (proning).

See procedure on Choosing Support Surfaces. When choosing a device, consider its effectiveness in decreasing pressure, its cost, and whether it will alter patient's abilities (e.g., make ADLs more difficult).

See procedures on Turning and Positioning. When bridging, check with your hand to be sure that bony prominence lies between pillows or blocks and receives no pressure.

4. Perform frequent skin checks:
   - After each turn and after sitting
   - At least twice a day for chronic conditions after tolerance is established
   - Bony prominences must be monitored more frequently than twice daily whenever there is a change in any part of skin program or in patient's risk factors or if any redness, heat, or swelling is noticed in area.

See procedure on Skin Check.

Patients must continue skin checks at home when risk factors persist.

If any change occurs, assess skin after each turn or transfer from wheelchair until you are certain that current tolerance (length of time lying or sitting without pressure relief) is acceptable.

Braden Scale for Predicting Pressure Sore Risk

Patient's Name _____   Evaluator's Name _____   Date of Assessment _____

	1	2	3	4
Sensory perception Ability to respond meaningfully to pressure-related discomfort	**1. Completely limited:** a. Unresponsive (does not moan, flinch, or grasp) to painful stimuli, due to diminished level of consciousness or sedation, OR b. Limited ability to feel pain over most of body surface.	**2. Very limited:** a. Responds only to painful stimuli. Cannot communicate discomfort except by moaning or restlessness, OR b. Has a sensory impairment which limits the ability to feel pain or discomfort over 1/2 of body.	**3. Slightly limited:** a. Responds to verbal commands but cannot always communicate discomfort or need to be turned, OR b. Has some sensory impairment wich limits ability to feel pain or discomfort in 1 or 2 extremities.	**4. No impairment:** Responds to verbal commands. Has no sensory deficit which would limit ability to feel or voice pain or discomfort.
Moisture Degree to which skin is exposed to moisture	**1. Constantly moist:** Skin is kept moist almost constantly by perspiration, urine, etc. Dampness is detected every time patient is moved or turned.	**2. Moist:** Skin is often but not always moist. Linen must be changed at least once a shift.	**3. Occasionally moist:** Skin is occasionally moist, requiring an extra linen change approximately once a day.	**4. Rarely moist:** Skin is usually dry; linen requires changing only at routine intervals.
Activity Degree of physical activity	**1. Bedfast:** Confined to bed.	**2. Chairfast:** Ability to walk severely limited or nonexistent. Cannot bear own weight and/or must be assisted into chair or wheelchair.	**3. Walks occasionally:** Walks occasionally during day but for very short distances, with or without assistance. Spends majority of each shift in bed or chair.	**4. Walks frequently:** Walks outside the room at least twice a day and inside room at least once every 2 hours during waking hours.
Mobility Ability to change and control body position	**1. Completely immobile:** Does not make even slight changes in body or extremity position without assistance.	**2. Very limited:** Makes occasional slight changes in body or extremity position but unable to make frequent or significant changes independently.	**3. Slightly limited:** Makes frequent though slight changes in body or extremity position independently.	**4. No limitations:** Makes major and frequent changes in position without assistance.
Nutrition Usual food intake pattern	**1. Very poor:** a. Never eats a complete meal. Rarely eats more than 1/3 of any food offered. Eats 2 servings or less of protein (meat or dairy products) per day. Takes fluids poorly. Does not take a liquid dietary supplement, OR b. Is NPO[1] and/or maintained on clear liquids or IV[2] for more than 5 days.	**2. Probably inadequate:** a. Rarely eats a complete meal and generally eats only about 1/2 of any food offered. Protein intake includes only 3 servings of meat or dairy products per day. Occasionally will take a dietary supplement, OR b. Receives less than optimum amount of liquid diet or tube feeding.	**3. Adequate:** a. Eats over half of most meals. Eats a total of 4 servings of protein (meat, dairy products) each day. Occasionally will refuse a meal, but will usually take a supplement if offered, OR b. Is on a tube feeding or TPN[3] regimen, which probably meets most of nutritional needs.	**4. Excellent:** Eats most of every meal. Never refuses a meal. Usually eats a total of 4 or more servings of meat and dairy products. Occasionally eats between meals. Does not require supplementation.
Friction and shear	**1. Problem:** Requires moderate to maximum assistance in moving. Complete lifting without sliding against sheets is impossible. Frequently slides down in bed or chair, requiring frequent repositioning with maximum assistance. Spasticity, contractures, or agitation leads to almost constant friction.	**2. Potential problem:** Moves feebly or requires minimum assistance. During a move skin probably slides to some extent against sheets, chair, restraints, or other devices. Maintains relatively good position in chair or bed most of the time but occasionally slides down.	**3. No apparent problem:** Moves in bed and in chair independently and has sufficient muscle strength to lift up completely during move. Maintains good position in bed or chair at all times.	
				Total score _____

[1]NPO: Nothing by mouth.
[2]IV: Intravenously.
[3]TPN: Total parenteral nutrition.
Source: Barbara Braden and Nancy Bergstrom. Copyright, 1988. Reprinted with permission.

Figure 4-1

- If any signs of damage are noticed, ensure that area receives no pressure until signs have resolved. Then revise program to decrease possibility of recurrence.

5. Minimize shearing forces by limiting amount of time patient sits in bed at greater than 30 but less than 90 degrees.

6. Support patient's feet against footplate or footboard to prevent sliding when sitting in bed.

7. Minimize friction:
   - Avoid sliding patient across sheets. Turning sheets should be used cautiously to minimize friction and trauma to the skin.
   - Avoid sliding bare skin against transfer sliding board.
   - Patients with spasticity may need careful positioning or padding to reduce friction.

Check site every 15 min. If signs of circulatory impairment do not resolve within 30 min, length of time sitting or lying without pressure relief must be reduced.

When patient sits in this position, sacrum and attached deep fascia slide downward while skin stays in same position (shearing). This action causes stretching and angulation of local blood vessels and contributes to tissue necrosis.

Friction increases potential for skin breakdown by applying mechanical forces to skin and can cause abrasion. A turning sheet may result in less friction when repositioning heavy patients who are difficult to raise off sheet during turns.

 DOCUMENTATION

1. Document the assessment of the skin condition and risk factors.
2. Note the skin care program, including tolerances, pressure reliefs, skin checks, and other interventions.
3. Note patient and family teaching and their ability to carry out the program.
4. Document the patient's response to the skin care program.

REFERENCES

Barbenel, J. Jordan, M., Nicol, S., and Clark, M. (1977) "Incidence of Pressure Sores in the Greater Glasgow Health Board Area" *Lancet* 2:548–550.

Bergstrom, N., Braden, B.J., Laguzza A., Holman, V. (1987) "The Braden Scale for Predicting Pressure Sore Risk" *Nursing* 36(4):205–210.

Bergstrom, N., Demuth, P., and Braden, B. (1987) "A Clinical Trial of the Braden Scale for Predicting Pressure Sore Risk" *Nursing Clinics of North America* 22:417–428.

Gosnell, D.J. (1973) "An assessment tool to identify pressure sores" *Nursing Research* 22–55.

Gosnell, D.J. (1987) "Assessment and evaluation of pressure sores" *Nursing Clinics of North America* 22:399–415.

Kosiak, M., (1991) "Prevention and Rehabilitation of Pressure Sores" *Decubitus* 4(2): 60–68.

Lowthian, P. (1979) "Pressure Sore Prevalence" *Nursing Times* 75:358–360.

Norton, D., McLaren, R., and Exton-Smith, A.N. (1962) *An Investigation of Geriatric Nursing Problems in Hospitals* London: National Corporation for the Care of Old People.

U.S. Department of Health and Human Resources (1992) *Pressure Ulcers in Adults: Prediction and Prevention. Clinical Practice Guideline, No. 3* AHCPR Publication No. 92-0047 Rockville, MD: Agency for Health Care Policy and Research.

Assessment of a Pressure Ulcer

PURPOSE

To accurately assess, to communicate, and to document skin breakdown

STAFF RESPONSIBLE

EQUIPMENT

1. Adequate lighting (overhead or flashlight)
2. Straight-edge ruler or other measuring device. (e.g., single-use measuring tools)
3. Sterile probe
4. Camera
5. Pressure Ulcer Assessment Form: (Fig. 4-2)

 ## GENERAL CONSIDERATIONS

1. Assessment and documentation should occur when skin breakdown or redness is initially noted. Assess a reddened area each time the person is repositioned and open areas with each dressing change.
2. Documentation includes all standard criteria applicable to pressure ulcer assessment. Objective terminology is used at all times.
3. If the pressure ulcer is not responding to treatment within 2 to 4 weeks, the plan of care and adherence to the plan should be reevaluated (Bergstrom et al., 1994).
4. Photographs of changes in the wound can document evidence of wound healing. Prior to taking photographs request permission in accord with facility policy or guidelines. Always respect patient's right to refuse.

PATIENT AND FAMILY EDUCATION

1. Patients and primary caregivers are taught to assess pressure ulcer before passes and if a pressure ulcer is present at discharge.
2. Emphasize the importance of contacting the clinical service if healing does not progress or if the ulcer deteriorates.

Procedure

Standard Criteria

1. *Size:* Measure length and width of pressure ulcer area with ruler or commercially available plastic measuring device.
2. *Depth of tissue involved:* If tunneled or deep wound, measure with sterile probe or cotton swab, then measure probe against ruler.
3. *Shape:* Photograph ulcer and place on form, or draw scaled-down version of shape in assessment chart form.
4. *Location:* Mark with "x" on figure, or describe in terms of nearest anatomic landmark.
5. *Color:* State percent that is red, yellow, black, or other.
6. *Heat:* Note whether heat is present over site or around sore.
7. *Edema:* Note whether edema is present and its extent.
8. *Edges and surrounding tissue:* Note whether edges are macerated, well- or poorly defined, rolled, undermined, or different in color.

 ### Additional Information

Do not contaminate ulcer with measurement tool. Measure largest diameter, then take another measurement perpendicular to largest diameter.

For shallow wounds, assessment of tissue involved (i.e., stage) is better than pure depth. Necrotic tissue results in inaccurate assessment.

For example, right medial malleolus or sacrum.

Describe changes in hue in relation to person's normal color.
Compare temperature to contralateral body part if possible.

If surrounding tissue is affected, describe color, extent, and stage if applicable. Deeper wounds have more distinct edges.

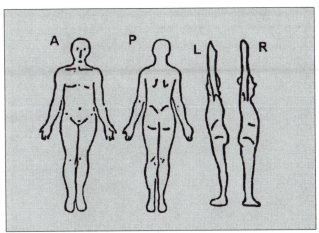

Patient Name Plate

Stage: 1   2   3   4   E

Stage 1 - nonblanchable erythema of intact skin
Stage 2 - partial-thickness skin loss involving epidermis and/or dermis
Stage 3 - full-thickness skin loss, may be down to but not through underlying
        fascia, undermining may be present
Stage 4 - full-thickness skin loss with necrosis or damage to muscle
Stage E - covered with eschar; unable to determine

Identify ulcer location on figure above

Date				
Size	☐ Superficial Width: _____cm Length:_____ cm Depth:_____cm Undermining:____ cm _____ cm	☐ Superficial Width: _____cm Length:_____ cm Depth: _____cm Undermining:____ cm _____ cm	☐ Superficial Width: _____cm Length:_____ cm Depth: _____cm Undermining:____ cm _____ cm	☐ Superficial Width: _____cm Length:_____ cm Depth:_____cm Undermining:____ cm _____ cm
Wound color (should total 100%)	Red: _____% Yellow: _____% Black: _____% Other: _____%	Red: _____% Yellow: _____% Black: _____% Other: _____%	Red: _____% Yellow: _____% Black: _____% Other: _____%	Red: _____% Yellow: _____% Black: _____% Other: _____%
Edges	☐ Macerated ☐ Well-Defined ☐ Poorly Defined ☐ Rolled ☐ Undermined	☐ Macerated ☐ Well-Defined ☐ Poorly Defined ☐ Rolled ☐ Undermined	☐ Macerated ☐ Well-Defined ☐ Poorly Defined ☐ Rolled ☐ Undermined	☐ Macerated ☐ Well-Defined ☐ Poorly Defined ☐ Rolled ☐ Undermined
Quantity of drainage	☐ None ☐ Scant ☐ Moderate ☐ Large	☐ None ☐ Scant ☐ Moderate ☐ Large	☐ None ☐ Scant ☐ Moderate ☐ Large	☐ None ☐ Scant ☐ Moderate ☐ Large
Drainage color				
Odor	☐ Yes ☐ No	☐ Yes ☐ No	☐ Yes ☐ No	☐ Yes ☐ No
Photo taken	☐ Yes ☐ No	☐ Yes ☐ No	☐ Yes ☐ No	☐ Yes ☐ No
Assessment		☐ Unchanged ☐ Improved ☐ Regressed	☐ Unchanged ☐ Improved ☐ Regressed	☐ Unchanged ☐ Improved ☐ Regressed
Signature				

Date:	**Comments**

Weekly Pressure Ulcer Assessment

01-033017-10

Figure 4-2A

Date of Photo:	Date of Photo:

Date of Photo:	Date of Photo:

Date:	Comments

Weekly Ulcer Assessment

Figure 4-2B

9. *Necrotic or healthy tissue:* Describe color, extent, and location of ulcer.

10. *Drainage:* Describe presence, color, opacity, and amount.

Describe anything that is not pink, healthy tissue, simply and objectively.

Measure soiled area on sponge or number of sponges soiled and length of time dressing was in place or state as: none, scant, moderate, or large. If there is no drainage, note whether ulcer is moist or dry.

11. *Odor:* Describe whether odor is present, strong, or recognizable.

12. *Classification of Pressure Ulcers*
    Stage I. Nonblanchable erythema of intact skin; the heralding lesion of skin ulceration
    NOTE: Reactive hyperemia can normally be expected to be present for one-half to three-fourths as long as the pressure occluded flow to the area. This should not be confused with a stage I pressure ulcer.
    Stage II. Partial-thickness skin loss involving epidermis and/or dermis. The ulcer is superficial and presents clinically as an abrasion, blister, or shallow crater.
    Stage III. Full-thickness skin loss involving damage or necrosis of subcutaneous tissue that may extend down to, but not through, underlying fascia. The ulcer presents clinically as a deep crater with or without undermining of adjacent tissue.
    Stage IV. Full-thickness skin loss with extensive destruction, tissue necrosis, or damage to muscle, bone, or supporting structures (for example, tendon or joint capsule)
    NOTE: Undermining and sinus tracts may also be associated with stage IV pressure ulcers.

Recommended by the National Pressure Ulcer Advisory Panel 1989 Consensus Conference as derived from staging systems proposed by Shea (1975) and the International Association for Enterostomal Therapy (1988) (Agency for Health Care Policy and Research, 1992).

DOCUMENTATION

1. All standard assessment criteria are recorded each time that the pressure ulcer assessment is documented.

2. Frequency of documentation is based on institutional policy.

3. Document any change in nursing interventions due to the assessment.

REFERENCES

French, E.T. and Lewell-Sifner, K. (1991) "A method of consistent documentation of pressure sores" *Rehabilitation Nursing* 4(16):204–207.

Gosnell, D.J. (1973) "Assessment and evaluation of pressure sores" *Nursing Clinics of North America* 22:399–415.

King, R.B. (1981) "Assessment and Management of Soft Tissue Pressure" In N. Martin, N.B. Holt, and D. Hicks (Eds.) *Comprehensive Rehabilitation Nursing* New York: McGraw-Hill; pp. 242–268.

Kosiak, M. (1991) "Prevention and Rehabilitation of Pressure Sores" *Decubitus* 4(2):60–68.

U.S. Department of Health and Human Resources (1992) *Pressure Ulcers in Adults: Prediction and Prevention. Clinical Practice Guidelines, No. 3.* AHCPR Publication No. 92-0047. Rockville, MD: Agency for Health Care Policy and Research.

Shea, J.D. (1975) "Pressure Sores: Classification and Management" *Clinical Orthopedics and Related Research* 112:89–100.

Young, J.S. and Burns, P.E. (1981) "Pressure Sores and the Spinal Cord Injured: Part II" *SCI Digest* 3:11–26.

Skin Check

PURPOSE

To assess skin areas (with emphasis on bony prominences) for the presence of potential or existing skin breakdown; to maintain skin integrity; to promote wound healing by providing a basis for decision making

STAFF RESPONSIBLE

EQUIPMENT

1. Mirrors. (Two mirrors are necessary for patients with high quadriplegia to do self-inspections. A long-handled mirror is issued to all patients who will learn the skin self-check procedure.)

2. Measuring tape if needed.

 ## GENERAL CONSIDERATIONS

1. Regular, systematic skin checks are essential for patients with decreased or absent sensation or impaired motor function as well as for those individuals assessed at risk for pressure ulcers on the basis of other risk factors.

2. Patients who are stable and low at risk, who maintain their turning and wheelchair tolerances, and who have intact, healthy skin require skin inspections twice a day (in the morning before dressing and at night when undressing).

3. In addition to routine twice-daily skin checks, inspection should be performed in the following circumstances:

- On admission
- Until sitting and turning tolerances are established by checking after wheelchair sitting or when the patient is recumbent, after each turn, until the patient is medically stable, and until high risk for pressure ulcers does not exist
- When upgrading turning tolerance (with each turn) and when upgrading wheelchair tolerance (after sitting)
- When decreasing wheelchair tolerance (after sitting) and when decreasing turning tolerance (with each turn)
- Every 15 min up to 1 h after the initial skin check if circulation to the skin shows signs of impairment until redness resolves—do not reposition on red area
- When changing the type of supportive cushion or mattress or adaptive equipment being used, when the patient is wearing new shoes (after sitting or turning, after removal of equipment, and after the patient has been wearing shoes for 1 to 2 h)
- After wheelchair sitting or turning if risk factors increase

PATIENT AND FAMILY EDUCATION

1. All patients with decreased or absent sensation or motor deficits should learn to check their own skin or how to direct or assist others in checking their skin.

2. Patients who are to be independent in skin checks are taught by the nurse and then supervised for each check until they regularly do self-initiated skin checks. After this point, periodic supervision is needed.

3. Patient education includes information about method of inspection, areas to be inspected, frequency of inspections (including upgrading of tolerance), and management when signs of alteration in skin integrity are noted.

Procedure

 ### Steps

1. Remove patient's clothing, and position patient to reveal areas to be checked with mirrors and light source.

 ### Additional Information

Many patients are able to do skin self-inspection (Fig. 4-3). Patient position for skin check and position of mirror for self-inspection will depend on patient's previous activity or position and indications on nursing care plan. When checking skin of patient with high quadriplegia, position first mirror at inspection site. Position second mirror at patient's head so that patient can check skin. Positioning of second mirror is important because patient may need to

2. Identify areas of the body to be checked (Fig. 4-4) based on patient status and risk factors.

teach and direct others regarding pressure points and management of alterations in skin.

All skin surfaces are checked, at minimum, at admission, before morning dressing, and when undressing in evening.

3. Visually check the skin for:
   • Signs of pressure (redness, blistering, open areas, areas of color or temperature changes)
   • Burns
   • Rashes
   • Excess moisture
   • Abrasions/bruises

Moisture between skin folds may result in maceration of skin. Tactile temperature checks are especially helpful if unable to detect redness in dark-skinned patients and can be crudely assessed by touching area with dorsum (back) of fingers.

4. If signs of pressure ulcers are present (e.g., hyperemia that persists for more than 30 min, increased heat, swelling, or open area), position patient to relieve all pressure over area.

Refer to positioning and bridging procedures if necessary. Attempt to identify cause of damage, and take necessary action to prevent further damage to skin.

5. Reassess reddened area in 15 min and again in 30 min if necessary. If redness is unresolved in 60 min, continue to monitor until resolution occurs.

Do not reposition patient on damaged areas.* Licensed nurse assesses pressure area after report of skin damage by staff member.

6. If signs of rash or moisture between skin folds are present, clean area with mild soap and water. Dry thoroughly and apply appropriate lotion/ointment.

Apply medicated ointments only as directed by physician. Cornstarch may be applied to clean and dry skin fold, after thorough drying of skin.

7. Inform physician of skin breakdown, unresolved red areas, rashes, bruises, edema, and other skin changes.

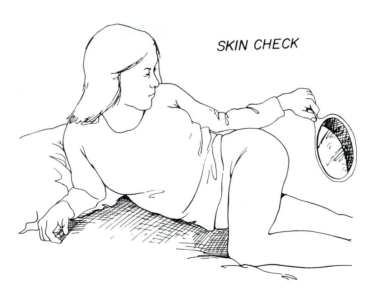

SKIN CHECK

Figure 4-3

Figure 4-4

BONY AREAS TO CHECK

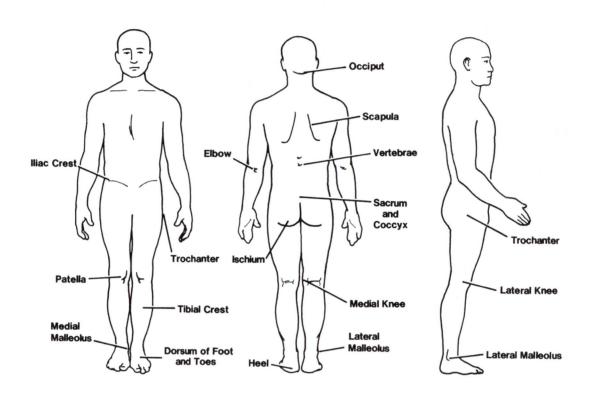

DOCUMENTATION

1. Document any unusual findings from the skin check (e.g., initial signs of pressure, resolution of pressure effects, rashes, edema, or any trauma to the skin).

2. Document changes in sitting and positioning tolerance, turning schedules, and local treatment of the skin area on the basis of the findings of the skin inspection.

3. Document the routine performance of the skin check according to institutional policy.

4. Document patient/caregiver teaching and results.

REFERENCES

Cardona, V. et al. (1994) *Trauma Nursing: From Resuscitation to Rehabilitation* Philadelphia: W.B. Saunders.

King, R.B., Boyink, M., and Keenan, M. (1977) *Rehabilitation Guide*. Chicago: Rehabilitation Institute of Chicago.

Prevention of Pressure Ulcers

Pressure Relief Activities

PURPOSE

To prevent pressure ulcers by providing regular intermittent relief of pressure over bony prominences

STAFF RESPONSIBLE

EQUIPMENT

See below under specific activities.

 GENERAL CONSIDERATIONS

1. Pressure is considered the primary factor contributing to soft tissue necrosis and pressure ulcers.

2. Unrelieved pressure interferes with circulation and thus with nutrition of tissues (Landis, 1930).

3. Pressure ulcers can be prevented by intermittent relief of pressure over bony prominences.

4. When the patient is in the recumbent position, the greatest pressures are exerted over the heels when supine and the trochanters when side lying. Therefore, these areas are at highest risk for skin breakdown. Few support surfaces reduce trochanteric and heel pressures to less than capillary pressure.

5. The greatest pressures over bony prominences occur when the patient is in the sitting position. In this position, pressure greater than 100 mmHg can be exerted over the ischia (Mooney, Einbund, Rogers, and Stauffer, 1971).

6. When mentation, sensation, and motor function are intact, persons change position in response to the discomfort of pressure. A deficit in any of these areas requires that the patient (or someone else) remember to relieve pressure.

7. When the patient is seated, pressure needs to be relieved for a minimum of 10 s every 15 to 30 min (King, 1981; Kling, 1983). When recumbent, a change of position is usually recommended every 2 h or more often, depending on the presence of risk factors.

8. Risk factors for the development of pressure ulcers may dictate more frequent pressure relief activity or the use of devices to distribute pressure evenly (see procedure on Assessment and Management of Pressure Ulcer Risk Factors).

9. Individualized assessment, goal setting, planning, reevaluation, and patient education are basic to the development of an effective pressure relief program.

PATIENT AND FAMILY EDUCATION

1. Teach the patient and primary caregiver:
   - Frequency of pressure relief activities required
   - Length of pressure relief
   - Methods (includes requesting assistance)
   - The rationale for pressure relief
   - Assessment of the adequacy of pressure relief
   - The rationale and methods for increasing or decreasing the frequency of pressure relief
   - Consequences of inadequate pressure relief

   All these points are taught before hospital discharge. The first five are taught before a pass, and the first three are taught when the patient initially sits for 30 min or longer. The presence of brain damage, aging, or anxiety associated with sitting for the first time or with transfer to a new facility can interfere with learning. Therefore, frequent assessment and reinforcement are required.

2. Physical therapists and occupational therapists may teach patients individualized techniques for push-ups and lean-overs. Nurses provide initial instruction and evaluation of compliance when they assist the patient to sit for the first time.

3. Evaluate the patient's compliance with pressure relief activity. Attempt to assess follow-through when the patient is off the unit (i.e., in therapy or on passes) as well as while he or she is on the nursing unit.

REFERENCES

U.S. Department of Health and Human Services (1992) *Pressure Ulcers in Adults: Clinical Practice Guideline No.3* AHCPR Publication No. 92-0047. Rockville, MD: Agency for Health Care Policy and Research.

U.S. Department of Health and Human Services (1994) *Treatment of Pressure Ulcers. Clinical Practice Guideline No.*

15. (AHCPR Publication No.95–0652.) Rockville, MD: Agency for Health Care Policy and Research.

King, R.B. (1981) "Assessment and Management of Soft Tissue Pressure" In N. Martin, N.B Holt, and D. Hicks (Eds.) *Comprehensive Rehabilitation Nursing* New York: McGraw-Hill.

Kling, C. (1983) "Integumental System" In S. Benda (Ed.) *Spinal Cord Injury Nursing Education Suggested Content* American Spinal Injury Association.

Landis, E. (1930) "Studies of Capillary Blood Pressure in Human Skin" *Heart* 5:209.

Mooney, V., Einbund, M., Rogers, J., and Stauffer, E. (1971) "Comparison of Pressure Distribution Qualities in Seat Cushions" *Bulletin of Prosthetic Research* Spring:129–143.

Wheelchair Pressure Relief

PURPOSE

To prevent pressure ulcers through regular relief of pressure while the patient is seated

STAFF RESPONSIBLE

EQUIPMENT

1. Wheelchair cushion
2. Optional equipment for patients with weak upper extremities: electric reclining wheelchair

GENERAL CONSIDERATIONS

1. Refer to general considerations of Pressure Relief Activities.

2. Patients with intact upper extremities (triceps) can do push-ups. If the upper extremities are weak, the patient can do forward or side leans, or another person can lift the patient.

3. Wheelchair cushions are necessary to redistribute pressure, but no cushion eliminates the need for regular pressure relief.

4. Wheelchair armrests and footplates must be properly adjusted for the person to promote pressure reduction.

PATIENT AND FAMILY EDUCATION

1. Method of pressure relief, frequency, and length of pressure relief are taught as soon as possible after the patient initiates sitting.

2. Teach the principles for increasing or discontinuing sitting time.

Procedure

Assessment and Teaching

 Steps

1. Assess patient knowledge about wheelchair pressure reliefs.

2. Inform patient of frequency for pressure relief (push-ups, leans). Demonstrate method or inform patient to request assistance every 15 to 30 min (depending on policy).

3. Limit sitting time to 30 min to 1 h the first time that patient sits.

 Additional Information

Do not assume that patients who are beginning to sit or those who are sitting when admitted to a unit will independently perform wheelchair push-ups or request assistance.

Sitting time depends on number and intensity of risk factors present as well as on other factors, such as fatigue and pain.

4. Examine patient's ischia, posterior trochanters, and sacro-coccygeal bony prominences for hyperemia when patient returns to bed to determine whether pressure relief activity was adequate.

5. Gradually increase sitting time (tolerance) by 30 min. Maintain increased tolerance time for 2 days before increasing sitting tolerance again. Examine skin each time patient returns to bed until satisfactory sitting tolerance is reached.

6. Regularly review with patient progress or problems in performing wheelchair pressure reliefs at prescribed intervals.

7. Remind patient to do pressure relief, or offer assistance if he or she is in your presence for 30 min and has not done a push-up or lean-over.

8. Consult with physical therapist (if needed) regarding specific pressure relief technique that patient should be using.

Specific Methods

1. *Push-up:* Patient places hands on both wheels or armrests and pushes up (Fig. 4-5).

2. *Side lean:* Patient places one arm under wheelchair push handle while leaning toward opposite side of wheelchair (Fig. 4-6).

3. *Forward lean:* Patient leans forward, resting forearms on thighs. To return to upright position, patient uses triceps or pectoral muscles to push upright. In presence of inadequate musculature, patient places one arm over wheelchair push handle while leaning forward and reaching forward with other arm. Alternatively, patient may be able to rest upper body on bed or low table.

4. For individuals who are unable to perform the foregoing maneuvers, a caregiver can shift weight by lifting person from behind or from front of wheelchair.

5. Motorized reclining wheelchair can be used to achieve recumbent position to decrease pressure over ischia.

Prolonged hyperemia (more than 30 min) is evidence of potential cellular damage. When this situation exists, time in position must be decreased and/or pressure reliefs must be increased (or both).

Goal for sitting tolerance should be established with patient. For most persons, tolerance of several hours or longer is required to resume important life activities. Hyperemia must resolve in less than 30 min to increase sitting tolerance. Frequent pressure reliefs can enable patient to achieve longer sitting tolerance.

Review reinforces importance of this preventive activity and provides opportunity for goal setting and mutual problem solving.

 Additional Information

Intact triceps are required to perform a stable push-up. Push-ups lift patient's weight off both buttocks.

Forward leans can be performed if trunk musculature, triceps, or strong pectoral muscles are present (Nixon, 1985). Patient safety is a factor for independent forward leans. This maneuver does not totally eliminate pressure but can decrease pressure by transferring weight to posterior thighs.

This is an impractical option for routine long-term pressure relief.

This is a more realistic option for individuals who are dependent in pressure relief activity.

 DOCUMENTATION

1. Document education and patient's performance of pressure relief as well as sitting tolerance.

2. Document the method of pressure relief.

REFERENCES

King, R.B., Boyink, M. and Keenan, M. (1977) *Rehabilitation Guide* Chicago, IL: Rehabilitation Institute of Chicago.

Nixon, Vickie (1985) *Spinal Cord Injury. A Guide to Functional Outcomes in Physical Therapy Management.* Rockville, MD: Aspen.

WHEEL CHAIR PUSH UP

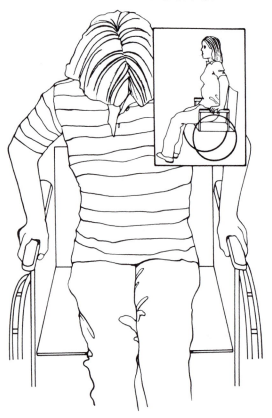

Figure 4-5

WHEEL CHAIR PRESSURE RELIEF BY LEANING TO ONE SIDE

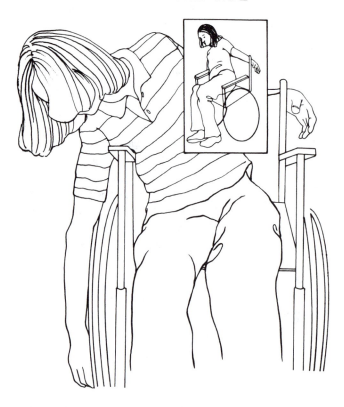

Figure 4-6

Turning and Positioning

PURPOSE

To prevent pressure ulcers; to maintain range of motion; to decrease the influence of pathologic reflexes and posturing; to prevent pooling of lung secretions through regular repositioning; to improve circulation

STAFF RESPONSIBLE

EQUIPMENT

1. Pillows, foam blocks, or small towels.
2. Optional:
   - Proning cart
   - Protective boots
   - Body wedges or foam blocks
   - Special mattresses, beds, or toppers that reduce or alternate pressures

GENERAL CONSIDERATIONS

1. Refer to General Considerations of Pressure Relief Activities.
2. Few products can reduce pressure to less than capillary pressure for all positions. Therefore, the major emphasis is relieving pressure by change of position.
3. All patients with reduced mobility or sensation need to be turned and positioned on an individualized schedule.
4. No two skin surfaces should rest together. A pillow or foam block is placed between the patient's legs so that one leg is not lying on top of the other.
5. Proper body mechanics must be practiced by the lifters during all turning and positioning procedures.
6. Patients are positioned for comfort as well as pressure relief.
7. Turning schedules are individualized according to the patient's skin tolerance. Most individuals can tolerate

turning every 2 h, but some may require more frequent repositioning. Turning or sitting time can be increased only when hyperemia over bony prominences resolves within 30 min after pressure relief.

8. Always increase time in one position gradually (i.e., usually no more than a half hour at a time). Evaluate a new schedule for 2 to 3 days.

9. Whenever possible, all positions are utilized. Prone, supine, side lying, and small shifts in position are encouraged.

10. The prone position assists with even distribution of weight and can promote extension of the hips and knees. This position is contraindicated in certain medical conditions (breathing problems), when it increases flexor or extensor tone, when there are limitations in ROM of hip and knee extension (elderly persons or persons with arthritis), and in the presence of increased intracranial pressure, unstable spine, or any condition in which increased intrathoracic pressure is to be prevented. Patients with sacral pressure ulcers use the prone position to mobilize themselves on a prone cart.

11. When side-lying, avoid positioning directly on trochanter (AHCPR, 1992).

12. At times, minor rotations in position are adequate to relieve pressure and may allow increased intervals between turning and increased patient comfort.

13. Inspect the skin when repositioning the patient.

14. Firm (not hard) standard mattresses that support the body are recommended. Foam mattress overlays over a regular mattress aid slightly in distributing pressure.

15. For patients who must be turned more frequently than every 2 h because of risk of pressure ulcers, consider using a special bed or mattress overlays that reduces pressures to less than capillary pressure (see "Guide to Choosing Bed and Mattress Toppers").

16. If spasticity occurs or if the patient moves out of position, commercial support boots or splints can be used. If spasticity continues with the foot support, remove it, increase the frequency of ROM to the ankle joint, and support the lower legs on a foam wedge or small pillows to decrease heel pressure.

17. Static positioning devices (e.g., pillows under a leg or placed to support side lying) may not stay in place if a patient is mobile.

18. Patients should be positioned so that they are able to call for assistance if needed (i.e., the call light should be within reach, or the patient should be on a monitor).

19. Caution with turning and positioning is necessary for patients with increased intracranial pressure (ICP). Evidence exists that turning from supine to side lying and proning can increase ICP. Consultation with the physician is indicated before using these positions for patients with ICP (Palmer and Wyness, 1988).

20. Nursing care plans should contain special positioning instructions if abnormal tone exists. If needed, physical and occupational therapists can be consulted regarding positioning approaches to control abnormal tone.

21. Patients should have a well-established turning tolerance before hospital discharge.

PATIENT AND FAMILY EDUCATION

1. Patients and primary caregivers are taught the following:
   - Positioning techniques for all position options
   - Principles for increasing tolerances or for decreasing tolerances if risk factors increase
   - Maintenance of equipment
   - Purchasing of equipment

2. Include the patient and primary caregiver in performing the procedure as much as possible to encourage independence at the patient's level of function.

Procedures

 Steps

1. Gather equipment, and keep it within reach.

2. Position bed at waist level with side rail closest to you in low position.

3. Assess patient's ability to assist.

4. Explain procedure to patient. Choose one of the following positions.

 Additional Information

Support equipment needed may be pillows or foam blocks, small towels, or foam wedges.

Consider patient's physiologic condition, mobility, strength, endurance, balance, understanding, and motivation.

Supine Position

1. Follow steps 1 through 4, previous procedure.

2. Position patient on his or her back in center of bed.

3. Position patient in proper alignment.

4. Place pillow under upper and lateral borders of scapulae, shoulders, neck, and head.

5. Place pillows or arm supports under involved upper extremities, positioning arm alongside body and forearm slightly supinated or in neutral position.

6. Place trochanter roll alongside involved hip and upper half of thigh, if external rotation of hip is problematic.

7. Position to maintain dorsiflexion of foot and to prevent pressure on heel. Place firm foam block between legs to prevent hip adduction and internal rotation when potential for these problems exists.

8. Apply equipment (e.g., casts or splints) as directed by care plan.

9. Place call light within reach. Raise side rails.

Side-Lying Position

1. Follow steps 1 through 4, previous procedure.

2. Move patient to edge of bed closest to you.

3. Position patient's arms at sides or across chest.

4. Cross leg closest to you over the other in direction to which patient will turn. Check contraindications before carrying out this step.

 Additional Information

When patient is positioned supine, heels should not rest on mattress. Foam wedge or small soft pillow under legs will free heels from pressure, or special support boots can be used. Pillows and foam blocks can be used for bridging to prevent pressure over bony prominences.

You can move patient in bed by moving one-third of body at a time unless logrolling is required for spinal precautions or other condition. Extra assistance of one or two staff may be needed if patient is heavy or has complications.

To be in correct alignment, the following should form a straight line: chin, suprasternal notch, and symphysis pubis. Both sides of body, including trunk, should be symmetric, and head should be in midline.

This position will help prevent flexion contracture of neck. For patients with hemiplegia, it may be necessary to position small pillow or rolled towel under scapula to protract it (Fig. 4-7).

This will help prevent internal rotation of shoulder and flexion of elbow as well as edema formation.

Placement of a small pillow or roll under distal thigh producing slight knee flexion can reduce extensor spasticity, which is commonly seen in presence of hemiplegia. Roll must not exert any pressure on popliteal space. Such pressure interferes with circulation and compresses nerves. Use foam block between legs when spasticity is present.

 Additional Information

When patient is positioned on his or her side (Fig. 4-8) avoid positioning directly on trochanter, ankles should be free of pressure. Do not rest one leg on top of the other. You can bridge trochanter, side of knee, and ankle. Angle of positioning can be altered slightly to change pressure. Alternate sides in side lying unless one side is contraindicated.

This step will help turn part of patient's body over to side.

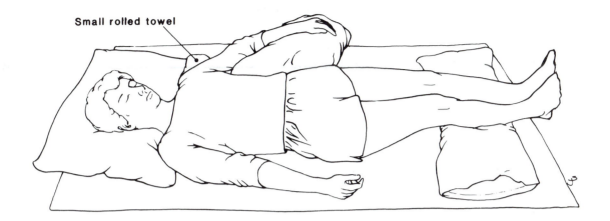

Small rolled towel

Figure 4-7   Supine

5. Put one hand on patient's shoulder/scapula closest to you and other hand on trochanter.

6. Roll patient. While rolling away is ideal, many persons may not have the upper arm strength to roll away and find it easier to roll the individual toward them.

7. Place pillow behind patient's back.

8. Place upper leg in flexed position away from bottom leg (hip flexed 55 to 60 degrees and knee flexed 0 degrees or position upper leg behind body with 30 degrees flexion at hip and 35 degrees at knee).

9. Position one or two pillows under top leg to support it from groin to foot.

10. Position upper arm on pillows to provide support for joints and to prevent edema.

11. Apply equipment as directed by nursing care plan (e.g., casts or splints).

12. Put call light within reach. Raise side rails.

Prone Position

1. Follow steps 1 through 4, previous procedure.

2. Move patient down in bed so that feet are beyond mattress.

3. Position patient supine on one side of bed, with arm toward which patient will roll positioned overhead or extended at side (can be slightly tucked under body).

Keep patient from rolling prone by keeping your hand on patient's shoulder and trochanter until pillows are placed.

This will help prevent patient from rolling onto his or her back.

Positioning upper leg behind body reduces trochanteric pressure (Garber, Campion, and Krouskop, 1982). Pillows between legs and attention to placing top leg in front of or behind bottom leg ensures that two skin surfaces are not in contact with each other and avoids excess pressure.

Do this to prevent internal rotation and adduction of hip and to maintain horizontal plane in line with hip, preventing pull on hip joint.

  Additional Information

When positioning prone, protect iliac crests, patellae, dorsum of feet, and toes. Position feet between mattress and footboard if possible (Fig. 4-9).

Discuss appropriateness of proning patients with physician if potential contraindications to proning exist (see General Considerations 10, p. 231).

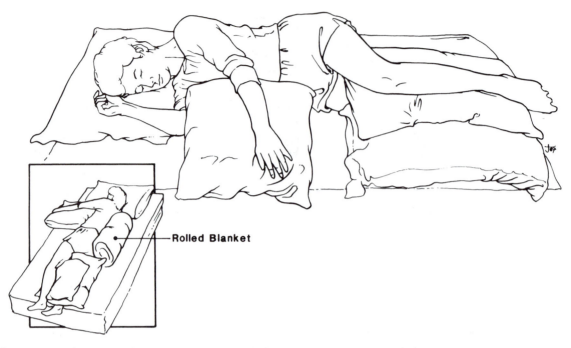

Figure 4-8 Side-Lying

4. When bridging, position pillows so that patient will roll onto them when rolled prone.

When bridging, pillows should be positioned to protect iliac crests, knees, and dorsum of feet as shown in Fig. 4-9. If patient will not be bridged, small, flat support is placed under abdomen to prevent hyperextension of lumbar curve, and chest is supported with flat pillow. Small foam supports are placed under lower legs.

5. Cross uppermost leg over body in direction to which patient will turn.

This step will help turn patient to prone position.

6. Roll patient to side toward pillows. For example, if turning patient toward right, position left leg across body. Place right arm over head or extended at side. Roll patient over on pillows.

7. Position patient's head on pillow that provides comfortable support, and maintain neutral position without promoting flexion or extension. Patient's head can be rotated to either side if this activity is not contraindicated.

8. Position upper extremities in comfortable position.

9. Check for effective pressure relief, when bridging, by running your hand under iliac crests, knees, and dorsum of feet. Check that undue pressure is not exerted over genitalia of males.

10. Arrange urinary equipment to promote effective drainage and to avoid undue pressure on skin tissue.

11. Leave patient in this position for one-half hour initially, and remain with patient during that time.

At first, attempt prone position during the day when patient is alert. Often, patient is fearful of positioning prone. Time can be increased after patient has established comfort level. Patient's skin can often tolerate longer periods of time in prone position than in other positions because this position tends to distribute pressure evenly.

12. Apply any equipment as directed by nursing care plan (e.g., splints).

13. Put call light within reach. Raise side rails.

DOCUMENTATION

1. Document the time in each position and redness over a bony prominence that does not resolve within 30 min of positioning off the site.

2. Document the effectiveness of specific positioning approaches (i.e., small rotations or bridging) to manage spasticity and to prevent excessive pressure.

3. Document any unusual occurrences during turning and positioning.

4. Document patient and family teaching and success.

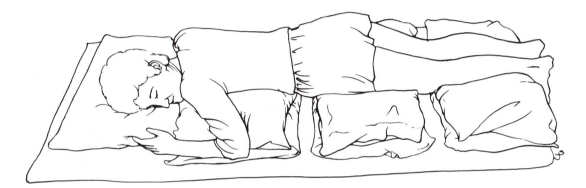

Figure 4-9 Prone

Three-Quarter Prone Position

Steps

Additional Information

When positioning three-quarter prone, protect iliac crest and trochanter; four to five foam blocks are needed and a full-length sheepskin. This should follow steps 1 to 4 in this procedure.

1. Place full-length sheepskin lengthwise under patient.

2. Position patient on his or her side on top of the sheepskin.

3. Position top leg in front of bottom leg, position on two to four horizontal pillows.

4. Turn patient over on to chest, facing away from you, supporting chest on pillow.

5. Lift up on sheepskin and slide foam blocks lengthwise underneath the sheepskin, above and below the iliac crest.

6. Assess for adequate bridging by sliding your hand under the trochanter between the foam blocks.

7. Pull patient's bottommost arm gently through towards his or her back.

8. Apply equipment as directed by nursing care plan (splints, casts, etc.).

9. Ensure patient is comfortable, side rails are up, and call light is in reach.

Head may rest on pillow if comfortable to patient.

More than two pillows may be needed to keep ankle, knee, and hip in same horizontal plane.

Placing top arm temporarily over side rail helps keep patient positioned while placing pillow under chest.

This will bridge iliac crest to protect it from pressure.

Additional foam blocks may be used to provide adequate bridging of trochanter.

This arm may be positioned bent at the elbow in a "Statue of Liberty" position.

30-Degree Oblique Position

 Steps

 Additional Information

This position greatly decreases pressure over the sacrum and trochanter (Seiler, Allen, and Stahlen, 1986). Protect ankles so they are free of pressure. Do not raise head of bed more than 30 degrees to prevent shearing (Braden and Bryant, 1990). Alternate sides unless contraindicated.

This should follow steps 1 to 4 in this procedure.

1. Pull the patient to the edge of the bed closest to you.

2. Position patient's arm at his or her side.

   See "Supine Positioning"–Additional Information–Step 1.

3. Cross leg closest to you over other leg in the direction to which the patient will turn. Check contraindications prior to this step.

   This step will help turn part of patient's body to his or her side.

4. Place one hand on patient's shoulder closest to you and other hand on the trochanter.

5. Roll the patient about 30 degrees to the side from a supine position.

6. Place a pillow behind the patient's back.

7. Place upper leg in a flexed position away from the bottom leg (hip flexed 55 to 60 degrees and knee flexed 80 degrees or position upper leg behind the body with 30 degrees flexion at the hip and 35 degrees at the knee).

   This will prevent the patient from rolling on his or her back.
   This ensures that the two skin surfaces of the legs are not in contact with each other and avoids excess pressure.

8. Position one or two pillows under top leg to support it from the groin to the foot.

9. Position upper arm on pillows to provide support for joints and to prevent edema.

10. Apply equipment as directed by nursing care plan (casts, splints, etc.).

11. Ensure patient is comfortable, side rails are up, and call light is within reach.

 DOCUMENTATION

In progress note :
1. Document time in position and redness over a bony prominence that does not resolve within 30 min of positioning off the site.
2. Document effectiveness of specific positioning approaches to manage spasticity and to prevent excessive pressure (i.e., small rotations, bridging).
3. Document unusual occurrences during turning and positioning.
4. Document patient/family teaching and success on teaching checklist/progress note.
5. Document care performed in medical record.

REFERENCES

U.S. Department of Health and Human Services (1992) *Pressure Ulcers in Adults: Prediction and Prevention* AHCPR Publ. 92-0047. Rockville, MD: Agency for Health Care Policy and Research.

U.S. Department of Health and Human Services (1994) *Pressure Ulcers in Adults: Prediction and Prevention* AHCPR Publ. 95-0653. Rockville, MD: Agency for Health Care Policy and Research.

Garber, S., Campion, L., and Krouskop, T. (1982) "Trochanteric Pressure in Spinal Cord Injury" *Archives of Physical Medicine and Rehabilitation* 63:549–552.

Gee, Z., and Passarella, P. (1985) *Nursing Care of the Stroke Patient: A Therapeutic Approach* Pittsburgh, PA: AREN.

Matthews, P., Carlson, C.E., and Holt, N.B. (Eds.) (1987) *Spinal Cord Injury: A Guide to Rehabilitation Nursing* Rockville, MD: Aspen.

Nixon, V. (1985). *Spinal Cord Injury: A Guide to Functional Outcomes in Physical Therapy Management* Rockville, MD: Aspen.

Palmer, M., and Wyness, M. (1988) "Positioning and Handling: Important Considerations in the Care of the Severely Head-Injured Patient." *Journal of Neuroscience Nursing* 20:42–49.

Seiler, W.O., Allen, S., and Stahlen, H.B. (1986) "Influences of the 30° Laterally Inclined Position and the "Super Soft" 3 Piece Mattress on Skin Oxygen Tension on Areas of Maximal Pressure—Implications for Pressure Sore Prevention" *Gerontology* 32:158–166.

Zejdlik, C. (1983) *Management of Spinal Cord Injury* Monterey, CA: Wadsworth.

Guideline for Selecting Pressure Management Surfaces for Bed Positioning

PURPOSE

To assist the clinician in selecting an appropriate support surface for individual clients in bed

STAFF RESPONSIBLE

EQUIPMENT

No equipment necessary

GENERAL CONSIDERATIONS

The selection of a support surface should be individualized to the particular patient. The purpose of a pressure management surface is to redistribute interface pressures between the surface and the body in such a manner as to minimize interference with blood flow, particularly over the bony prominences. To aid in the selection of an appropriate surface the clinician needs to assess:

1. Skin integrity—including site, number, and severity of pressure ulcers if any
   - Risk factors for skin breakdown. An assessment tool such as the Braden or Norton scale may be used
   - Cost
   - Ease of maintenance and use of recommended option
   - Appropriateness of option for environment of use. Some devices, particularly powered ones, may have operational requirements that make them inappropriate or unsuitable for home use. Others may have maintenance and upkeep issues that make them cost-prohibitive for institutional use.
   - Impact on functional level

CATEGORIES OF SURFACES

Surfaces can be divided into several categories based on mechanism and method of action (Table 4-1). The first major divi-

sion is into mattress toppers or mattress replacements. Toppers are designed to be used as an adjunct to a standard mattress. They are typically the least expensive option, although there are some relatively expensive products in this group. Mattress replacements are intended to completely replace the standard mattress. They may come as stand-alone items or as a part of a complete bed system. Specialty beds tend to be the most expensive option. Mattress replacements are commonly available for rental or lease, as well as purchase.

The second major division is between static or dynamic products. Static surfaces depend on construction materials and methodology to redistribute pressure as evenly as possible throughout all contact points. They may be made of foams, gels, liquids, or gases contained within a supporting skin of some type—usually fabric or plastic. There are a few combination products made with foam and some combination of one of the other materials. Use a static support surface if a patient can assume a variety of positions without bearing weight on a pressure ulcer and without "bottoming out" (AHCPR).

Dynamic surfaces, as the name implies, function by shifting the points of application of pressure under the patient or by moving the patient through space. Due to the moving parts and circuitry required, they tend to be among the more expensive options. There are also upkeep requirements that go along with maintaining the surface at optimal function and ensuring patient safety. Use a dynamic support surface if the patient cannot assume a variety of positions without bearing weight on a pressure ulcer, if the patient fully compresses the static support surface, or if the pressure ulcer does not show evidence of healing. If a patient has large stage III or stage IV pressure ulcers on multiple turning surfaces, a low-air-loss bed or an air-fluidized bed may be indicated (AHCPR Guidelines).

REFERENCES

Bell, J.C., Matthews, S.D. (1993) "Results of a Clinical Investigation of Four Pressure-Reduction Replacement Mattresses" *Journal of Enterostomal Therapy Nursing* 20:204–210.

Conine, T.A., Choi, A.K., Lim, R. (1989) "The User-Friendliness of Protective Support Surfaces in Prevention of Pressure Sores" *Rehabilitation Nursing* 14(5):261–263.

Table 4-1   Wound Care: Product Categorization

Material	Pros	Cons	Examples	Manufacturer
Mattress Toppers: Static				
Foam	• Least expensive • Minimal interference with mobility • Easy to transport • Low maintenance	• Varying levels of effectiveness • Durability • Absorbent; can contribute to maceration • Loses fire retardancy if laundered	• Eggcrate • Biofloat • GeoMatt	• Eggcrate • Bioclinic • SpanAmerica
Gel	• Low maintenance	• Weight • Temperature		
Air	• Lightweight • Cost	• Leaks • Can be overinflated or underinflated • Must be checked periodically for proper inflation	Safkare	Gaymar
Water	• Inexpensive • Modular forms allow focusing area of pressure redistribution	• Weight • Leaks • Temperature sensitive		
Combination	Varies with combination of materials used			
Mattress Toppers: Dynamic				
Alternating Air	• Lightweight • Can decrease need to reposition patient • Cannot be over- or underinflated	• Maintenance • Can interfere with emergency procedures and patient mobility	• Grant	• Grant
Low air loss	• Lightweight • Can decrease need to reposition patient • Cannot be over- or underinflated	• Maintenance • Can increase fluid loss • Can interfere with emergency procedures and patient mobility	• Accucair	• Support Systems International
Mattress Replacements: Static				
Foam	• Cost • Comfort	• Durability • Varying levels of effectiveness	• Therarest • DeCube	• Kinetic Concepts • Comfortex
Air	• Cost	• Leaks • May need periodic reinflation		
Water	• Comfort	• Weight • Interfere with mobility	• Lotus	• Lotus
Combination	Varies with combination of materials used			
Mattress Replacements: Dynamic				
Foam	• Some designs minimize need to manually reposition patient • Can assist pulmonary toilet	• Maintenance • Motion may be distressing to patient • Noise	• Theraturn • Rotorest	
Air	• Very low contact pressures can be achieved • Most designs have quick deflate mode for emergency procedures and overinflate mode to assist with mobility	• Some fluidized air use beads which can spill or become entrapped in body tissues • Some designs are extremely heavy • Prolonged use may lead to vascular deconditioning and orthostatic hypotension with some designs	• Pegasus Airwave • Clinitron • Restcue	• Pegasus • Support Systems International
Low-Air-Loss	• Very low contact pressures can be achieved • Most designs have quick deflate mode for emergency procedures and overinflate mode to assist with mobility	• May increase fluid loss • Cost	• Mediscus DFS • Flexicair	• Mediscus Group • Support Systems International
Combination	Varies with combination of materials used			

Ferrell, B.A., Osterweil, D., Christenson, P. (1993) "A Randomized Trial of Low-Air-Loss Beds for Treatment of Pressure Ulcers" *Journal of the American Medical Association* 269(4):494–497.

Fowler, E.M. (1987) "Equipment and Products Used in Management and Treatment of Pressure Ulcers" *Nursing Clinics of North America* 22:449–461.

Jackson, B.S., Chagares, R., Nee, N., Freeman, K. (1988) "The Effects of a Therapeutic Bed on Pressure Ulcers: An Experimental Study" *Journal of Enterostomal Therapy* 15(6):220–226.

Krouskop, T., Williams, R., Krebs, M., et al. (1985) "Effectiveness of Mattress Overlays in Reducing Interface Pressure during Recumbency" *Journal of Rehabilitation Research and Development* 22:7–10.

Lilla, J.A., Friedrichs, R.R., and Vistnes, L.H. (1975) "Flotation Mattresses for Preventing and Treating Tissue Breakdown" *Geriatrics* 30:71.

Maklebust, J., Mondoux, L., and Sieggreen, M. (1986) "Pressure Relief Characteristics of Various Support Surfaces Used in Prevention and Treatment of Pressure Ulcers" *Journal of Enterostomal Therapy* 14:8.5–8.9.

Smoot, E.R. (1986) "Clinitron Bed Therapy Hazards" *Plastic and Reconstructive Surgery* 77(1):165.

Warner, D.J. (1992) "A Clinical Comparison of Two Pressure-Reducing Surfaces in the Management of Pressure Ulcers" *Decubitus* 5(3):52–55.

Wells, P., and Geden, E. (1984) "Paraplegic Body-Support Pressures on Convoluted Foam, Waterbed and Standard Mattresses" *Research in Nursing and Health* 7:127–133.

Whittemore, R. (1998) "Pressure-Reduction Support Surfaces: A Review of the Literature" *Journal of Wound Ostomy and Continence Nurses* 25:6–25.

Wound Care

General Wound Care

PURPOSE

To prevent wound infection, promote healing, and protect peri-wound tissues

WOUND TYPES

All

STAFF RESPONSIBLE

EQUIPMENT NEEDED

1. Nonsterile examination gloves
2. Solution for cleansing wound, usually normal saline
3. Sponges for cleaning, blotting wound
4. Bag for disposal of used equipment and soiled dressings
5. Prescribed dressing
6. Sterile gloves

OPTIONAL EQUIPMENT

1. Wound irrigation setup (Low-pressure irrigation may be used instead of sponges to clean wound.)
2. Wound irrigating solution—usually normal saline
3. Topical agent
4. Culture collection equipment
5. Skin protectant for use under tape or at wound margins

 ### GENERAL CONSIDERATIONS

1. Wound care in the institutional setting should generally be provided using sterile technique. Clean technique may be used, although not routinely recommended, in the home care setting based on an assessment of the patient, the environment, and associated risk factors. Appropriate barrier precautions to prevent transmission of micro-organisms between provider and recipient of care must be maintained throughout irrespective of setting (Simmons et al., 1990).

2. Wound care should always begin with an assessment of the wound. This is to verify that the current treatment plan is appropriate or identify the need for it to be modified. At minimum, assessment of the wound should include:
   1. Anatomic location of the wound
   2. Stage of wound if appropriate
   3. Size of wound
   4. Shape of wound
   5. Color of wound bed
   6. Description of periwound tissues
   7. Presence, color, description, and quantity of exudate

3. Periodic assessments should also look for signs and symptoms of clinical infection—purulent exudate, local inflammation, odor, streaking. On a weekly basis there should be an evaluation of treatment effectiveness—whether or not the wound has improved, regressed, or remains unchanged (AHCPR Pressure Ulcer Treatment Guidelines).

4. Hands should be washed using soap and water (waterless sanitizers such as Purell Hand Sanitizer or Alkare may be used in settings where running water is not available) before and after removing old dressing and applying new dressing. Gloves should be changed between removing old dressing and applying new dressings.

5. Privacy should be provided for patient by closing door or clearing area of extraneous persons. Only the area to be treated should be exposed.

PATIENT AND FAMILY EDUCATION

The patient and primary caregivers should be instructed in proper wound care procedures. Opportunity for return demonstration of technique will help to assure patient/caregiver ability to perform procedure independently.

Procedure

Steps

1. Remove soiled dressing if present.

2. Set up equipment (open containers and kits, remove caps, cut tape, etc.).

3. Clean wound with gentle pressure using appropriate solution. Use fresh gauze sponge for each pass over wound. Work from center of wound to exterior margins in a spiral direction.

4. If multiple-use solution containers are used, they should be labeled with date and time they are initially opened.

5. Blot wound margins using dry gauze.

6. Apply prescribed topical agents.
7. Apply prescribed dressing.
8. Secure dressing using tape or self-adhering topper dressing as indicated.

9. Discard used supplies per facility protocol.

10. Document assessment and dressing change per established procedure.

Additional Information

Soiled dressings should be discarded in accordance with facility procedures for disposal of medical waste. Normal saline solution may be used to loosen dressing if needed.

Low-pressure irrigation may be used instead of sponge cleaning to minimize trauma to wound bed.

Single-use containers are preferred in the institutional setting. Even bacteriostatic agents such as povidone-iodine can support bacterial growth if contaminated and subsequently provide a source of infection.

Moisture at periwound area may retard adherence of occlusive dressings and tape.

Clean wound bed before applying topical agents.

Montgomery straps or a binder may be used as an alternative to tape for securing dressings in patients with adhesive sensitivity.

Used supplies should be discarded in accordance with facility procedures for disposal of medical waste.

Standardized forms may be used for documentation of wound assessment instead of routine progress notes. This may help to insure that all appropriate assessment parameters are addressed.

REFERENCES

Afilalo M., Dankoff J., Guttman A., Lloyd J. (1992) "DuoDERM Hydroactive Dressing versus Silver Sulphadiazine/Bactigras in the Emergency Treatment of Partial Skin Thickness Burns" *Burns* 18(4):313–316.

Agren MS. (1996) "Four Alginate Dressings in the Treatment of Partial Thickness Wounds: A Comparative Experimental Study" *Journal of Plastic Surgery* 49(2):129–134.

Alvarez, O., Rozint, J., Meehan, M. (1990) "Principles of Moist Wound Healing: Indications for Chronic Wounds" in Krasner, D., (Ed.) *Chronic Wound Care: A Clinical Sourcebook for Healthcare Professionals* King of Prussia PA: Health Management Publications.

Bale, S. and Harding, K.G. (1990) "Using Modern Dressings to Effect Debridement" *Professional Nursing* 5(5):244–245.

Berry, D.P., Bale, S., Harding, K.G. (1996) "Dressings for Treating Cavity Wounds" *Journal of Wound Care* 5(1):10–17.

Bolton, L., van Rijswijk, L., (1991) "Wound Dressings: Meeting Clinical and Biological Needs" *Dermatology Nursing* 3(3):146–161.

Brown, L.L., Shelton, H.T., Bornside, G.H., Cohn, I., Jr. (1978) "Evaluation of Wound Irrigation by Pulsatile Jet and Conventional Methods" *Annals of Surgery* 187(2):170–173.

Bryant, R.A., (Ed.) (1992) *Acute and Chronic Wounds: Nursing Management* St Louis, MO: Mosby Year Book.

Carr, R.D., Lalagos, D.E. (1990) "Clinical Evaluation of a Polymeric Membrane Dressing in the Treatment of Pressure Ulcers" *Decubitus* 3(3):38–42.

Colwell, J.C., Foreman, M.D., Trotter, J.P. (1993) "A Comparison of the Efficacy and Cost-Effectiveness of Two Methods of Managing Pressure Ulcers" *Decubitus* 6(4):28–36.

Cuzzell, J. (1997) "Choosing a Wound Dressing" *Geriatric Nursing* 18(6):260–265.

Daltrey, D.C., Rhodes, B., Chattwood, J.G. (1981) "Investigation into the Microbial Flora of Healing and Non-Healing Decubitus" Ulcers *Journal of Clinical Pathology* 34(7):701–705.

Dunavant, M. K. (1982) "Wound and Fistula Management" In D. Broadwell and B. Jackson (Eds.) *Principles of Ostomy Care* St. Louis, MO: Mosby; pp. 658–686.

Hall, C.M. (1997) "Wound Dressings: Use and Selection" *Geriatric Nursing* 18(6):266–267.

Hall, S.D. and Ponder, R.B. (1992) "Nonwoven Wound Care Products" *Ostomy and Wound Management* 38(6):24–30.

Hess, C.T. and Thomas, D.R. (Eds.) (1998) *Wound Care Communications Network, Resources in Wound Care:1998 Directory* Springhouse, PA: Springhouse.

Iffgang, S. (1987) "Topical Treatment of Pressure Ulcers" *Home Care* 9:44–52.

Kemp, M.G., Krouskop, T.A. (1994) "Pressure Ulcers: Reducing Incidence and Severity by Managing Pressure" *Journal of Gerontology Nursing* 20(9):27–34.

Lineaweaver, W., McMorris, S., Soucy, D., and Howard, R. (1985) "Cellular and Bacterial Toxicities of Topical Antimicrobials" *Plastic and Reconstructive Surgery* 75:39.4–39.6.

Lineaweaver, W., et al. (1985) "Topical Antimicrobial Toxicity" *Archives of Surgery* 120(3):267–270.

Novotny-Dinsdale, V. and Miller, M. (1993) "Evaluation of Two Reusable Wound Irrigation Systems" *Journal of Emergency Nursing* 19(4):329–331.

Nurses' Drug Alert (1987, June) "Avoid Use of Hydrogen Peroxide and Povidone-Iodine in Open Wounds" *American Journal of Nursing* 11:41.

Oberg, M., and Lindsey, D. (1987) "Do Not Put Hydrogen Peroxide or Povidone Iodine into Wounds" *American Journal of Diseases of Children* 141:27–28.

Ohlsson, P., Larsson, K., Lindholm, C., Moller, M.A. (1994) "Comparison of Saline-Gauze and Hydrocolloid Treatment in a Prospective, Randomized Study" *Scandinavian Journal of Primary Health Care* 12(4):295–299.

Rudolph, R., and Noe, J.M. (1983) *Chronic Problem Wounds* Boston: Little, Brown.

Rund, C.R. (1990) "Alternative Treatments-Alternative Settings" in Krasner, D. (Ed.) *Chronic Wound Care: A Clinical Sourcebook for Healthcare Professionals* King of Prussia PA: Health Management Publications.

Sayag, J., Meaume, S., Bohbot, S. (1996) "Healing Properties of Calcium Alginate Dressings" *Journal of Wound Care* 5(8):357–362.

Schneider, D., and Hebert, L. (1987) "Subcutaneous Gas from Hydrogen Peroxide Administration under Pressure" *American Journal of Diseases of Children* 141:10–11.

Shanon, M.L. (1982) "Pressure Sores" In C.M. Norris (Ed.) *Concept Clarification in Nursing* Rockville, MD: Aspen.

Simmons, B., et al. (1990) "Infection Control for Home Health" *Infection Control and Hospital Epidemiology* 11(7):362–370.

Stevenson, T.R., et al. (1976) "Cleansing the Traumatic Wound by High Pressure Syringe Irrigation" *JACEP* 5(1):17–21.

Surgical Materials Testing Laboratories "Dressings for Management of Different Wound Types" World Wide Wounds, Jan 1998: http://www.smtl.co.uk/WMPRC/DataCards/dressings-data-cards-by-wound-type.html/.

Teepe, R.G.,et al. (1993) "Cytotoxic Effects of Topical Antimicrobial and Antiseptic Agents on Human Keratinocytes in Vitro" *Journal of Trauma* 34(1):8–19.

Thomas, S., (1992) "Hydrocolloids" *Journal of Wound Care* 1(2):27–30.

Thomas, S., et al. (1996) "The Effect of Dressings on the Production of Exudate from Venous Leg Ulcers" *Wounds* 8(5):145–150.

Thomas, S. and Loveless, P. "A Comparative Study of Twelve Hydrocolloid Dressings" World Wide Wounds, July 1998: http://www.smtl.co.uk /World-Wide-Wounds/1997/july/Thomas-Hydronet/hydronet.html/.

Thomas, S., et al. (1993) "A Comparison of the Wound Cleansing Properties of Two Hydrogel Dressings" *Journal of Wound Care* 2(5):272–274.

U.S. Department of Health and Human Services. (1994). *Pressure Ulcers in Adults: Prediction and Prevention* AHCPR Publ. 95-0653 Rockville, MD: Agency for Health Care Policy and Research.

Selecting a Dressing

PURPOSE

To facilitate the selection of an appropriate dressing for individuals based on assessment of the individual and the wound to be treated

 GENERAL CONSIDERATIONS

1. No one dressing is appropriate for all persons in all situations. There are various methods of action and support

provided by different categories of dressings that should be considered in the context of the entire person before a dressing is recommended or applied.

2. It is well documented that a moist environment provides the best enhancement of wound healing. Excessive moisture, however, may interfere with tissue repair and promote bacterial colonization or infection. The presence of slough and eschar will also delay wound healing.

3. Generally, dressing selection should be prioritized by (Hall, 1997; Cuzzell, 1997):
   1. Removal of slough and eschar to provide a clean wound bed
   2. Identify and treat infection
   3. Exudate control to minimize maceration
   4. Provide and maintain a moist clean environment
   5. Protect the wound

4. Dressings may be grouped in several categories based on formulation and mechanism of action. Although there may be subtle differences between dressings in a category from different manufacturers, the general indications will be consistent for all products in a group. Many types and categories of dressing are available for the clinician in wound care. Dressings have been designed and developed to absorb exudate, remove slough, facilitate granulation and reepithelialization, or provide the desired moist environment. Some dressings can provide more than one clinical effect simultaneously, others have a single specialized purpose and subsequently fewer clinical applications. Dressing selection requires an understanding of the wound healing and tissue repair process combined with an understanding of the properties of individual categories of dressings.

5. The following tables are intended to illustrate the categorization schema used in this section. Table 4-2 lists categories of dressings with the wound attributes that they are designed to manage along with examples of commercially available products in the listed categories. Tables 4-3 and 4-4 identify wound types and attributes in a grid with the intersection identifying categories of dressings intended to manage that wound type. A specific category of dressing may appear in multiple positions in Tables 4-3 and 4-4.

6. The routine use of antimicrobials is not recommended for wound management, and they are not included in this section. It is not uncommon for wound beds, particularly chronic wounds, to be colonized with one or more microorganisms. In the absence of infection, antimicrobial use to eliminate colonization is not generally recommended. Many antimicrobial solutions used to clean wounds particularly such as povidone-iodine solution, Dakin's solution, and hydrogen peroxide are known to impair wound healing and are not recommended for routine or long-term use. Clinical infection as evidenced by purulent drainage, local inflammation, or systemic symptoms must be resolved with appropriate antimicrobial therapy for wound healing to progress.

REFERENCES

Doughty, D.B. (1992) "Principles of Wound Healing and Wound Management" in Bryant RB (Ed) *Acute and Chronic Wounds: Nursing Management* St Louis, MO: Mosby Year Book.

Maklebust, J., and Sieggreen, M. (1996) *Pressure Ulcers: Guidelines for Prevention and Nursing Management*, 2d ed. Springhouse, PA: Springhouse

Thomas S. (1997) "A Structured Approach to the Selection of Dressings" *World Wide Wounds* July.

Wound Care Communications Network (1998) *Wound Care Products by Defined Categories, Resources in Wound Care:1998 Directory* Springhouse, PA: Springhouse.

Table 4-2   Wound Care—Product Categorization Table

Product	Type	Special Considerations	Example (Brand Name)	Manufacturer	Wound Type
Gauze: Generally used as topper dressings. May also be used to wick exudate from wound bed or to protect wound. Readily available and generally lowest cost (plain). Additives and specialty types will increase cost. Caution when used as packing; may inhibit wound contraction when packed too tightly.	Plain	Coarse mesh; will adhere to wound bed—recommended for debriding wounds	12 ply	Various	Debriding Packing
			8 ply Kerlix Kling	Kendall	
		Fine mesh; not appropriate for debridement		Johnson and Johnson	Topper wrapping

Table 4-2   Wound Care—Product Categorization Table (*continued*)

Product	Type	Special Considerations	Example (Brand Name)	Manufacturer	Wound Type
		Nonwoven; not appropriate for debridement	NuGauze	Johnson and Johnson	
			Sof-Kling	Johnson and Johnson	
	Specialty		Packing strips	Various	Packing,
			Drain sponge	Various	Stomas, IVs
		Nonadherent pad	Telfa	Kendall	Skin tears
			Kerlix	Kendall	Packing large wound
	Impregnated: dry	Saline	Mesalt	Monlycke	Moderate to heavy
			Curasalt	Kendall	drainage; packing, absorption
		Charcoal			Odor control; moderate to heavy drainage
	Impregnated: moist	Petroleum jelly	Adaptic	Johnson and Johnson	Burns; abrasions; skin tears
		Medicated— antimicrobial	Xeroform	Kendal	Burns; donor sites; grafts; abrasions
			Xeroflo	Sherwood	
			Scarlet Red	Smith and Nephew	
		Hydrogel	Curafil Gauze	Kendall	
Polymers: Synthetic dressings usually prepared as foams or membrane films. Films can be obtained in sheets or as spray-on products. Spray-on products are generally used as protectants rather than dressings.	*Membranes*—may be used as topper dressing or as a primary dressing. By design are nonabsorbent though some formulations are vented to allow wicking of exudate. Not recommended for wounds surrounded by fragile skin. May be difficult to apply and remove.	Moisture vapor permeable	Opsite	Smith and Nephew	Abrasions; IV sites; skin tears
			Carra Film	Carrington	
			Tegaderm	Johnson and Johnson	
			Polyskin II	Kendall	
		Impermeable	Opraflex		
			Blisterfilm	Sherwood	
		Spray or wipe-on	Incontinence Barrier Spray, Barrier Wipes	Bard	Rashes; skin protection
			Skin-prep Barrier Spray	United	
	Foams: Nonlinting and absorbent. May have adhesive border otherwise need a secondary dressing.		Lyofoam	Acme United	Drainage control; excoriation; stomas; moderate to heavy drainage; minor autolytic debridement
			Epilock	Convatec	
			Tielle	Johnson and Johnson	
			Flexzan	Dow Hickam	
			Allevyn	Smith and Nephew	
Hydrocolloids—occlusive or semi-occlusive dressings of varying composition and formulation. Provide a moist environment that supports autolytic debridement, exudate absorption, and granulation.	Wafers		Duoderm	Convatec	Abrasions; pressure ulcers; vascular ulcers
			Comfeel	Coloplast	
			Hydrocol	Dow Hickam	
			Ulcer Dressing	Johnson and Johnson	
	Flakes/granules provide additional exudate control. Requires topper.		Absorption dressing	Bard	Pressure ulcers; vascular ulcers; infected or clean wound filler
			Duoderm granules	Convatec	

Table 4-2   Wound Care—Product Categorization Table (*continued*)

Product	Type	Special Considerations	Example (Brand Name)	Manufacturer	Wound Type
	Pastes—provide additional exudate control and wound filling. Must be used with a topper.		Duoderm paste Comfeel	Convatec Coloplast	Pressure ulcers; vascular ulcers; infected or clean wound filler
Hydrogels: water- or glycerin-based gels. Help maintain a moist environment, support autolytic debridement, rehydrate eschar, fill dead space, and may provide some pain control. Water-based dry more rapidly.	*Pastes:* may cause some maceration of wound edges. Topper dressing always required		Intrasite Carrasyn Nu-Gel Bioclusive Curafil Curasol Gel	Smith and Nephew Carrington Johnson and Johnson Kendall Healthpoint	Vascular ulcers; pressure ulcers; burns
	Wafers		Vigilon Flexderm Curagel Nu-Gel	Bard Dow Hickam Kendall Johnson and Johnson	Burns; scant to moderate drainage
Alginates: soft nonwoven absorbent fibers derived from seaweed. Conform well to wound bed and margins and interact with exudate to maintain moist environment. Require a topper dressing.	Sponges and ropes		Kaltostat AlgiSite Sorbsan Carra Sorb Seasorb Curasorb	Convatec Smith and Nephew Dow Hickam Carrington Coloplast Kendall	Moderate to heavy drainage; pressure ulcers; burns; packing filler (ropes)
Combination products: usually a combination of two or more physically distinct products.	Nonwoven gauze and foam		ExuDry	Frastec	Burns; scant to moderate drainage
	Alginate and collagen		Fibracol	Johnson and Johnson	Packing filler; moderate to heavy drainage
Other	*Hydrofiber:* Nonwoven pad or ribbon of cellulose fibers		Aquacel	Convatec	Exudate control
	Amino acid membranes		Inerpan	Sherwood	
Moisture Barrier	Creams		Bard Incontinence		Skin protectant from urinary, fecal incontinence; scant wound drainage
			Skin Moisture Barrier	Hollister	
	Sprays and wipes	(see also polymers)	Incontinence Spray	Bard	Skin protectant; minor draining of wounds
			Granulex Dermagran Skin Protect Skin-Prep	Dow Hickam Derma Sciences Smith and Nephew	Skin protectant
Wound Cleaners	*Sprays and solutions*		Puri-Clens Cara-Klenz Ultra-Klenz Constant Clens Saf-Clens Normal saline	Coloplast Carrington Sherwood Calgon-Vestal Many	Any Recommended for most wounds

Table 4-2   Wound Care—Product Categorization Table (*continued*)

Product	Type	Special Considerations	Example (Brand Name)	Manufacturer	Wound Type
Antiseptic solutions: Used to control bacterial growth, treat local infection and colonization. Not recommended for routine cleansing or extended use as they impair fibroblast formation and will impede wound healing.	*Povidone-iodine* *Acetic acid* *Hypochlorite solution*		Betadine Dakin's Burrow's	Many	

Table 4-3   Pressure Ulcers, Vascular Ulcers, Burns

	Stage I 1st-degree Burns	Stage II 1st-degree Burn	Stage III 2d-degree Burn	Stage IV 3d-degree Burn
Drainage Heavy			Alginate, impregnated medicated gauze (burn)	Alginate
Moderate		Alginates, hydrocolloid wafer, and granules	Alginate; hydrogel; hydrocolloid flakes, paste, granules; impregnated medicated gauze, burns—polymer urethane foam	Alginate; hydrocolloid paste, flakes, granules
Scant to none	Membrane film, moisture barrier (spray/wipe or cream), burn, impregnated gauze, moist	Hydrocolloid wafer	Hydrocolloid wafer, hydrogel, moist or dry, burn-impregnated medicated gauze	Hydrogel, wet-to-wet saline
Slough Scant Moderate to heavy		Polymer, hydrocolloid Wet-to-dry	Hydrogels, hydrocolloid Wet-to-dry, hydrogels	Hydrogels, dry; hydrocolloid Wet-to-dry, hydrocolloid—dry
Eschar		Wet-to-dry	Enzymatic debridement, surgical debridement	Enzymatic debridement, surgical debridement
Clean dry	None Protective dressing	Protective dressing Membrane film dressing Hydrocolloid wafer	Hydrocolloid Hydrogel Foam	Hydrocolloid Hydrogel wafer Burn Impregnated gauze

Table 4-4   Skin Tears, Abrasions, Stomas, Surgical, and Other Miscellaneous Wounds

	Skin Tears, Abrasions, Avulsions, Incisions, Excoriation		Stomas	Other Rectal Tears, Abscesses, Fistulas
Drainage Heavy		Absorptive pads (ABD)	Polymer (urethane) foam	Packing, pouching
Moderate	Polymer	Absorptive pads (ABD)	Polymer (urethane) foam, nonwoven gauze	
Scant to none	Impregnated gauze, moist; polymer; nonwoven gauze	Nonwoven gauze	Nonwoven gauze; no dressing	
Eschar		Wet-to-wet to soften; wet-to-dry to remove; enzymatic debridement		
Clean dry	Protective dressing; membrane film	Protective gauze dressing; membrane film dressing	Protective or no dressing	

Changing a Hydrocolloid Paste Dressing

PURPOSE

To provide a moist environment for a healing wound through correct use, application, and removal of a hydrocolloid paste dressing; to promote wound healing

WOUND TYPES

	Stage	Color	Exudate
Use for	II, III, IV	Red, yellow	Scant to moderate to copious

EQUIPMENT NEEDED

1. Cleaning solution: normal saline recommended
2. Hydrocolloid paste
3. Mixing solution: normal saline or as provided by manufacturer
4. Sterile container for mixing paste
5. Sterile tongue blade or applicator

GENERAL CONSIDERATIONS

1. Hydrocolloid dressings are designed to interact with the wound fluid and provide a moist environment to protect the wound, promote cell migration, vascularization, and reepithelialization. Pastes can be used as wound fillers under an occlusive dressing topper or independently under a gauze topper for exudate control when an occlusive dressing is contraindicated or not desired.

2. Hydrocolloid pastes are available in a variety of formulations—flakes or granules to be mixed at time of use or pre-mixed in tubes or single-use pack. For deep wounds without tunneling, a hydrocolloid paste may be used to fill the wound bed and provide additional exudate control to prolong wear time of an occlusive dressing (Surgical Materials Testing Laboratories, 1998).

3. The wound should be cleaned with normal saline prior to dressing application to remove excess wound drainage and any remnants of the previous dressing. Frequency of change and appropriate topper should be included as part of initial prescription. When used with a nonocclusive topper this will be changed once daily. If used with an occlusive dressing topper this will be changed once every 3 to 7 days.

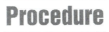

Procedure

 Steps

1. Remove old dressing and discard appropriately.
2. Irrigate wound to remove excess exudate and/or remnants of previous dressing according to low-pressure irrigation procedure.

3. Blot wound margins dry with sterile 4 × 4 gauze sponge.

4. If using flakes or granules, mix paste to desired consistency.

5. Gently apply paste to wound using sterile tongue blade.

6. Cover with appropriate topper dressing.

7. Seal borders of dressing with tape.

 Additional Information

Use of gauze sponge to remove residue may disturb wound bed. Low-pressure irrigation is preferable.

Adhesion may be impaired if topper dressing is placed on wet skin.

Some pastes come in premeasured portions of flakes and solute. If mixed too thin, paste may leak out prematurely and absorptive capacity will be reduced. If too thick, paste may be difficult to manipulate.

Do not attempt to force wound pack or fill beyond wound margins.

An occlusive topper can be used for extended wear. Plain gauze can be used if more frequent changes and inspection are required. If gauze topper is used, dressing must be changed frequently enough to prevent drying of paste.

This will minimize leakage of paste as exudate is absorbed.

8. Collect and discard used dressing supplies.

9. Date and initial tape border.

10. Document dressing change according to established procedure.

Used dressings and supplies should be discarded in accordance with facility medical waste disposal policy.

Changing a Hydrocolloid Wafer Dressing

PURPOSE

To provide a moist environment for a healing wound through correct use, application, and removal of a hydrocolloid wafer dressing; to promote wound healing

WOUND TYPES

	Stage	Color	Exudate
Use for	II, III, IV burns vascular ulcers	Red, yellow	None to moderate

EQUIPMENT

1. Gloves
2. Normal saline
3. Syringe for wound irrigation or irrigation set
4. Tape
5. Hydrocolloid wafer
6. Bag for disposal of used supplies, soiled dressing

GENERAL CONSIDERATIONS

1. Hydrocolloid dressings are designed to interact with the wound fluid and provide a moist environment to protect the wound, promote cell migration, vascularization, and reepithelialization. They may be used for autolytic debridement. This autolytic debridement effect may cause the wound to appear to have worsened on first dressing change due to lysis of tissue that was no longer viable but may have appeared healthy to the naked eye when dressing was applied. Hydrocolloid wafers have been used successfully with diabetic ulcers as well as those identified in the table above. However, in one study when applied to diabetic ulcers that contained necrotic tissue, the wounds deteriorated further (Surgical Materials Testing Laboratories, 1998).

2. Hydrocolloid wafers are available in a variety of sizes. The size should be selected to provide a 1-in. margin between the wound edges and the dressing on all sides. Hydrocolloid wafer dressings are occlusive and designed to be left in place for up to 7 days. Dressings should be changed prior to that point if leakage occurs. For deep wounds without tunneling, a hydrocolloid paste may be used to fill the wound bed and provide additional exudate control to prolong wear time of dressing. Translucent wafers are also available for use on stage I ulcers or as topper dressings (Thomas, 1992).

3. The wound should be cleaned with normal saline prior to dressing application to remove excess wound drainage and any remnants of the previous dressing.

Procedure

 Steps

1. Irrigate wound to remove excess exudate and/ or remnants of previous dressing according to low-pressure irrigation procedure.

2. Blot wound margins dry with sterile 4 × 4 gauze sponge.

3. Remove backing from dressing.

4. Center dressing over wound.

 Additional Information

Use of gauze sponge to remove residue may disturb wound bed. Low-pressure irrigation is preferable.

Adhesion may be impaired if wafer placed on wet skin.

Hold dressing by edges to maintain sterility.

A 1-in. margin should be left around wound on all sides. The dressing does not adhere to wound bed. An inadequate margin may cause premature lifting of dressing and decrease wear time.

5. Apply dressing and press with palm of hand for 10 to 15 s.	*Body heat from your hand helps conform the dressing to the patient and promote adhesion.*
6. Seal all four edges with tape.	*Will further assist adhesion, minimize edge rolling and premature lifting of dressing to extend wear time.*
7. Date and initial tape border.	*Ensures that dressing does not exceed maximum recommended wear time.*
8. Document dressing change according to established procedure.	

Changing a Hydrogel Paste Dressing

PURPOSE

To promote wound healing by supporting a moist wound environment and assisting exudate control

STAFF RESPONSIBLE

WOUND TYPES

	Stage	Color	Exudate
Use for	II, III, IV burns	Red, yellow, black	None to moderate

EQUIPMENT

1. Sterile gloves
2. Normal saline or other wound cleansing solution
3. Hydrogel paste
4. Normal saline or other solute

5. Sterile container for mixing dressing
6. Sterile applicator or tongue blade
7. Fine-mesh or nonwoven gauze or other topper dressing
8. Tape
9. Bag for soiled dressings and used supplies

OPTIONAL EQUIPMENT

1. Montgomery straps or binder

 ## GENERAL CONSIDERATIONS

1. Hydrogel pastes are provided in a number of formulations and packages. They can be obtained premeasured or premixed. They are designed to be used as stand-alone dressings but require some sort of topper dressing. They can be used to provide fluid for the softening of eschar in a wound or to absorb fluid and provide exudate control in a draining wound. They may completely liquefy in heavily draining wounds requiring more frequent dressing changes than hydrocolloid pastes (Thomas et al., 1993).

Procedure

 Steps

1. Prepare hydrogel.
2. Cleanse wound per standard procedure.

3. Apply mixed hydrogel using sterile applicator.

4. Cover wound with topper dressing.

5. Tape dressing.

 Additional Information

Skip this step if using a product that is provided premixed.

Irrigation is the best means of removing residue of old dressings and other debris from wound bed without damaging wound bed.

Dressing should be applied to cover surface of wound from margin to margin. Overlap is not required.

Plain gauze, membrane film, or hydrocolloid wafers may be used as a topper. Generally plain gauze is preferable for frequent changes.

Montgomery straps or binder may alternatively be used to secure dressing.

6. Discard used supplies per protocol.

7. Document per established procedure.

Used dressings and supplies should be disposed in accord with infection control and medical waste policy for your facility. Once bagged, they may be placed in the general waste stream for home care.

Applying a Hydrogel Wafer Dressing

PURPOSE

To promote wound healing and patient comfort

WOUND TYPES

	Stage	Color	Exudate
Use for	II, III, burns and abrasions	Red	Scant to moderate

EQUIPMENT

1. Gloves
2. Wafer dressing
3. Normal saline or other cleansing solution for wound
4. Topper sponges or gauze wrap, fine-mesh or nonwoven gauze recommended
5. Tape

OPTIONAL EQUIPMENT

1. Topical antimicrobial

GENERAL CONSIDERATIONS

1. Hydrogel wafer dressings are frequently used as a means of exudate control for burns, donor graft sites, severe abrasions, and minor pressure ulcers. Some formulations have a bonus effect of providing limited pain relief and cooling sensation to denuded skin. Hydrogel wafers are not designed to be used as a complete dressing. Some type of topper dressing, generally a plain gauze sponge or wrap, is recommended. Some newer formulations have an antimicrobial substance embedded to aid in the control and treatment of bacterial contamination and colonization (Alvarex et al., 1990).

Procedure

 Steps

1. Remove soiled dressing and discard.

2. Cleanse wound using normal saline according to standard procedure.

3. Apply topical antimicrobial if ordered using sterile gauze or sterile applicator.

4. Apply wafer dressing over wound.

5. Cover dressing with designated topper.

6. Secure topper with tape.

7. Collect and discard used supplies according to established procedure.

8. Document dressing change per established procedure.

 Additional Information

Soiled dressings should be disposed of in accordance with facility medical waste disposal policy.

Irrigation or gauze sponges with saline may be used to clean wound. See procedure: General Wound Care.

Wafer size should be selected to allow dressing to extend at least one-half inch beyond wound margins. Dressings may be slightly overlapped if need to provide larger coverage area.

Gauze wrap may be used instead of sponges to secure large dressings, dressings in awkward body parts, or dressings/wounds that circumscribe body parts.

If the wound/dressing circumscribes a body part, the tape should be applied to the topper only and not to damaged skin.

Used supplies should be discarded in accordance with facility medical waste disposal policy.

Alginate Dressings

PURPOSE

To promote wound healing via exudate control

WOUND TYPES

	Stage	Color	Exudate
Use for	II, III, IV	Red, yellow	Moderate to copious

EQUIPMENT NEEDED

1. Sterile gloves
2. Normal saline
3. Topper dressing (gauze, membrane film, hydrocolloid wafer)
4. Tape

OPTIONAL

1. Protectant skin barrier for periwound margins

GENERAL CONSIDERATIONS

1. Alginate dressings are made from naturally occurring polysaccharides found in seaweed. They are generally distributed as ropes or mats made of nonwoven fiber. Some alginate dressings require trimming to fit entirely within the wound margins. As they absorb exudate they form a soft hydrogel. In addition to exudate control they have been found to control odor and there are subjective reports of analgesic effect.

2. Frequency of change will be determined by amount of exudate and should be included as part of dressing prescription. The dressing should be changed when saturated and fiber has been converted to gel. This may vary between 1 and 4 days (Surgical Materials Testing Laboratories, 1998).

Procedure

 Steps

1. Remove old dressing and discard.

2. Irrigate wound to remove any alginate residue.

3. Trim alginate to fit wound per manufacturer direction.

4. Apply skin protectant to periwound margins if ordered and allow to dry.

5. Apply alginate wafer or rope.

6. Pat down dressing to conform to wound surface.

7. Secure dressing with appropriate topper dressing.

8. Discard used supplies per established procedure.

9. Document dressing change per standard procedure.

 Additional Information

Soiled dressings should be discarded in accordance with facility medical waste disposal policy.

Low-pressure irrigation using syringe and angiocath or commercial wound irrigation set is preferred method of cleaning wound.

Not all alginate formulations require trimming to fit wound margins.

Protective barrier may be indicated particularly when exudate is copious and wound margins become macerated between dressing changes.

Rope is indicated only for deep wounds or those with some undermining but no tunneling.

Do not pack wound tightly. This may impede contraction of wound.

Gauze toppers are generally recommended. Hydrocolloid wafers or membrane films have been used to increase wear time. They may also significantly increase cost. If a hydrocolloid topper is desired, combination alginate-hydrocolloid dressings are available which may be more cost-effective.

Used dressings and supplies should be discarded in accordance with facility medical waste disposal policy.

Changing a Wet-to-Dry Dressing

PURPOSE

To remove necrotic debris from a wound through correct application of a wet-to-dry dressing

WOUND TYPES

	Stage	Color	Exudate
Use for	III, IV	Yellow, black	Scant to copious

EQUIPMENT

1. Tape
2. Sterile normal saline
3. Woven coarse-mesh gauze/sponge or fluff
4. Prescribed wetting solution (Normal saline is the solution of choice; Betadine, Dakin's, or Burrow's solution may be prescribed for short-term use on infected wounds.)
5. Gauze sponges for topper dressing

OPTIONAL EQUIPMENT

1. Skin prep
2. Binder or Montgomery straps

GENERAL CONSIDERATIONS

1. Wet-to-dry dressings are indicated for wound debridement only. They typically have the lowest materials cost of all dressings. However, when done properly they require frequent changes and consequently are a labor-intensive method of wound management. In the hospitalized patient, once labor costs are included they may become cost-prohibitive. The wetting solution and frequency of change should be included in initial prescription. An antimicrobial solution may be used for a limited time to facilitate control of bacterial growth, reduce colonization, or provide local treatment for infection. For optimal effect, wet-to-dry dressings should be changed four to six times per day at evenly spaced intervals. It is critical that the dressing be changed shortly after it dries and that a coarse-mesh woven gauze be used. A fine-mesh or nonwoven gauze does not provide the necessary adhesion to remove necrotic tissue. A dressing that is changed before it dries also may not adequately remove necrotic debris. A dressing left in place too long will not debride the wound as rapidly and delay healing (Colwell et al., 1993).

Procedure

 Steps

1. Remove soiled dressing and discard per established procedure.
2. Set up equipment.

3. Moisten coarse-mesh gauze.

4. Fill wound bed with moistened gauze.

5. Cover filled wound with topper sponge.

6. Tape topper in place.

7. Discard used supplies according to established procedure.

8. Document dressing change according to established procedure.

Additional Information

Soiled dressings should be discarded in accordance with facility medical waste disposal policy.

If multiple-dose solutions are used, containers should be labeled with date and time of opening and name of patient.

Gauze should thoroughly moistened but not so wet it can not dry between changes.

Gauze needs to contact all of wound bed but should not be packed tightly, which would impede wound contraction or blood flow.

Moistened gauze needs to be kept in contact with wound bed to ensure contact with slough and debris. ABD pads may be used for large wounds, regular gauze sponges for smaller wounds.

Montgomery straps or binder may be used to secure dressing and minimize tape irritation from frequent dressing changes.

Used supplies should be discarded in accordance with facility medical waste disposal policy.

Changing a Wet-to-Wet Dressing

PURPOSE

To remove softened eschar over a wound or provide exudate control through correct application of a wet-to-wet (continuous moist) dressing

WOUND TYPES

	Stage	Color	Exudate
Use for	III, IV	Red	Moderate to copious

EQUIPMENT

1. Tape
2. Sterile normal saline
3. Nonwoven or fine-mesh gauze
4. Prescribed wetting solution (Normal saline is the solution of choice; Betadine, Dakin's, or other antiseptics may be prescribed for short-term use on infected wounds.)
5. Gauze toppers (ABD pads may be used for large wounds.)

OPTIONAL EQUIPMENT

1. Skin prep
2. Binder or Montgomery straps

GENERAL CONSIDERATIONS

1. Wet-to-wet (continuous moist) dressings are indicated for exudate control and softening eschar in preparation for debridement. They typically have the lowest materials cost of all dressings. However, when done properly they require frequent changes and consequently are a labor-intensive method of wound management. In the hospitalized patient, once labor costs are included they may become cost-prohibitive.

2. It is critical that the dressing be changed before it dries and yet not be applied so wet that it causes maceration of periwound tissues. A fine-mesh or nonwoven gauze is recommended as these are less likely to adhere to the wound bed and, hence, will not remove granulating tissue. The frequency of change and solution to be used should be indicated as part of the initial prescription but are generally done every 8 h with normal saline.

Procedure

 Steps

1. Remove soiled dressing and discard per established procedure.
2. Set up equipment.

3. Moisten sponges.

4. Gently fill wound or cover eschar with moistened sponges.
5. Cover with appropriate topper dressing.
6. Tape dressing in place.

7. Discard used supplies.

8. Document dressing change per established procedure.

Additional Information

If multiple-dose solutions are used, containers should be labeled with date and time of opening and name of patient.

Gauze sponges should be left moist enough to not dry between changes but not moist enough to drip beyond wound margins or when gauze is lifted.

Do not pack tightly as this may impede wound contraction.

Montgomery straps or binder may alternatively be used to secure dressing and minimize tape irritation.

Disposal of used dressings and equipment should be done in accordance with facility medical waste disposal policy.

Wound Irrigation: Low-Pressure

PURPOSE

To remove exudate, slough, and other debris from wound bed in preparation for dressing application

WOUND TYPES

	Stage	Color	Exudate
Use for	II, III, IV, burns; vascular ulcers; diabetic ulcers; surgical wounds	Red, yellow	Any

EQUIPMENT

1. Gloves
2. 30-cc Syringe or commercial irrigation kit
3. 18- to 19-Gauge angiocatheter
4. Irrigating solution (normal saline)
5. Sterile container for irrigating solution
6. Gauze sponges
7. Plastic medicine cup or commercial splash shield
8. Disposable eyeshields or goggles
9. Disposable underpads
10. Plastic bag for waste disposal
11. Prescribed dressing

 GENERAL CONSIDERATIONS

1. Low-pressure wound irrigation is an effective method of removing exudate, slough, and other debris from the wound bed. It can be performed using a commercial irrigation kit or a 30-cc Luer-Lok tip syringe with an 18- to 19-gauge needle. Routine wound cleaning should be performed with irrigation to minimize damage to wound bed while maximizing removal of undesirable materials. Low-pressure irrigation is an effective method of wound cleaning, providing less disruption to granulating tissue in the wound bed than cleaning with gauze and friction. A larger stream such as with a bulb syringe or a gravity stream through intravenous infusion tubing will not deliver adequate pressure to remove exudate, bacteria, and cellular debris. Pressures achieved by these methods are less than 4 psi. A smaller needle than a 19-gauge may deliver pressures greater than 30 psi and cause tissue damage. Target pressures are 5 to 20 psi with 8 psi considered adequate (Stevenson et al., 1976; Rund, 1990). Wound irrigation should be done with each dressing change when used as the primary mode of cleaning the wound bed.

Procedure

 Steps

1. Remove soiled dressing and discard.

2. Place disposable underpad in proper position to collect runoff from wound.

3. Set up equipment—connect commercial irrigation set or pour solution into sterile container and fill syringe.

4. Attach splash shield to syringe or inverted medicine cup.

5. Don protective eyewear.

6. Place syringe and shield over wound and gently irrigate with slow, consistent pressure applied to the barrel of the syringe.

 Additional Information

Soiled dressings should be discarded in accord with facility medical waste disposal policy.

Minimize patient discomfort by protecting bed linens.

If commercial set is used, verify that solution is safe to use. Most solutions should be discarded after 24 to 72 h of opening.

The bottom can be removed from a plastic medicine cup and taped inverted to the distal end of the syringe to provide a splash shield.

As exudating wounds will generally be colonized with one or more microorganisms, eyewear can help protect the provider from potential infection.

Too rapid compression of the barrel will increase the pressure.

7. Gently blot wound margins dry with gauze sponge.

8. Discard used supplies in accordance with established procedure.

9. Apply prescribed dressing.

Wound margins should be dry to facilitate adherence of final dressing.

Reusable kits should be clean and stored according to manufacturers instructions. Disposable equipment should be discarded in accordance with facility medical waste policy.

Refer to procedure for specific dressing.

Packing a Wound with Gauze

PURPOSE

To pack a wound with gauze strips or pads to facilitate wound healing

STAFF RESPONSIBLE

EQUIPMENT

1. Gauze strip per physician's order
2. Prescribed cleansing agents
3. Sterile suture removal kit (use for first packing, and keep scissors as reusable item)
4. Dressing pack, including:
   - Sterile gloves
   - Sterile dressings or fluffs
   - Forceps
   - Plastic bag and tie
   - Tape
   - Folding basin
5. Sterile field
6. Waste bag

 ## GENERAL CONSIDERATIONS

1. Patients on isolation or precautions should be treated per infection control guidelines.

2. Gauze should reach the active depths of the wound but should not be packed tightly. Tight packing can create additional tissue damage.

3. The distal end of the gauze strip should extend beyond the opening of the wound to allow easy removal. Use only one strip.

4. Scissors need not be sterile but must be clean for each packing procedure.

5. Label gauze bottle and solutions with name, date, and time opened.

6. Iodoform gauze is active as long as its odor can be detected in the bottle.

7. Wound packing can be used with stages III and IV pressure ulcers to achieve healing from the tissue depths to the skin surface and to aid in the debriding of necrotic tissue. In most situations, surgery will eventually be done to close stages III and IV ulcers.

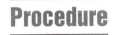 **Procedure**

 Steps

1. Refer to General Wound Care for steps of routine wound care.

2. Open dressing pack and scissors. Prepare sterile field.

3. Remove old gauze while wearing sterile gloves or using forceps.

4. Observe amount, color, and odor of drainage and condition of wound tissue.

 Additional Information

Note length of gauze or number of pads removed.

5. Discard dressing and forceps or gloves.

6. Don sterile gloves.

7. Cleanse wound, working from middle to outside edges. Irrigate wound if necessary.

Deep-tunneling wounds may require irrigation to cleanse.

8. Gather amount of gauze needed into sterile gloved hand.

Amount needed can be approximated from previous packing. Cut close to mouth of bottle to prevent contamination.

9. Hold gauze taut between thumb and fingers, and cut it cleanly with scissors.

10. Pack slowly into wound with sterile forceps held in other hand. Do not touch edges of wound.

If diameter of wound is small, wooden end of sterile cotton-tipped applicators may be used to introduce gauze instead of forceps.

11. Apply dressing over wound and adhere with tape or binder.

Remove gloves before applying tape, and discard them in plastic bag. Tape all four sides of dressing.

12. Close plastic waste bag and dispose of it.

Discard waste according to infection control procedures.

13. Store wound care supplies.

14. Wash hands.

15. Wash scissors with soap and water, and then clean scissors with Betadine, alcohol, or chlorine solution.

16. Store dry scissors in clean, covered container such as suture kit tray.

DOCUMENTATION

1. Document the treatment and description of the wound in the appropriate records.

2. Document any problems found in removing the old dressing and in packing the wound.

3. Document the patient's and family's ability to follow-through safely.

Skin Tears: Prevention and Management

PURPOSE

To prevent and manage skin tears, a traumatic injury to the skin of older adults

STAFF RESPONSIBLE

EQUIPMENT

1. Sterile normal saline

2. Sterile gauze dressings

3. Sterile cotton swabs

4. Kerlix

5. Clean and/or sterile gloves

6. Dressing as ordered by physician (e.g. Adaptic, Telfa, Op-Site, or Tegaderm)

7. Petroleum or antibacterial ointment if indicated

8. Skin protectant barrier wipes or sprays.

GENERAL CONSIDERATIONS

1. Skin tears occur most commonly on the extremities of older adults and are the result of a shearing or friction force which separates the epidermis from the dermis (Payne and Martin, 1990). Minor friction, shearing, or even a firm grasp can result in a skin tear.

2. Healing is significantly delayed in older adults, and the incidence of wound infections is much higher than for younger patients (Payne and Martin, 1990).

3. Prevention of skin tears is key. Safe moving, lifting, and transferring, along with elbow and shin protectors for the frail elderly, will prevent most skin tears.

4. The type and frequency of dressing changes will be ordered by the physician. Common options are:
   • Nonadherent dressing, such as Adaptic or Telfa, and Kerlix instead of tape. This works well for skin tears where the skin flap remains, and is usually changed daily.

- Adhesive (butterfly) strips, which are changed only as needed.
- Semipermeable membrane dressing, which may be used if no skin flap exists to cover the area. These are changed only every 5 to 7 days, but may be difficult to remove without damaging frail skin.

5. The nutritional status of the patient plays an important role in the risk of skin tears. Assess the nutritional status of elderly patients throughout their stay, using both clinical and laboratory findings.

6. Skin protectant barrier spray or wipes can be applied to intact fragile skin before adhesive tape is applied. Allow protectant barrier to dry thoroughly before applying tape. When the tape is removed, the protectant barrier is removed rather than skin. This is a preventative measure.

PATIENT AND FAMILY EDUCATION

Patient/patient caregiver should be taught the procedure prior to pass, or prior to discharge if no pass. Instructions include prevention, assessment, and treatment of skin tears.

Procedure

 Steps

 Additional Information

1. Set up necessary equipment.

    Set up disposal bag within close proximity.

2. If dressing currently in place, remove with nonsterile gloves and place in bag for disposal.

    Be sure to loosen dressing carefully, pulling in the direction of the skin tear.

3. Don sterile gloves.

4. If this is an initial dressing or the wound appears unclean, cleanse the wound with normal saline, moving in the direction of the skin tear only so as not to disrupt the epidermal flap.

    Cleansing too often may dissolve the fibrin clot holding the epidermal flap in place.

5. Pat wound margins dry with sterile gauze.

6. If there is a piece of viable skin (flap) partially attached, gently move it back into position.

    If skin flap is not viable, notify MD for debridement.

7. Apply a thin layer of petroleum or antibacterial ointment over wound with sterile cotton swab, according to MD orders.

    Apply in direction of skin tear only, to keep flap in place.

8. Cover wound with nonadhesive sterile dressing, according to physician order.

    Adaptic, Telfa, or butterfly straps are preferred methods when skin flaps are present. Semipermeable transparent dressing may be used on a wound with no protective skin flap.

9. Cover Adaptic, Telfa, or butterfly straps with Kerlix gauze.

    Use Kerlix, not tape, to hold dressing in place, as tape may further damage fragile skin.

10. Remove gloves.

11. Dispose of materials according to infection control guidelines.

 DOCUMENTATION

1. Document in progress notes the initial presentation of skin tear, any significant changes (at least weekly), and when skin tear is resolved.

2. Document any signs or symptoms of infection in progress notes and notify physician.

3. Document patient/family teaching and its success in progress notes or teaching checklist if indicated.

REFERENCES

Krasner, D. (1991) "An Approach to Treating Skin Tears" *Ostomy Wound Management* 32:56–58.

Payne, R.L. and Martin, M. (1990) "Skin Tears . . . The Epidemiology and Management of Skin Tears in Older Adults" *Ostomy Wound Management* 26:26–37.

Skin Rashes Caused by Urinary Incontinence

PURPOSE

To prevent and/or manage skin rashes caused by urinary incontinence

STAFF RESPONSIBLE

EQUIPMENT

As appropriate:
1. Cleanser or bath additive: pH compatible
2. Moisturizing cream/lotion: pH compatible
3. Moisture barrier ointment

 GENERAL CONSIDERATIONS

1. Patients at risk for moisture skin rashes include:
   - Patients incontinent of urine or stool
   - Diaphoretic patients
   - Elderly patients
   - Patients with dry skin
2. Skin should be assessed at least twice daily. At the first sign of a moisture/incontinence rash, a plan of care should be devised and implemented.
3. Proper moisturizing and cleansing of skin helps to keep it healthy (Hollingsworth, 1990), as well-hydrated skin acts as a barrier defense (Friers, 1996) and regulates the pliability of the epidermis.
4. Excessive moisture in contact with skin causes moisture buildup in the skin, which makes it more susceptible to breakdown (Panel for Prevention and Prediction of Pressure Ulcers, 1992). Macerated skin is more permeable to irritants (Friers, 1996). Stool and urine together lead more quickly to skin breakdown and must be dealt with quickly.
5. The pH of healthy skin is approximately 5.5. This acid mantle helps prevent infection. Urine pH can be as high as 8, and both urine and stool have caustic enzymes which may be harmful to skin (Hollingsworth, 1990).
6. Excessive bathing with soap and hot water may dry skin.
7. Alterations in skin integrity may be prevented by gentle cleansing after incontinence with a pH balanced cleanser (pH of 4 to 7) and followed if needed by a pH balanced moisturizer or barrier.
8. Adequate fluid intake is necessary to maintain good skin hydration.
9. As rashes may be due to a number of etiologies, assessment and treatment of rashes should be done in consultation with a physician. A rash of unknown etiology or that does not respond to nursing treatment measures should be diagnosed by a physician.

PATIENT AND FAMILY EDUCATION

The patient and/or family should be taught methods to prevent moisture rashes and to promote healthy skin, proper recognition and treatment of moisture rashes.

 Steps

1. Assess skin daily for signs of moisture rash.
2. Keep skin warm.
3. Keep skin clean and dry.
4. Use skin moisturizers/lubricants to prevent dry skin, but use in moderation.
5. Minimize/eliminate urinary incontinence (use toileting programs, incontinence devices, etc.).
6. Minimize/eliminate fecal incontinence through toileting/bowel programs. Eliminate causes of diarrhea.

 Additional Information

If rash present, determine if due to moisture.

Promotes vasodilation.

Excessive moisture can irritate skin.

Moisturizers help prevent dry skin, but too much lotion may cause skin breakdown.

Assess cause of change in incontinence (medication, UTI, increased disorientation, etc.).

If diarrhea is frequent, consider use of external collection device.

7. If diapers/incontinence pads must be used, change often, cleanse skin, and apply moisture barrier.

8. Cleanse after each incontinent episode with a gentle cleanser.

9. Pat dry (do not rub) and allow to air dry as much as possible.

10. Follow cleansing, if appropriate, with a barrier product.

11. Avoid use of talcum powders—if powders are necessary use refined cornstarch.

12. Encourage adequate oral fluid intake and a well-balanced high protein diet.

13. Avoid friction/shearing when moving patient.

Diapers/pads hold in heat and moisture, leading to skin breakdown.

Urine/stool left on skin and excessive use of soap will lead to skin breakdown.

The friction of washing can denude macerated skin.

These help keep moisture and irritants from contact with skin.

Talc can irritate skin.

DOCUMENTATION

1. Document skin assessment, incontinence assessment, and risk of acquiring moisture rashes.

2. Document plan of care regarding management of incontinence and other risk factors.

3. Document any changes in skin status and response to treatment plan.

REFERENCES

Friers, S.A. (1996) "Breaking the Cycle: The Etiology of Incontinence Dermatitis and Evaluation and Using Skin Care Products" *Ostomy Wound Management* 42(3):32–43.

Hollingsworth, M.B. (1990) "First Things First: Prevention and Treatment of Skin Irritation Caused by Urinary Incontinence" *Journal of Urological Nursing* 9(2):869–882.

Kramer, D. (1988) "Diaper Dermatitis in the Hospitalized Child" *Journal of Enterostomal Therapy* 15(4):167–170.

U.S. Department of Health and Human Services. (1992) *Pressure Ulcers in Adults: Prediction and Prevention. Clinical Practice Guideline No.3* AHCPR Publication No. 92-0047. Rockville, MD: Agency for Health Care Policy and Research.

U.S. Department of Health and Human Services. (1994) *Treatment of Pressure Ulcers. Clinical Practice Guideline No. 15* AHCPR Publication No. 95-0652. Rockville, MD: Agency for Health Care Policy and Research.

Care of Wounds/Skin in the Burn Patient

PURPOSE

To heal any skin/soft tissue areas caused by burns. To teach the burn patient long-term skin care management.

STAFF RESPONSIBLE

EQUIPMENT

1. Sterile dressings as needed

2. Topical agents as ordered by MD

3. Non-perfume, non-deodorant soap and lotion

GENERAL CONSIDERATIONS

1. Burns are classified as: superficial (1), partial thickness (2), full thickness (3), and electrical burn.

2. Burn patients are generally admitted to RIC following escharotomy, surgical debridement, &/or skin grafting with autographs or cultured epithelium.

3. The goals for wound care are as follows:
   • Continue wound healing using methods prescribed by the referring burn unit.
   • Prevent infection.
   • Protect new skin from further trauma, focusing attention on healed areas and donor sites.

4. The most common method of wound care is the close technique gauze dressing. This helps to limit evaporative fluid loss and prevent infection. Coarse mesh traps serous exudate and liquified eschar. Fine mesh protects vascular tissue and newly formed epitheilial buds.

5. Nursing observations include checking for signs/symptoms of:
   • Impaired circulation (e.g., pain, numbness, tingling).
   • Infection (e.g., odor, erythema, fever, tachycardia).

6. Topical agents help to prevent infection and hasten healing of burns. Agents include:
   • *Sulfamylon:* bacteriostatic for gram (+) and (−) organisms. Side effects may include metabolic acidosis.
   • *Silver Sulfadine (Silvadone):* affects gram (+), (−), and candida albicans. Grayish appearance in wound may simulate an infection. Side effects may include sensitivity reactions, leukopenia.
   • *Silver Nitrate:* applied wet to burn surface. Retains moisture and heat, decreases evaporation. Stains on contact.
   • *Neomycin/Bacitracin:* bacteriocidal. Prolonged use may lead to toxic effects.

7. Hydrotherapy is often used with burn patients as a less painful method of dressing removal. It cleanses the wound by loosening eschar and debris. Hydrotherapy also facilitates range-of-motion exercises by minimizing energy expenditure and discomfort. Hydrotherapy is performed 1-2 times daily for no more than 30 minutes to prevent chilling. Sterile technique is followed as possible until wounds are healed.

8. Long-term skin care of the burn patient after wound healing includes:
   • *Bathing:* daily with a non-deodorant, non-perfume soap. Use tepid water, avoid extreme temperatures, prevent chilling.
   • *Skin care:* As dry flaking skin is common, use a non-perfume water-based lotion (Lubriderm, Eucerin, Nutraderm) several times daily to mimic natural lubrication.

   • *Itching:* often accompanies dry skin. Avoid scratching which may tear new skin. Medications may help, including Benadryl and Atarax.
   • *Blisters:* commonly develop over healed areas. Protect and keep clean using a non-adherant dressing. Avoid constriction.
   • *Sensitivity:* Skin is thinner and more fragile until the scar matures. Avoid direct sunlight by covering all burns, wear light colored clothes and a hat. Compensate for increased sensitivity to cold by wearing several layers of clothing. As skin toughens, sensitivity will decrease.

9. Contractures are the most serious long-term complication of burns. Procedures to minimize contractures of the scar and joint include: proper wound and skin care, proper positioning, splinting, exercising, and use of pressure dressings. These measures must be instituted early, and continued until the scar matures (about 1 year).

10. Pressure dressings aid in circulation, cover and protect scars, and minimize hypertrophic scarring. Types include elastic wrap (Ace), tubular support bandages, custom made garments, and foam padding (Elastomer). Protective dressings are worn 24 hours a day until the scar matures, and weight gain or loss will require refitting of the dressing. Dressings may be removed 1 hour per day for hygiene. Two sets of garments are often ordered to allow for continuous wear and cleaning. For pediatric patients garments may be ordered in special colors or designs. Nursing management includes evaluating tolerance and blister formation, monitoring weight gain/loss, educating the patient and family, and evaluating their compliance with the dressing.

11. Other areas of concern to be addressed in the burn patient area: nutrition, pain management, psychosocial adjustment, body image, and sexuality. Please see references for further information on these topics.

PATIENT AND FAMILY EDUCATION

Educate the patient and family regarding the treatment of burns and prevention of complications.

DOCUMENTATION

1. Document any changes in the burn sites, signs/symptoms of infection, untoward reactions, or complications.

2. Document patient/family teaching and its success in the medical record or teaching checklist.

See attached chart of burn characteristics.

REFERENCES:

Artz, C., Moncrief, J., & Pruitt, B. (1979). Burns: A Team Approach. Philadelphia: W.B. Saunders Co. pp. 500–571.

Malik, M.H. & Carr, J.A. (1982). Manual on Management of the Burn Patient. Pittsburgh: Harmarville Rehabilitation Center.

(1983). Application of Biochemical Approach. In C.A. Trombly, Ed.: Occupational Therapy for Physical Dysfunction. Baltimore: Williams & Wilkins, pp. 399–408.

CHAPTER 5

Procedures to Manage Respiratory Function

Introduction

Approximately one of five Americans has some form of respiratory disease. A history of premorbid respiratory disease coupled with a neurologic disability, as is commonly seen in the rehabilitation setting, can put the individual at risk for respiratory complications.

Respiration involves mechanical, neurologic, and chemical controls. Respiration involves delivery of oxygen to the cells and removal of carbon dioxide. Air moves in and out of the lungs by means of a mechanical process called ventilation. Ventilation is regulated by neurologic centers in the brainstem and chemoreceptors in the vascular system. The neurologic centers and chemoreceptors regulate the rate, rhythm, and depth of inspiration. Ventilation consists of two phases: inspiration and expiration. Inspiration is an active process in which the diaphragm and intercostal muscles contract and create a negative intrapulmonary pressure that draws air into the lungs. Expiration under normal circumstances is a passive process that occurs when the intrapulmonary pressure is greater than atmospheric pressure. A forceful expiration is required to produce a cough or sneeze; this requires muscular effort from the abdominal and internal intercostal muscles (Stevens, 1987).

Injuries to the brainstem that might occur with stroke or head injury, can damage neuroregulatory centers and produce an irregular respiratory pattern. Damage to the cranial nerves, in particular IX (glossopharyngeal) and X (vagus), will interfere with the gag reflex and airway protection, thus putting the individual at great risk for aspiration (see Chap. 1).

After a spinal cord injury, an impairment of respiratory function may also occur. If the damage to the cord occurs at C3 or above, mechanical ventilation will be necessary. This may be accomplished with a mechanical ventilator or with phrenic nerve stimulators. Damage to the cervical and upper thoracic levels of the cord can result in decreased vital capacities and a weak, ineffective cough.

Brain damage and spinal cord injury are disabilities commonly encountered in rehabilitation that affect respiratory function. Nursing procedures address measures to optimize respiratory function, to maintain a patent airway, to prevent potential injury, and to utilize equipment associated with respiratory function.

When discussing procedures in rehabilitation, it is important to keep in mind some basic tenets of rehabilitation:

Rehabilitation is goal directed, and goals are mutually set with the patient and family.

Mobility is encouraged, and as the patient becomes more mobile (either ambulatory or in wheelchair) special adaptations of procedures may be necessary.

Patient and family education is a major goal. Educating the patient and family about procedures is an ongoing process.

Programs for care in the home must be able to be performed safely by caregivers, and necessary equipment must be available to the patient and family.

The procedures in this chapter address these issues as they pertain to respiratory care for the patient in rehabilitation and were developed in conjunction with the respiratory therapy staff.

Oxygenation: Measurement and Management

Pulse Oximetry (Single Determination)

PURPOSE

To measure and assess oxygen saturation via noninvasive means to guide treatment or evaluate patient oxygen saturation response to changes in activity

STAFF RESPONSIBLE

EQUIPMENT

1. Pulse oximeter
2. Probe compatible with oximeter (adult finger, child finger, ear probe)

GENERAL CONSIDERATIONS

1. Pulse oximetry is a useful tool in conjunction with other respiratory assessments in guiding and directing respiratory therapy care. A pulse oximeter reading is only one aspect of a patient's respiratory status.

2. The handheld pulse oximeter is intended for "spot checks or single reading determinations" only. If a patient requires continuous monitoring of pulse oximetry, the physician must order "continuous oximetry".

3. A physician order is required to perform a single determination or spot check pulse oximeter reading. The physician order may be entered as a prn order to obtain a reading when a change in patient condition is noted. Signs and symptoms of changes in respiratory status include, but are not limited to: tachypnea, cyanosis, respiratory distress, cardiac symptoms, change in mental status, dizziness, change in vital signs, seizures. A single determination spot check may also be ordered to evaluate patient response to changes in oxygen prescription.

4. For all newly admitted patients on oxygen therapy (F_{IO_2} > 21%) the nurse can be directed by a standing order to obtain a pulse oximetry reading as part of an initial assessment. It is not necessary to obtain readings on patients with high humidity collars on room air.

5. There are conditions when an incorrect reading may occur such as peripheral vascular disease, nail polish, dark skin tones, and cold extremities.

Procedures

 Steps

1. Gather equipment. Wash hands. Explain procedure to the patient.
2. Wipe sensor with alcohol pad. Allow to dry.
3. Turn machine on and wait for machine to perform internal self-check. When internal self-check is complete the machine will beep.
4. Place probe on appropriate body part (finger probe will be most commonly used), with sensor facing toward the fleshy part of the skin (Fig. 5-1).

 Additional Information

If machine fails to perform or problems occur with the self-check process, do not use the machine.

For patients with dark skin it may be necessary to place the sensor facing the nail bed rather than fleshy part of the finger. It may be necessary to remove nail polish.

5. The machine will take a few seconds to read out pulse rate and oxygen saturation (%). Allow time for both to stabilize. When reading stabilizes record the result.

6. Leave sensor on for one full minute and note any variation that occurs.

7. Remove probe. Clean probe with alcohol and allow to air dry.

Excessive movement can create motion artifact. Document the stabilized numbers but note the lowest reading obtained in the process.

If readings are suspect in terms of accuracy, move sensor probe to a second site and repeat steps 4 to 6.

For patients on special precautions clean probe with cleaning agent approved by Infection Control at your institution.

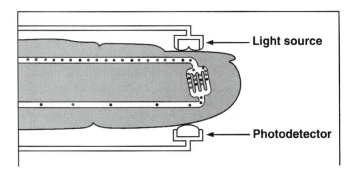

Figure 5-1   A sensor device that contains a light source and a photodetecter is placed around a pulsating arteriolar bed, such as the finger, great toe, nose, or earlobe. Red and infrared wavelengths of light are used to determine arterial oxygen saturation. (Reprinted with permission from *Principles of Pulse Oximetry*, Hayward, CA: Nellcor, Inc. 1988.)

DOCUMENTATION

1. Document in the appropriate record:
   - Result of readings and notify physician if reading is less than 95% or in accordance with parameters written by physician.
   - Respiratory condition changes, making note to indicate signs and symptoms exhibited by the patient and pulse oximeter reading.
   - Circumstances necessitating the procedure, current FIO_2 and respiratory rate to assist in interpretation and to correctly identify source of measurement.

PATIENT AND FAMILY EDUCATION

1. Explain rationale and procedure to patient and family, including significance of proper sensor placement.

2. Encourage cooperation in consistent placement of probe to assist in decreasing movement artifact.

3. Explain conditions that may interfere with light source and readings (nail polish, poor peripheral circulation, etc.).

REFERENCES

American Society for Testing and Materials (1992) *Standard Specification for Pulse Oximeters* Philadelphia, PA.

APIC (1996) *Infection Control and Applied Epidemiology, Principles, and Practice* St. Louis, MO: Mosby.

Gilboy, N. and McGaffigan, P. (1989) "Noninvasive Monitoring of Oxygenation with Pulse Oximetry" *Journal of Emergency Nursing* 15(1):26–31.

Grap, M.J. (1996) *Pulse Oximetry, Technology Series* American Association of Critical Care Nurses.

Noninvasive Pulse Oximeter Product Information Handout, (1997) Nellcor Inc. Hayward, CA.

Stevens, K. (1987) "Autonomic Regulation and Respiratory Function: Section 2 Respiratory Function: Alterations in Airway Clearance" in Matthews, P.J. and Carlson, C.E. (e   ds.) *Spinal Cord Injury: a Guide to Rehabilitation Nursing* Rockville, MD: Aspen.

Technology Assessment Task Force. "A Model for Technology Assessment Applied to Pulse Oximetry" *Critical Care Medicine* 21(4):615–624.

Oxygen Therapy

PURPOSE

To reverse and prevent tissue hypoxia; to treat or correct arterial hypoxemia; to decrease the work of breathing; to increase the efficiency of myocardial work

STAFF RESPONSIBLE

EQUIPMENT

1. Oxygen source (i.e., H. tank, E. tank, compressor, liquid oxygen, wall unit)
2. Flow meter
3. Humidifier (if flow is greater than 4 L/min or if patient at risk of dry mucous membranes)
4. Oxygen delivery device prescribed
5. "No Smoking" sign (not necessary in a nonsmoking environment)

GENERAL CONSIDERATIONS

1. The need for oxygen therapy must always be based on sound clinical judgment aided by arterial blood gas measurement or pulse oximetry (pulse ox) and a physician's order. Hypoxemia may elicit a compensatory increase in ventilatory and cardiac work; thus, the cardiopulmonary system works harder and total oxygen requirements are increased at times (Shapiro, Harrison, & Trout, 1979).

2. All oxygen therapy orders must be written by a physician and should include delivery device, flow rate, and approximate concentrations and parameters for use.

3. Pulse oximetry and arterial blood gas measurements provide a clinical means of assessing and evaluating the physiologic effects of oxygen and documenting the need for continued oxygen therapy. It is suggested that the physician order a pulse ox or arterial blood gas measurements before initiating therapy and periodically during treatment to evaluate the effectiveness of the therapy. A recent (2 days prior to transfer) pulse ox or arterial blood gas measurement will be needed to get oxygen supplied for home use.

4. Using the correct oxygen delivery device is critical to provide proper oxygen concentrations. Oxygen delivery devices are not interchangeable. Table 5-1 lists the most common delivery devices, flow rates, and fraction of inspired oxygen (F_{IO_2}) concentrations provided. An F_{IO_2} of 21% is equivalent to room air oxygen concentration.

5. It is critical to ensure that an adequate volume of oxygen is available to the patient at all times. Special attention to volume available must be considered when oxygen is needed during transport, off-unit procedures, therapies, or showers.

6. Patients with a documented history of chronic obstructive pulmonary disease may need to be regulated on lower concentrations of oxygen.

7. Care should be exercised when handling equipment; refer to infection control guidelines. A good rule of thumb is to keep the oxygen at least 5 feet away from a source of ignition (cigarettes, hair dryers, etc.). Consult the safety engineer regarding oxygen safety requirements at your facility.

8. Respiratory equipment including oxygen may be necessary after discharge. Planning must start early. Consult available resources for additional information about equipment ordering.

Procedures

 Steps

1. Check physician order for method of delivery and flow rate.
2. Call orders to respiratory therapy department.

3. Gather equipment, wash hands, and explain procedure to patient.

 Additional Information

Respiratory therapy may be responsible for initial assembly of oxygen delivery system and for equipment checks each shift.

Anxiety can increase oxygen demand.

4. Assess patient's current respiratory status. Consider rate, effort, pulse, color, rhythm, pattern, and endurance.

5. Check patient room for safety:
   * All electrical equipment must be within acceptable limits as set by your agency.
   * "No Smoking" sign must be placed appropriately. Explain safety precautions to patients and visitors.

6. Apply specific delivery system.

7. Turn on oxygen and set flow rate.

Do not allow smoking or use of electrical equipment within 5 feet of oxygen source.

Table 5-1	Comparison of Oxygen Delivery Devices and Flow Rates		
Oxygen Delivery Device	**Flow Rate**	**F_{IO_2}**	**Comments**
Nasal Cannula	1L/min	24%	No humidity needed at rates of
	2L/min	28%	less than 4L/min.
	3L/min	32%	F_{IO_2} will vary considerably with
	4L/min	36%	changes in respiratory rate and
	5L/min	40%	tidal volume.
	6L/min	44%	Humidity is recommended.
Simple Face Mask	5L/min	40%	
	6L/min	50%	
	7L/min	60%	
High-Humidity Trach Collar	5–8L/min	28–30%	F_{IO_2} is set on nebulizer dial.
	10L/min	>35%	Concentrations range from 35–100%

At times physicians will order a nasal cannula at meals to replace a face mask. The equivalents are:

Simple Face Mask at 5L/min = Nasal Cannula at 5L/min
6L/min   6L/min
7L/min   7L/min

High-Humidity Mask at 35% = Nasal Cannula at 4L/min
40%   5L/min
60%   6L/min

Nasal Cannula Oxygen Therapy

 Steps

 Additional Information

1. Check nasal patency and condition of nares before inserting cannula initially and daily.

2. Check for reddened areas under nose and over ears.

3. Provide good nose and mouth care twice daily.

4. Verify correct flow rate and adequate volume in tank each shift. Replace/refill tank if volume is low.

5. Position cannula by inserting nasal prongs into each nostril so that curve follows natural contour of nostril.

6. Pass cannula tubing over both ears, and position it under chin.

7. Slide adaptor cinch to adjust fit.

Common hazards include obstructed nostrils, dryness, nasal trauma, bleeding, tissue necrosis, and mucosal drying.

Use water-soluble lubricant as needed.

See Liquid Oxygen Procedure for procedure on refilling tanks.

Simple Oxygen Mask

 Steps

 Additional Information

1. Check pressure points on face and over ears for redness or irritation.

2. Wash and dry patient's face thoroughly.

   Humidified air will create excess moisture on the face so it may be necessary to dry face every 1 to 2 h.

3. Provide mouth care once per shift.

4. Verify flow rate and adequate volumes in tank. Replace/refill tank if volumes are low.

   See Liquid Oxygen Procedure for procedure on refilling tanks.

5. Replace mask, and secure it with elastic strap around patient's neck at level of tragus of ear or around head above ear.

6. Adjust nose clip and strap so that mask fits snugly.

High-Humidity Tracheostomy Collar (HHTC)

 Steps

 Additional Information

1. Check patient's skin at tracheostomy site and posterior neck for signs of irritation or pressure.

2. Wash and dry patient's neck thoroughly, prn.

   High-humidity collars will cause accumulation of moisture on the skin.

3. Check nebulizer and, if necessary, attach new prefilled nebulizer container.

4. Plug in heater.

   Always attach nebulizer to heater before plugging heater into electrical outlet. Make certain hands are dry before plugging in heater. Warm air is less irritating to tracheobronchial lining. Cold air can induce bronchospasm, so heater should be used as much as possible.

5. Verify prescribed settings.

   Settings are prescribed by the physician. Check flow rate and setting on the nebulizer. With a HHTC the prescribed F_{IO_2} is set on the nebulizer. The flow rate from oxygen source to nebulizer is determined by standards in your institution.

6. Empty tubing of excess fluid every 1 to 2 h.

   Always disconnect tubing at junction as close to collar as possible and drain away from the patient into appropriate receptacle.

7. Place collar over tracheostomy and secure strap around patient's neck.

   Allow adequate slack on strap to prevent pressure on neck, but keep collar in proper alignment. Make sure trach is not corked.

8. Throughout administration, periodically assess respiratory status (rate, work of breathing, endurance, color, nature of secretions, and ability to mobilize secretions).

   Notify physician of changes.

9. Check oxygen delivery settings and oxygen volume every shift.

10. Maintain oxygen delivery system at all times as prescribed. Notify therapists of need for oxygen.

    Assure adequate volume of oxygen is present and settings are correct prior to transporting patient.

11. When oxygen therapy is discontinued, remove oxygen equipment and discard any disposable equipment.

    Disposal is according to infection control procedures.

DOCUMENTATION

1. Document in the appropriate record:
   - Assessment of the patient's status before initiation of therapy
   - Assessment of the patient's status each shift when active respiratory problem exists
   - When oxygen therapy is discontinued, including the patient's response
   - Any changes in the patient's status, tolerance to therapy, or ability to keep the device in place
2. Note the care performed each shift.
3. Document patient and family teaching on the progress note or teaching checklist.

PATIENT AND FAMILY EDUCATION

1. Teach the patient and family about the type of oxygen therapy ordered, oxygen precautions, flow rate, therapeutic value, and flammable hazard.
2. Instruct the family on how to obtain and maintain necessary equipment.
3. Teach other specific procedures (i.e., pulse oximetry, tube changes, etc.) as appropriate.

REFERENCES

Shapiro, B., Harrison, R. and Trout, C.A. (1979) *Clinical Application of Respiratory Care*, 2d ed. Chicago: Year Book Medical Publishers.

Liquid Oxygen Therapy

PURPOSE

To provide an individual with a portable form of supplemental oxygen via cannula; to provide oxygen as prescribed for an individual's need

STAFF RESPONSIBLE

EQUIPMENT

1. Oxygen cannula
2. Liquid oxygen stationary unit
3. Stroller (portable liquid oxygen tank) (Fig. 5-2*C*)

GENERAL CONSIDERATIONS

1. Liquid oxygen is nonflammable; however, it will rapidly support and accelerate combustion. Common sense should prevail when using liquid oxygen.
2. A good rule of thumb is to keep the oxygen at least 5 feet away from a source of ignition (cigarettes, hair dryers, etc.). Consult the safety engineer regarding oxygen safety requirements at your facility.

3. The oxygen units are designed to be stored and operated in the upright position, otherwise leaking can occur. A loud screech is heard when unit is placed horizontally.
4. The liquid canister should be kept in a well-ventilated area. If it is used in a car, a window should be open slightly.
5. The walls of the canister are insulated, resembling a thermos, to keep the oxygen on the inside at a cold temperature. This is necessary to keep it in its liquid form.
6. When the flowmeter attached to the canister is turned on, the oxygen is warmed and delivered in the form of a gas without color, odor, or taste.
7. Keep hands away from the oxygen outlets while the portable tank is filling. The liquid oxygen temperature is far below freezing and may cause skin injuries similar to a burn.
8. Do not place any objects in the oxygen stream from the vent valve when filling the portable unit.
9. The unit should be checked for volume of oxygen once per shift or more frequently if flow rate is greater than 2 L/min, and prior to the patient leaving the unit.
10. Arrangements should be made with the home care vendor supplying the equipment for patient/family education prior to discharge when liquid oxygen will be used at home.

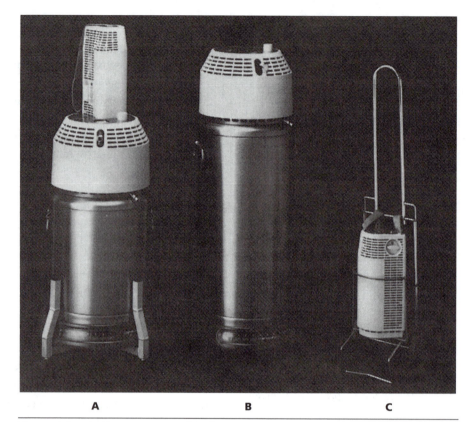

Figure 5-2 Liquid oxygen systems. (**A**) Filling Process, (**B**) Liberator, (**C**) Stroller. (*Source:* Courtesy of Mallinckrodt Inc. St. Charles, MO.

Procedures

(based on systems shown in Fig. 5-2)

To Fill Portable Unit from Stationary Unit

 Steps

 Additional Information

1. Clean connectors of moisture and dirt with a clean, dry, lint-free cloth.

2. Turn the flow valve selector off.

3. Hold the portable unit with both hands and position the contoured case over the matching recessed area on the cover of the stationary unit.

4. Lower the portable unit carefully into place taking care to assure proper engagement of quick connectors.

5. Place one hand on top of the portable unit directly over the quick connector and press straight down.

6. While holding the unit in the fill position, move the vent valve lever straight out to the open position (90 degrees from the normal off position).

7. With one hand maintain a slight downward pressure on the unit during filling to assure stability and proper fitting position.

Moisture can cause the portable and stationary units to freeze together.

This will lower the portable unit approximately ⅜ in. and assure proper engagement of the fill connectors.

This will result in a loud hissing noise. Note the time at start of fill.

8. Approximately 30 to 40 s into the filling procedure, close the valve for 5 s and reopen the vent valve one or more times.

9. Close the vent valve when the portable unit is full. A full unit is detected by a noticeable change in the sound of the venting gas or by the presence of dense white vapor around the cover of the stationary unit.

This will break up any ice that may have begun to form around the valve stem and serve to avoid any problems with the vent valve freezing open.

Though fill time may vary according to the temparature of the container being filled, anticipate fill time to be approximately 1 min and 30 s.

NOTE: *For any reason should the vent valve fail to close and the hissing continue, remove the portable unit by depressing the portable release button. The portable unit will stop venting in a few minutes.*

10. Disengage the portable unit from the stationary unit by holding the carrying strap above the unit and depressing the release button.

Should the units not disengage easily, it may have become frozen. DO NOT USE FORCE. *Simply allow a few moments for the frozen parts to warm and disengage when the ice has melted.*

WARNING: *Should liquid oxygen leakage occur when the portable unit is disengaged, proceed to reengage and disengage the unit again. This will help dislodge any ice or other obstruction. If liquid leakage is still present, notify supplier of stationary unit.*

11. Check the liquid oxygen contents indicator by lifting the portable unit by the end of the strap nearest the scale built into the top of the unit.

The liquid contents is indicated on the color-coded gauge.

 ## DOCUMENTATION

1. Document in appropriate record:
   - Assessment of the patient's status before initiation of therapy
   - Use of liquid oxygen, the time when the unit was filled, and routine equipment checks
   - When therapy is discontinued, and the patient's response

2. Document patient and family education in use of the equipment.

PATIENT AND FAMILY EDUCATION

Patient and family education for use at home should be arranged with the home care vendor supplying the equipment.

REFERENCES

Liquid Oxygen Systems. Mallinckrodt Inc. St. Charles, MO.

Self-Nebulizing Therapy

PURPOSE

To describe method of self-administration of nebulizer therapy using a home nebulizer unit; to describe role of the nurse in supervising patient performance

STAFF RESPONSIBLE

EQUIPMENT

1. Bedside nebulizer unit as prescribed (Pulmo-aide, Medimist, Schuco-mist). Units available from respiratory equipment vendor.

2. Prescribed medication.

3. Clean plastic bag.

4. Sterile saline (0.45 or 0.9 as prescribed).

5. Tissues.

6. Syringe.

 ## GENERAL CONSIDERATIONS

1. Goals of aerosol (nebulizer) therapy are:
   - To aid bronchial hygiene by restoring mucous blanket continuity; hydrating dry, retained secretions; and promoting expectoration
   - To humidify inspired gases
   - To deliver medications

2. Equipment brought in from home must be checked for electrical safety according to institute policies.

3. Nebulizers may run off oxygen source or compressed air provided by bedside unit.

4. Disposable nebulizers should be changed in accordance with infection control policies (usually every 24 h). For inpatients using their own reusable nebulizers from home, the nebulizer cups are to be sterilized in sporicidin solution or other approved solution every Monday, Wednesday, and Friday in the area approved by your institutional policy.

5. A physician order is necessary to initiate treatment and should include treatment, frequency, and prescribed medication.

6. Assess for the following symptoms:
   - Shortness of breath
   - Increased tightness in chest
   - Dyspnea
   - Headache
   - Chest pain
   - Shakiness or tremors
   - Dizziness

   NOTE: If any of these occur, stop treatment, notify physician, and resume treatment ONLY WITH PHYSICIAN APPROVAL.

7. Treatments should be spaced with a minimum of 4 h between sessions.

Procedures

 Steps

 Additional Information

1. Gather equipment. Verify physician order.

2. Explain purpose, method of treatment and side effects of medication to the patient.

   This procedure will be performed by the patient under the supervision of the nurse.

3. Wash hands.

4. Take baseline pulse.

   Note rate and rhythm. Do not start treatment if resting pulse is greater than 100 without physician approval.

5. Place prescribed medication dose in nebulizer and mix with saline (0.45 or 0.9) as prescribed.

   Generally 2 to 3 cc of saline is needed. Too much saline will dilute the solution.

6. Assist patient to comfortable position which allows for good chest expansion.

   Patient's posture should be relaxed and upright (Fowler's position) as much as possible.

7. Reinstruct patient in deep breathing techniques (diaphragmatic and lateral costal expansion) with an inspiratory pause on each breath.

8. Turn machine on and instruct patient to insert mouth piece and take slow deep breaths.

9. Check pulse 1 min after procedure is initiated.

   If significant change in rate or rhythm occurs, notify physician.

10. Monitor for side effects of medication. Instruct patient to report any adverse effects.

    See General Considerations # 6.

11. Continue treatment until medication is completely dispersed.

    Usually 10 to 15 min.

12. Wash nebulizer with water to remove excess medication.

13. Dry the nebulizer and store in clear plastic bag in well-lighted area.

14. Take pulse and check breath sounds.

DOCUMENTATION

1. Document medication administered, route, and time.
2. Document initial treatment, and periodically throughout patient stay:
   - Patient response to treatment: baseline pulse and pulse changes which occur; type, amount, consistency, and patient effort required to mobilize secretions; breath sounds before and after treatment; any adverse effects of treatment.
   - Patient participation in performing procedure and taking care of equipment.
3. Document any adverse effects which occur during treatment and actions taken for follow-up.

Use of Metered-Dose Inhalers (MDI)

PURPOSE

To facilitate the distribution and the effectiveness of the medication administered via metered-dose inhalers

STAFF RESPONSIBLE

EQUIPMENT

1. Inhaler
2. Delivery device

GENERAL CONSIDERATIONS

1. The effectiveness of the inhaled medication depends on how the inhaler is used.
2. There are three types of metered-dose inhalers available:
   - Bronchodilators [i.e., beta agonists; metaproterenol (Alupent), and albuterol (Ventolin, Proventil)]:
     - Produce both bronchodilation and cardiac stimulation.
     - Provide quick relief (in 5 to 15 min) and are used during an acute episode of breathlessness or routinely as prevention.
     - Enhances mucociliary transport.
     - Most common side effects: tachycardia and shakiness.
   - Corticosteroids (i.e., beclomethasone):
     - Reduce lung inflammation.
     - Used as a preventive measure, does not provide fast relief.
     - Most common side effects: hoarseness and dry mouth.

   - Mast cell inhibitors: [i.e., Intal (cromolyn)]:
     - Prevent mast cells in the lungs from releasing histamine and SRS-A (slow-reacting substance of anaphylaxis) after exposure to specific antigens.
     - Prevent bronchospasm induced by inhalation of specific antigens or by exercise.
     - Therapeutic benefit may not occur until 1 to 4 weeks after initiation of therapy .
     - They do *not* have direct bronchodilation, antihistamine, or anti-inflammatory effects.

     Most common side effects: bronchospasm, cough, nasal congestion, and wheezing.
3. The inhaler provides an exact dose of medication, so each dose must be inhaled completely.
4. Discourage use of any over-the-counter inhalants unless the patient checks with his/her physician. Most of these inhalants contain epinephrine, which is effective for only a short time and can cause excessive cardiac or CNS stimulation. In an attempt to maintain relief, the patient may use these inhalers too frequently, thereby overdosing and causing rebound bronchospasm.
5. Initiate patient/family education early and involve them in procedure as soon as possible.
6. If patient is to take a bronchodilator and a corticosteroid, administer the bronchodilator first. This dilates the airways so the corticosteroid can be inhaled more deeply into the lungs.
7. If using beclomethasone, patient should rinse mouth or gargle with water or mouthwash after use. This helps prevent fungal infections in the mouth and throat.
8. Most canisters contain 200 to 300 puffs of medication. The patient need not spray a dose into the air to see how much medication is left. Amount left in canister can be estimated when closed canister is floated in water. An empty canister floats (Fig. 5-3).
9. Use of a spacer must be considered for each MDI. Some inhalers have spacers built into device.

Place your canister in a bowl of water to determine the approximate number of doses remaining.

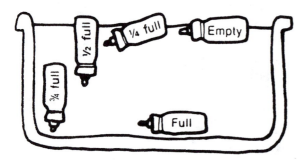

Refill your prescription when the canister is ¼ full.

Figure 5-3 How do I know when I need a refill?

Procedure

 Steps

 Additional Information

1. Put the inhaler parts together.

2. Shake the inhaler to mix the medication and propellant.

Insert into spacer, if using spacer.

Otherwise dosage may be inadequate.

3. Remove the cap from the device and the mouthpiece.

4. Hold the canister with your index finger and third finger on top and your thumb on the bottom.

5. Instruct patient to exhale completely through mouth at end of normal breath.

If patient is unable to perform own administration, cue patient to exhale through the mouth before administering medication.

6. Place the mouthpiece of the spacer in mouth, keeping tongue below the opening of the inhaler. KEEP MOUTH OPEN.

Inhalation should be slow for 3 to 5 s. If no spacer, place inhaler two fingers away from mouth.

7. Have patient inhale slowly and deeply while depressing the top of the canister.

8. Close mouth.

9. Have patient hold breath as long as he/she can comfortably (10 s is good).

This allows medication to be absorbed into bloodstream.

10. If two puffs are prescribed, wait 1 min before the second puff. If practical, it is optimal to take the second puff 10 to 15 min after the first.

This allows the first puff to dilate the airways, which will allow the second puff to penetrate more deeply into the bronchial tree.

11. Clean inhaler daily:
    • Remove the metal canister by pulling it up firmly
    • Rinse the plastic container under warm water
    • Dry it thoroughly

DOCUMENTATION

1. Document metered-dose inhaler and number of puffs administered.
2. Document initial administration, effectiveness of the procedure and any adverse reactions experienced.
3. Document patient/family education.

PATIENT AND FAMILY EDUCATION

1. Initiate patient and family education early, and involve the patient and family in the procedure as soon as possible.
2. See procedural steps related to patient and family education.

RESOURCES

Asthma and Allergy Foundation of America
1125 15th Street, NW Suite 502
Washington, DC 20005
(202) 466-7643, (800) 727-8462

Allergy & Asthma Network
Mothers of Asthmatics, Inc.
3554 Chain Bridge Road, Suite 200
Fairfax, VA 22030
(703) 385-4403, (800) 878-4403

National Asthma Education & Prevention Program
National Heart, Lung, and Blood Institute
1200 Wisconsin Avenue, Suite 500
Bethesda, MD 20854-0105
(301) 251-1222

American Academy of Allergy, Asthma, and Immunology
611 East Wells Street
Milwaukee, WI 53202
(800) 822-2762

National Jewish Center for Immunology and Respiratory Medicine
1400 Jackson Street
Denver, CO 80205
(800) 423-8891

American College of Allergy, Asthma, and Immunology
85 West Algonquin Road
Arlington Heights, IL 60005
(800) 842-7777

American Lung Association/American Thoracic Society
1740 Broadway
New York, NY 10019
(212) 315-8700, (800) 586-4872 (to contact local chapter)

Cough Enhancement

Cough Assist/Assistive Cough

PURPOSE

To loosen pulmonary secretions and force them into the upper respiratory tract where they can be expectorated or suctioned

CONTRAINDICATIONS

Procedure is contraindicated in patients with known or history of abdominal aortic aneurysm, pneumothorax, lung hemorrhage, tuberculosis, lung cancer.

SPECIAL CONSIDERATION

The presence of a vena cava filter may be considered a contraindication to subdiaphragmatic pressure during assistive cough. Others do not consider it a contraindication due to the risk of complications such as pneumonia without cough assist. The increase in abdominal pressure while performing abdominal thrusts may cause displacement or distortion of the filter. Placement and condition of the filter should be checked when able to be visualized on x-rays.

STAFF RESPONSIBLE

EQUIPMENT

1. Pillows
2. Kleenex
3. Emesis basin
4. Specimen cup (if culture ordered)
5. Gloves
6. Eye shields (as needed)
7. Suction equipment (as needed)

GENERAL CONSIDERATIONS

1. The cough is a reflex or voluntary action.
2. The mechanics of the cough involve:
   - Deep inspiration
   - Closure of the glottis

   - Contraction of the muscles of the chest wall, abdomen, and pelvic floor, which increase intrathoracic and intraabdominal pressure
   - Opening of the glottis
   - Rapid expulsion of air in the exhalation phase
3. Any disruption of the above steps in the cough mechanism may produce a need for assistive cough.
4. Several aspects of the patient's condition should be assessed:
   - Energy source for the cough
   - Ciliary movement
   - Structural abnormalities in airways or lung parenchyma
   - Neurologic function
   - Abdominal conditions (i.e., recent surgery) that would limit performance of procedure.
5. An effective cough should be low pitched and deep.
6. The patient will generally be able to cough more effectively following respiratory treatments but may require assistive coughing at other times throughout the day, i.e., position change, after eating or drinking. Exercise caution when performing cough assist within 1 h after a meal.
7. Assistive coughing is indicated on a prn basis for all patients with T6 or higher spinal cord injury or chronic lung disease and every 2 h or more in patients with active respiratory problems or a tracheostomy. Patients with a lesion as low as T11 may need assistive cough.
8. Technique and indications for assistive cough should be demonstrated and taught to patients and primary caregivers before first weekend pass.
9. An abdominal binder is often issued to patients with spinal cord injury who have loss of abdominal musculature, e.g., high paraplegia and quadriplegia, to increase intraabdominal pressure as adjunct to this procedure.
10. A "counter-rotation" method of assistive cough may be utilized for patients who are unable to follow instruction for taking a deep breath and coughing. This method is effective when patient is side-lying and trunk rotation is allowed.
11. Exercise caution in patients with sensation to minimize discomfort.
12. For patients with an implanted electrophrenic pacemaker make certain hand position is below level of pacer electrodes.

Procedure

 Steps

1. Explain procedure and rationale to the patient. Gather equipment.
2. Position patient.

3. Place hands
   - One- or two-handed abdominal thrust (Fig. 5-4)
   - Lateral costal border: two-handed with hands on diaphragm and thumbs meeting xiphoid process. (Fig. 5-5)
   - If side-lying, place one hand along the lower border of the rib cage on the side uppermost or use the one-handed abdominal thrust.

4. Instruct patient to take several deep breaths and try to hold breath for several seconds before coughing.
5. Instruct patient to turn head away form you and cough while you are pushing upward and inward against the diaphragm.
6. Steps 3 to 5 are repeated until secretions are expelled or patient is unable to produce secretions.
7. Check patient's respiratory status:
   - Color
   - Breathing rate
   - Breath sounds
   - Character of secretions
   - Ability to breathe alone
   - Ability to phonate

Additional Information

Sitting up straight or leaning forward pushes the diaphragm upwards and puts the patient in a position that facilitates exhalation. Consider each patient individually. For maximum comfort and to work with gravity other positions may be used including:
- *Side-lying*
- *Head down*
- *Supine*

Similar to subdiaphragmatic thrusts or Heimlich maneuver.

Patient may do this independently by placing wrists one on top of the other under the xiphoid process. Hand placement is critical in order to prevent injury to underlying organ.

For counter-rotation method, place one hand on topmost hip and one hand on topmost shoulder. When patient inhales, move hip forward and shoulder back. When patient exhales and coughs, move hip back and shoulder forward.

High volumes are necessary to generate a high expiratory flow to clear secretions.

EXCEPTION: *Lateral costal border cough assist in which hands push medially and inferiorly.*

Cough may prove ineffective if patient becomes tired or is unable to exert necessary force for cough.

Based on assessment, a plan should be instituted to:
- *Discontinue assist cough, let patient rest*
- *Suction secretions*
- *Request further respiratory treatment*
- *Increase hydration*
- *Implement other measures to loosen secretions.*

 DOCUMENTATION

Document:
1. Method and frequency of assistive cough.
2. Effectiveness of assistive cough, patient tolerance of procedure, need for suctioning, and unusual occurrences.

3. Patient teaching checklist and instruction or demonstration provided.
4. Implementation of procedure.

REFERENCES

Matthews, P.J., Carlson, C.E., and Holt, N.B. (1987) *Spinal Cord Injury: A Guide to Rehabilitation Nursing* Rockville, MD: Aspen.

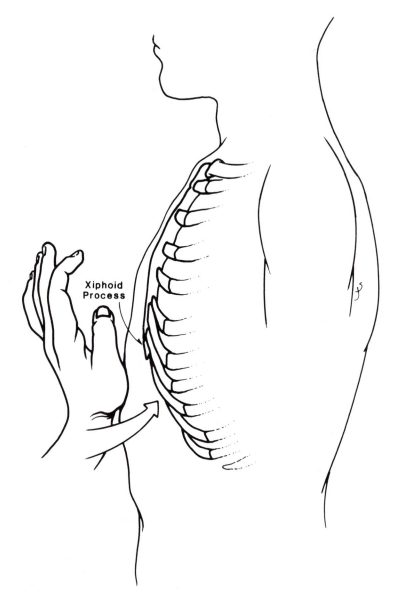

Figure 5-4 Assistive cough: Hand cupped over xiphoid process. Place hand (cupped) over xiphoid process. On exhalation, hand should move in and upward, assisting the diaphragm. [*Source:* From *Spinal Cord Injury: A Guide to Rehabilitation Nursing* (p. 227) by P.J. Matthews, C.E. Carlson, and N.B. Holt, 1987, Rockville, MD: Aspen Publishers, Inc. Copyright 1987 by Aspen Publishers, Inc.

Postural Drainage with Chest Percussion/Vibration

PURPOSE

To prevent the accumulation of secretions and possible infection; to mobilize and drain secretions

STAFF RESPONSIBLE

EQUIPMENT

1. Stethoscope

2. Pillows and/or positioning aids

3. Tissues

4. Emesis basin or sputum cup

5. Suction equipment (as needed)

6. Gloves

7. Eye shields

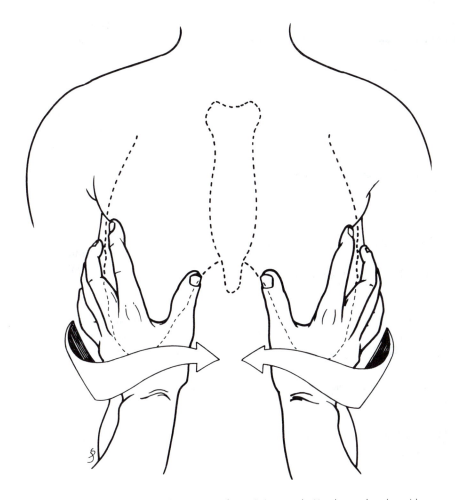

Figure 5-5 Hand location and movement for assistive cough. Hands are placed on side of rib cage. On exhalation, push inward and up following normal anatomic movement. [*Source:* From *Spinal Cord Injury: A Guide to Rehabilitation Nursing* (p 227) by P.J. Matthews, C.E. Carlson, and N.B. Holt, 1987, Rockville, MD: Aspen Publishers, Inc. Copyright 1987 by Aspen Publishers, Inc.]

GENERAL CONSIDERATIONS

1. Postural drainage is the use of specific positions to drain specific lung segments and bronchi by gravity. Percussion and vibration is the use of tapping and vibrating the chest wall to assist in mobilizing secretions.

2. In the acutely ill and/or injured patient modified positions may be used since the general condition of the patient frequently may not allow for a great amount of patient manipulations. If this is the case, specific rotational positions for the particular patient should be discussed with the physician.

3. Postural drainage is indicated when there is an accumulation of secretions which may occur with:
   • Atelectasis
   • Obstructive lung disease (asthma, bronchitis, bronchiectasis)
   • Cystic fibrosis
   • Post-op or bedridden patient with retained secretions
   • Prophylactic in patients with high cervical injuries, multiple sclerosis, or cerebral palsy prone to aspiration

4. Contraindications:
   • Unstable cardiovascular system
   • Fractured ribs or flail chest
   • Hemorrhagic conditions
   • Empyema
   • Increased intracranial pressure
   • Unstable spine
   • Recent skin grafts
   • Recent spinal fusion
   • Recent craniotomy
   • Untreated tension pneumothorax
   • Hemoptysis

- Diagnosed or suspected pulmonary embolus
- Abdominal aortic aneurysm

5. Respiratory therapy treatments if ordered (IPPB aerosol or nebulizer) should precede postural drainage for maximal effectiveness.

6. The effectiveness of postural drainage is enhanced when combined with percussion and vibration.

7. The following conditions represent situations in which consultation with physician is advised before performing postural drainage:
   - Metastatic cancer
   - Pulmonary embolus and anticoagulant therapy
   - Osteoporotic changes
   - Empyema
   - Possible pneumothorax.

8. Areas to consider in decreasing frequency or stopping treatments include:
   - Ability to adequately mobilize secretions with cough assist
   - Breath sounds
   - Activity level: if up and about this may be adequate enough to mobilize secretions
   - Sputum production: is it absent, decreased in amount, easily mobilized
   - Mental state: can follow instructions and maintain own bronchial hygiene
   - Absence of signs of respiratory infection or retained secretions (elevated temperature, elevated white blood count, color of sputum).

9. Auscultate breath sounds prior to and following procedure.

10. Do not perform for 1 to 2 h after administering tube feeding unless order obtained from physician for concurrent treatment with feedings.

11. A patient who is in pain should have treatment coordinated with pain medication.

12. In the acutely ill or injured patient, percussion and vibration must be ordered by the physician.

13. If unable to raise the front of the bed, place pillows under the hip to achieve a head-down position.

14. Percussion should be done only over the rib cage. Areas on the clavicle, scapula, and vertebrae should be very gently percussed. Areas over the breasts and kidney should not be percussed.

15. Cough alone is of limited value beyond sixth and seventh generation of bronchial branching. Percussion and vibration move secretions from narrow passages to wider ones where cough is effective.

16. The four positions—right side lying, left side lying, supine, and prone with pillows under the hips—will facilitate overall drainage of the lung and can be taught to patients who will need postural drainage at home.

17. Generally it is best done early in the morning as decreased mobility at night may increase secretion retention.

18. Percuss and vibrate the bases and apex of the lungs to center of the chest. Cough assist or suctioning may be needed to help expel secretions.

Procedure

 Steps

1. Explain procedure to the patient. Gather equipment.
2. Place patient in proper position for drainage (Fig. 5-6).

3. Maintain position at least 5 to 10 min. Do not leave patient when in postural drainage.

4. If ordered, perform percussion 5 to 10 min to specific area being drained while in position. Cup hands (finger and thumbs together) and rhythmically and alternately strike the chest wall.

 Additional Information

Area of lung to be emphasized should be assessed through looking at chart; chest assessment, especially breath sounds; x-rays; and consultation with the physician. If bed does not allow for Trendlenburg positioning, pillows may be used to achieve a head-down position. For children, procedures may be done most effectively with child on lap.

Maintain position longer if it is productive.

Cupping of the hands provides a cushion of air between the hands and the chest to eliminate irritation or pain. Sound produced is a muffled clap not slap. Use thin sheet or piece of clothing between your hand and patient.

5. If ordered, perform vibration for three to five breaths. Ask patient to take a deep breath. Perform vibration on exhalation only. Keep elbows straight and gently shake chest wall.

6. Cough and/or suction following treatment.

7. Repeat steps 3, 4, 5, and 6 in all positions. Evaluate which positions are productive and discontinue unproductive positions.

Pressure from vibration on inhalation will limit chest expansion. The vibration technique entails short, quick, fine jerking movements. The power comes from the shoulder of the person doing the technique.

Secretions may continue to be expectorated 1 h later.

 DOCUMENTATION

1. Document frequency of procedure.

2. Document procedure performed.

3. In progress notes:
   - Indications for procedure
   - Effectiveness of treatment
   - Any unusual occurrences

4. Document patient/family education.

REFERENCES

Matthews, P.J., Carlson, C.E., and Holt, N.B. (1987) *Spinal Cord Injury: A Guide to Rehabilitation Nursing* Rockville, MD: Aspen.

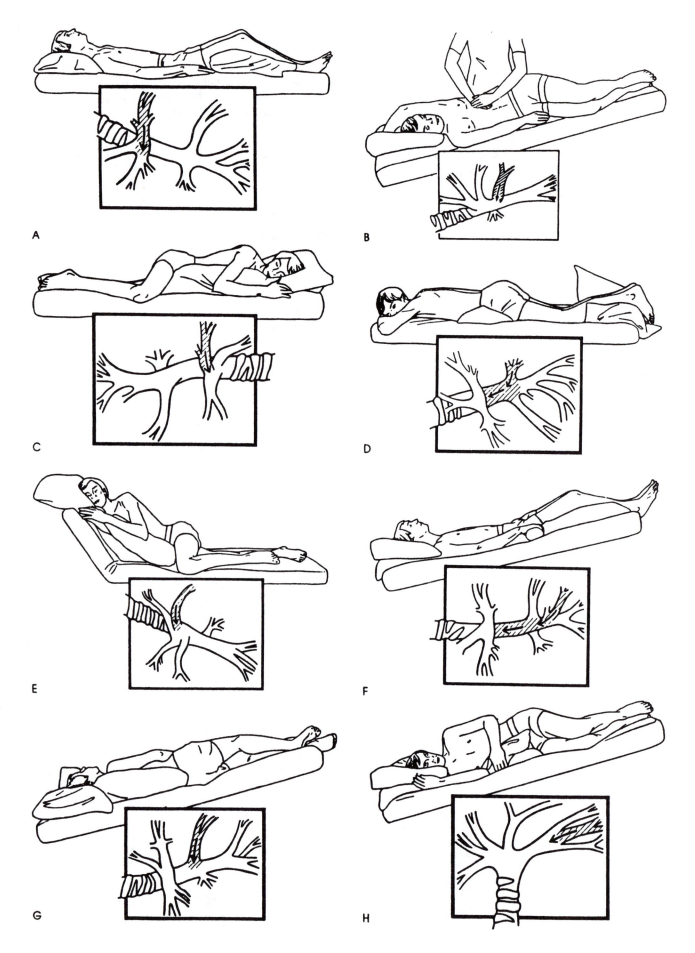

A

B

C

D

E

F

G

H

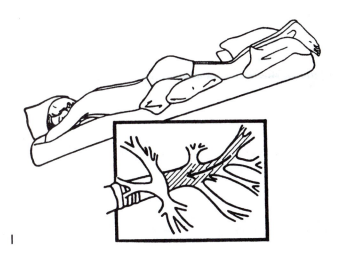

Figure 5-6 Positions for complete postural drainage (in sequence). (*A*) Upper lobes, anterior segments. (*B*) Upper lobe, posterior segment, right posterior bronchus. (*C*) Upper lope, posterior segment, left posterior bronchus. (*D*) Right middle lobe. (*E*) Left lingula. (*F*) Lower lobes, apical segment. (*G*) Lower lobes, anterior basal segment. (*H*) Lower lobe, lateral basal segment. (*I*) Lower lobes, posterior basal bronchus. [Figure adapted from M.L. Morrison (ed.), *Respiratory Intensive Care Nursing*, 2d ed. Boston. Little Brown, 1979. Reproduced by permission.]

Incentive Spirometry
(Sustained Maximal Inspiratory Therapy)

PURPOSE

To optimize lung inflation, optimize cough mechanism and early detection of acute pulmonary disease

STAFF RESPONSIBLE

EQUIPMENT

1. Incentive spirometer
2. Kleenex
3. Soap/water

GENERAL CONSIDERATIONS

1. The incentive spirometer promotes sustained maximal inspiration, a technique used for prophylactic bronchial hygiene. Several models are available but all work on same principle.

2. Studies indicate that inflated alveoli remain open for at least 1 h after treatment.

3. Advantages of incentive spirometry therapy include:
   - Effective prophylactic technique
   - Patient able to do therapy frequently without supervision once skill has been learned
   - Acute pulmonary disease is reflected in changes in performance (decreased volume and timing)
   - Minimal staff time is required

4. A physician's order is needed to initiate therapy.

5. Criteria for incentive spirometry include:
   - Patient must be cooperative and able to take voluntary deep breaths
   - Inspiratory capacity greater than 12 mL/kg
   - Respiratory rate under 25 per min
   - Patients should be without acute atelectasis, pneumonia, or obvious retained secretions

6. For patients with an open tracheostomy tube, a tracheostomy adaptor is used so that the spirometer is attached to the tracheostomy tube.

Procedure

Steps

Additional Information

1. Gather equipment. Explain procedure to patient and wash hands.

2. Position patient.

   Semi-Fowler's is advantageous for lung expansion. Avoid restrictive clothing or bed linens.

3. Rinse mouthpiece with warm water.

4. Connect mouthpiece to end of tubing.

5. Slide flow rate indicator to prescribed level.

   Inspiratory goal should be twice patient's tidal volume.

6. Instruct patient to take four slow easy breaths.

7. After fourth inhalation have patient let out all air until he or she can exhale no more.

8. Position unit in upright position and put mouthpiece into mouth.

   Tilting the device toward the patient at 30 to 45 degrees can reduce the amount of work required.

9. Instruct patient to make a tight seal on mouthpiece.

10. Instruct the patient to take a *slow* deep breath on spirometer.

    Do not blow into the unit. It works on inspiration not expiration.

11. Patient should try to inhale and hold breath for 3 to 5 s or as tolerated.

    Note how high patient raises ball and length of time it is held in place.

12. Have patient exhale totally.

13. Take a moment to relax then resume exercise.

    With rapid use sustained maximal inspiratory effort cannot be attained and may lead to hyperventilation.

14. Repeat steps 6 to 13 as prescribed.

    Generally, four to five breaths every 1 to 2 h unless otherwise indicated. For patients with T6 or higher level of injury, routine use should be at least three times a day.

15. Encourage cough and deep breathing.

16. Clean mouthpiece with soap and warm water and store unit in its bag.

DOCUMENTATION

1. Document initial use and changes. Information should include the following:
   - Respiratory status
   - Current performance: volume, frequency
   - Position of patient and unit
   - Signs and symptoms of fatigue, respiratory distress

2. Document prescribed frequency of treatment.

3. All staff documents procedure performed.

4. Document patient/family education and competence.

REFERENCES

Shapiro, B. A., Harrison, R. A., and Trout C. A. (1979) *Clinical Application of Respiratory Care* Chicago: YearBook Medical Publishers, Inc.

P-Flex Inspiratory Muscle Trainer

PURPOSE

To improve diaphragmatic strength and endurance through resistive training exercises using P-Flex trainer (Fig. 5-7) and protect against muscle fatigue

STAFF RESPONSIBLE

EQUIPMENT

1. P-Flex Trainer
2. Nose clips (as needed)
3. Oxygen (as needed)
4. Oxygen adaptor (as needed)

 ## GENERAL CONSIDERATIONS

1. Studies regarding use of P-Flex Trainer are currently in progress. This device is most frequently used with chronic obstructive pulmonary disease (COPD) patients as part of the pulmonary rehabilitation program. It is also used to improve respiratory function for patients with spinal cord injury.

2. P-Flex Trainer is based on the principle that as patient inhales the resistance provided by the training device, the respiratory muscles work harder.

3. A physician's order is required to initiate treatment. The order should include the length of the training session, frequency, and setting.

4. Current respiratory status to include:
   - Respiratory rate and effort
   - Vital capacity
   - Pulse

5. If improperly used or training time is not adhered to, diaphragmatic fatigue can occur. Characteristic signs of fatigue include:
   - Abdominal paradoxing
   - Tachypnea
   - Intercostal retraction or use of accessory muscles
   - Subjective complaints of increased work of breathing

6. An oxygen adaptor port can be added between mouthpiece and body of device. The oxygen adaptor should be used with flow rate of oxygen prescribed by the physician.

7. It is generally recommended to use the device at the same time, at least two times each day and no sooner than 2 h after meals.

8. Any change in respiratory status (including increased secretions, infection, changes in airway) will mandate a change in training regimen.

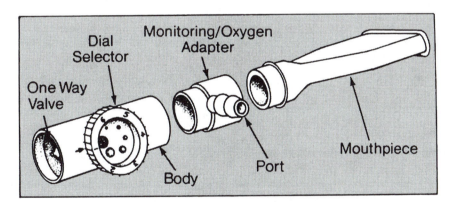

Dial Setting				1																		
Training Period			Week 1							Week 2							Week 3					
Day	1	2	3	4	5	6	7	1	2	3	4	5	6	7	1	2	3	4	5	6	7
Training Record ✓when completed each day																					
Performance Record: (walking distance, exercise tolerance, etc.)	Baseline: _____ _____																				

Figure 5-7 P-Flex Inspiratory Muscle Trainer and Flow Sheet to Monitor Progress. Each patient should have a copy to track his or her progress. (*Source:* Courtesy of Respironics *Healthscan Asthma & Allergy* Products, Cedar Grove, NJ.)

Procedure

 Steps

 Additional Information

1. Gather equipment.

2. Rinse mouthpiece with water and dry before using.

3. Explain procedure to patient.

4. Have patient sit in position which promotes good lung expansion. Semi-Fowler's is recommended.

5. Assess respiratory status and pulse rate before starting training session.

   If physician has advised oxygen use, connect oxygen tubing to adaptor.

6. Apply nose clips provided with trainer per patient comfort with nose clips.

   This assures maximum benefit as the individual then breathes solely through the device.

7. Insert mouthpiece into patient's mouth and encourage him or her to make a tight seal around device.

8. Set dial at selector 1 or prescribed setting.

9. Instruct patient to inhale and exhale through the trainer in a relaxed manner.

10. Maintain mouthpiece in place and continue until signs of respiratory fatigue are noted, 10- to 15-min training session is completed, or patient discomfort occurs.

    Initially training should be limited to 10 to 15 min a day. Slowly increase time as tolerated by patient over the course of a week until patient can tolerate two 15-min sessions per day.

11. Increase degree of resistance on dial selector as directed per order.

    When patient tolerates two 15-min training sessions per day for a period of at least 3 days, notify clinician directing the program as resistance may now be increased. When resistance is increased, training time should be reduced to 10 to 15 min until patient tolerates two training sessions per day.

12. Measure pulse post-training.

13. Clean device by washing with soap and then shake dry and store in bag.

    Because breath is inhaled via trainer, clean in hot soapy water and rinse once a week. Then soak in ½ strength white vinegar/water solution for ½ h. Rinse dry.

DOCUMENTATION

1. Document initial performance including respiratory status prior to training, pulse pretraining, degree of resistance, length of training session, post-training respiratory status and pulse, patient response to training session in progress note in medical record.

2. Indicate training parameters—degree of resistance, length of training, and functional level.

3. Document training session and outcome.

4. Encourage patient to track own progress on P-Flex flow sheet provided with training device (see Fig. 5-7).

REFERENCES

P-Flex inspiratory muscle trainer and flow sheet, Respironics Healthscan Asthma & Allergy Products, Cedar Grove, NJ.

Airway Management

Ambu and Inflation Hold

PURPOSE

To manually provide a sustained maximal inflation to prophylactically loosen secretions in patients with an artificial airway; to provide manual ventilatory support and oxygenation for patients with an artificial airway

STAFF RESPONSIBLE

EQUIPMENT

All equipment is considered emergency equipment to be kept at the bedside of any patient with an artificial airway.

1. Manual resuscitator bag (ambu bag)
2. Oxygen source
3. Oxygen connecting tubing (may be part of bag)
4. Oxygen flowmeter

 GENERAL CONSIDERATIONS

1. Ambu with inflation hold is used to preoxygenate patients requiring suctioning. For patients receiving oxygen therapy or on mechanical ventilation, ambu and inflation hold must be performed with supplemental oxygen flow (10 L/min) before and after suctioning. For patients with known chronic obstructive pulmonary disease, check with the physician regarding the recommended flow rate.

2. Ambu and inflation hold should be performed prophylactically on all patients with an artificial airway at least once per shift if they are unable to perform sustained maximal inspiration on their own.

3. When ambu and inflation hold is performed to provide manual ventilatory support for patients on mechanical ventilation, the number of breaths should be consistent with the ventilator rate or the typical respiratory rate.

4. The volume of air delivered with each breath depends on how the bag is compressed. Generally, a one-hand technique is adequate. Additional volume (two-hand technique) may be necessary for large individuals or those with significant retained secretions. Obtain the proper size bag for children.

5. All patients on mechanical ventilation *must* have an ambu bag on their person at all times, and the staff assigned must be familiar with use of the bag in emergency situations.

6. Before and after the procedure, the nurse should assess the patient's respiratory status, including:
   - Respiratory rate
   - Depth of respirations
   - Pattern of breathing
   - Symmetry of breathing
   - Breath sounds

7. Infection control measures should be followed with use of equipment. Position the ambu bag to avoid any contact with surfaces that are grossly contaminated (i.e., the floor, linen by urinary drainage devices, and the like).

Procedure

 Steps

1. Check order for frequency and need for supplemental oxygen.

2. Assemble necessary equipment.

Additional Information

A physician order for supplemental oxygen and emergency equipment should be obtained with admission orders for all patients with an artificial airway.

3. Identify patient. Introduce yourself and procedure to be performed.

4. Wash hands. Apply gloves and apply eye shields.

Nonsterile gloves should be used if hands are likely to come in contact with body secretions. Eye shields are recommended to prevent contact with secretions during procedure.

5. Attach connective tubing of ambu bag to flowmeter. Turn oxygen on at rate of 10 L/min.

Oxygen is required for patient on supplemental oxygen therapy (over 21%) or on mechanical ventilation.

6. Verify that airway cuff is inflated.

7. Connect adaptor of ambu bag to patient's tracheostomy tube. For cuffless tracheostomies, have patient close mouth and breathe in as you give the breath and hold breath until bag is released.

If mouth is open and pattern is not synchronized, benefits of procedure may be negated by air loss through upper airway.

8. Instruct patient to breathe in as you compress bag. Hold bag in compressed position for 3 to 5 s, and then release.

Manual inhalations should be synchronized with patient's own respiratory rate as much as possible.

9. Observe for any adverse reactions.

Procedure should loosen secretions.

10. Repeat steps 7, 8, and 9.

When suctioning, give three breaths before and after each pass of the catheter. For prophylactic treatment perform five repetitions.

11. Suction or cough assist if necessary.

12. Disconnect ambu bag from tracheostomy tube.

13. Check cuff inflation orders, and set cuff accordingly (see procedure on cuff inflation/deflation).

Physician order should include cuff instructions for inflation/deflation.

14. Reconnect mechanical ventilator tubing or supplemental oxygen to tracheostomy tube as prescribed.

15. Turn off oxygen, and return equipment to appropriate storage place.

If continual oxygen is not needed.

 ## DOCUMENTATION

1. Document the procedure and frequency of care provided in the appropriate medical record.

2. Document efficacy of the procedure and patient's tolerance of procedure.

3. Document any unusual findings.

4. Record patient/family education as appropriate.

PATIENT AND FAMILY EDUCATION

1. Explain the methods and actions to reduce anxiety.

2. Teach the procedure as necessary.

REFERENCES

Shapiro, B.A., Harrison, R.A., and Trout, C.A. (1979) *Clinical Application of Respiratory Care* Chicago: YearBook Publications.

Care of Patient with a Tracheostomy Tube

PURPOSE

To describe activities to maintain patent airway, prevent infection, ensure emergency care and education of patient/caregivers prior to discharge

STAFF RESPONSIBLE

EQUIPMENT

1. Manual resuscitator bag (ambu bag)

2. Adaptor for tracheostomy tubes

3. Suction machine and suction kits

4. Spare trach (required for vent-dependent patients)

GENERAL CONSIDERATIONS

1. A tracheostomy tube is an artificial airway which is surgically placed and bypasses the upper airway and glottis (Fig. 5-8). It is the most permanent and desirable of all artificial airways.

2. Indications for tracheostomy tube include:
   - Relief of upper airway obstruction
   - Protect airway (prevent aspiration)
   - Facilitation of bronchial hygiene and suctioning
   - Prolonged mechanical ventilation

3. Outer cannulas are generally inserted and removed by the physician or respiratory therapist. Adult trach tubes are generally changed every 6 weeks while children may have tubes changed as often as three times per week. Indications for change include:
   - Stoma is infected
   - Different style or size is required
   - Trach is grossly dirty or damaged
   - Cuff is damaged and no longer functional
   - Ineffective airway exchange
   Outer cannulas may be changed more frequently (daily to three times per week) in children to reduce opportunity for granulation tissue growth.

4. DO NOT LET STOMA CLOSE. IF THE PATIENT IS ON MECHANICAL VENTILATION AND YOU ARE UNABLE TO REINSERT TRACH TUBE, OCCLUDE STOMA WHILE PROVIDING MASK/BAG VENTILATION. Ask second person to insert one size smaller trach tube. Notify physician and respiratory therapy immediately to evaluate patient.

5. Obturator and spare trach should be kept with any patient on mechanical ventilation at all times. For all other patients a spare trach should be kept on each unit for emergencies.

6. Inner cannulas are to remain in place at all times except during cleaning and prescribed corking schedule. For patients on ventilator, a spare Shiley inner cannula can be inserted for a maximum of 10 min for cleaning procedures.

7. Inner cannulas are not interchangeable. The inner cannula is fitted to the exact length of a particular tube's outer cannula.

8. Physician orders for patients with a tracheostomy tube should include:
   - Suctioning: frequency and preoxygenation needed
   - Tracheostomy tube order (preferably with type and size)
   - Treatment regimen: trach care, humidity
   - Duration to be corked/cuffed
   - Precautions in therapy areas and need for on-unit therapy

9. For tracheostomy tubes used to prevent aspiration it is recommended that the cuff be inflated during meals and for 1 h after meals, tube feedings, when vomiting occurs, and other high risk times.

10. During resuscitation cuffed tracheostomy tubes should be inflated. For fenestrated trach, insert inner cannula and inflate balloon and ventilate patient. When cuffless trach is in place ambu via trach but compensate for air loss through upper airway by increasing ventilatory rate or depth. For Kistner buttons or Montgomery tube, occlude trach with appropriate cork/cap or your hand. Begin mouth-to-mask breathing via upper airway. When sufficient help is available remove trach and insert cuffed tube.

11. Whenever humidity, ventilators, ambu bags, aerosol or oxygen therapy is prescribed, respiratory therapy will set up and maintain equipment. When breathing through a tracheostomy tube, the air bypasses the normal humidification centers and therefore can lead to drying of the mucosal lining within the trachea. For this reason breathing through open trach tube for prolonged periods without humidification should be avoided. Alternative sources of humidity include artificial nose and high-humidity trach collar. Care must be taken to follow infection control procedures with this equipment.

12. Infection control procedures are to be followed when working with all respiratory equipment. On the unit

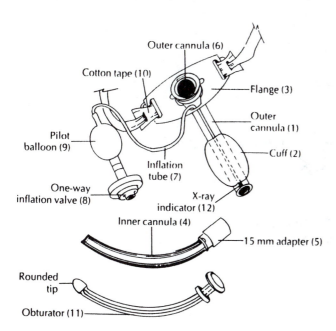

Figure 5-8 Parts of a tracheostomy tube. (Reproduced with permission from D.H. Eubanks and R.C. Bone, *Comprehensive Respiratory Care: A Learning System*, 2d ed. St. Louis, Mosby, 1990, p. 570.)

nurses are responsible for careful use and storage of equipment which includes:

- Manual resuscitation bags: should be stored at bedside, and tracheostomy adaptor should not come in contact with grossly contaminated areas. If grossly contaminated wipe adaptor with alcohol pad before using.
- Humidification tubing: routinely the water which collects in the tubing must be emptied as it can be a source of bacterial growth. The tubing should be disconnected from humidity source and emptied into appropriate receptacle (trash can, sink, toilet). To drain the tubing elevate the piece which connects with patient and allow water to drain out in the opposite direction. NEVER DRAIN WATER BACK INTO HUMIDITY SOURCE.
- Spare cannulas and corks should be stored in dry, clean, closed containers at the bedside. After use they should be cleaned with normal saline. If secretions are present hydrogen peroxide and saline may be needed. Then wipe dry with sterile 4 × 4 gauze.

13. Patients with tracheostomy tubes are considered priority patients for transport to appointments and should be carefully assessed prior to transport. If there is a significant risk of airway obstruction a nurse should accompany patient and bring portable suction. Factors to consider include:
    - Current respiratory status: stable or changing
    - Frequency/intensity of suctioning needed
    - Cough adequacy
    - Duration of time off unit

Tracheostomy Tube—Catheter Size Chart

Recommended Trach Size	Suction Catheter Size
0	4
1	5
2	6
4	10
6	12 or 14
8	12 or 14
10	14

- Age of patient
- Cognition
- Communication ability
- Nature of the disability
- Patient ability to manage own trach care
- Availability and competence of family to accompany patient and perform suctioning procedure
- Patient level of anxiety

A physician order is required for patients to be transported unescorted outside of the facility.

14. Respiratory equipment for home care is ordered by nursing based on physician prescription. See equipment section of discharge planning manual for specific information. The respiratory therapy home care vendor is available for information on product options and patient/family teaching prior to weekend pass or discharge. The family is to practice these skills.

15. The person responsible for extubation must be knowledgeable of airways and able to reinsert airway if airway obstruction occurs. Common complications associated with extubation include:

Ulceration Tracheal Mucosa	Tracheal Stenosis
Vocal Cord Paralysis	Obstructive Granulation Tissue
Tracheomalacia	

Procedure

Steps

1. Bring suction machine and oxygen delivery device, ambu bag, and catheters to bedside.

2. Note on admission form:
   - Type and size of trach
   - Reason for trach
   - Frequency of suctioning and catheter size
   - Airway management: medications, fluids, cough assist
   - Swallowing ability
   - Bronchial hygiene: USN, CPT, incentive spirometry, ambuing, and humidification
   - Oxygen therapy
   - Corking program
   - Breath sounds and complete respiratory assessments

Additional Information

For information on catheter size for suctioning see chart (above). Include assessment of patient's functional level with management of respiratory care.

3. Have physician write necessary orders.

4. Notify respiratory therapy for evaluation and to obtain necessary equipment.

5. Evaluate patient use of call system and order alternative system if necessary.

6. Determine method of communication and list in care plan.

7. Assess patient need for room near nurses' station.

See General Considerations.

Verbal communication is limited with trach tube.

DOCUMENTATION

1. Document routine care as appropriate.

2. Document patient/family education.

PATIENT AND FAMILY EDUCATION

Patient/family teaching prior to pass/discharge should include:
- Anatomy and physiology of respiratory system
- Effects of injury on respiratory status
- Measures to maintain patent airway
- Measures to improve vital capacity
- Tracheostomy care and suctioning procedures
- Recognition of complications
- Emergency equipment and actions

- How to do routine trach change
- Equipment cleaning

Teaching must be documented in progress note in the medical record. Respiratory therapist or physician should teach family trach change procedure.

REFERENCES

Eubanks, D.H., and Bone, R.C. (1990) *Comprehensive Respiratory Care: A Learning System*, 2nd ed. St. Louis, Mosby.

Mathews, P.J., Mathews, L.M., and Mitchell, R.R. (1992) "Artificial Airways Resuscitation Guidelines You Can Follow" *Nursing92* 12(1):53–58.

Shapiro, B.A., Harrison, R.A., and Trout, C.A. (1979) *Clinical Applications of Respiratory Care* Chicago: YearBook Publications.

Tracheostomy Cleaning and Stoma Care

PURPOSE

To clean the inner cannula and stoma of accumulated secretions; to maintain a patent airway; to prevent infection; to describe hygienic care of the stoma and tracheostomy tube

STAFF RESPONSIBLE

EQUIPMENT

1. Tracheostomy cleaning kit (brush, pipe cleaners, sterile drape, two sterile containers)

2. Hydrogen peroxide (3%)

3. Sterile normal saline

4. Plastic bag

5. Precut gauze dressings (as needed)

6. Two sterile gloves

7. Two nonsterile gloves

8. Spare inner cannula (may be cleaned and reused)

9. Ambu bag

10. Disposable inner cannula for tracheostomy tube (as needed)

11. Reusable Velcro trach ties

GENERAL CONSIDERATIONS

1. Tubes with no inner cannula (Portex, Kamen-Wilkinson, Montgomery) require good humidification and routine suctioning to maintain patency. No attempt is made to clean the internal lumen of these tubes. Tracheostomy care in this instance is limited to cleaning the stoma site and changing the dressing.

2. Tracheostomy care is recommended every shift and as needed. If infection of the airway or stoma is present or if secretions are profuse, the nurse should increase the frequency of tracheostomy care until the problem is resolved.

3. With Olympic buttons, or Shiley fenestrated tracheostomy tubes that are corked 24 h per day, routine tracheostomy care can be reduced to one or two times per day. Store the inner cannula when not in use in a dry, clean, capped container.

4. If the patient requires suctioning, do this before initiating tracheostomy care.

5. With long-term use of a tracheostomy tube, a dressing may not be required if secretions are minimal and if the stoma is clean. Factors to consider before discontinuing a dressing include:
   • Amount and type of secretions
   • Condition of the stoma and surrounding skin (if irritation is present, do not discontinue the dressing)
   • Environment (does it predispose the individual to infection?)

6. When the inner cannula is removed, a spare Shiley inner cannula (red top) can be inserted to maintain the airway in patients requiring positive-pressure ventilation. Whether the temporary cannula is used or not, the inner cannula should not be removed for a period longer than 10 min. Secretions can collect in the outer cannula and lead to obstruction of the airway. The temporary inner cannula is usually shorter than the outer cannula and if left in for extended periods of time can result in irritation or trauma to the trachea with suctioning.

7. Inner cannula care requires aseptic techniques.

8. The most common complication associated with tracheostomy care is accidental decannulation while changing tracheostomy ties.

Procedure

 Steps

 Additional Information

1. Gather all equipment and prepare work surface.

2. Wash hands.

3. Explain procedure to patient.

4. Position patient comfortably so that you have access to tracheostomy tube and stoma.

   Generally, supine or semi-Fowler's position is recommended. If patient has sternal occipital mandibular immobilizer brace, position patient supine. It may be necessary to remove chin piece to gain access to tube. Maintain spinal precautions and procedures while chin piece is off.

5. Open tracheostomy cleaning kit.

6. Remove sterile drape by grasping outer edge and open onto flat surface with plastic side down.

   This forms sterile field.

7. Without touching inside contents, turn tray over so that contents empty onto sterile field.

8. Place sectioned tray on work surface but not on sterile field and pour sterile saline solution for stoma care.

   You may choose to pour solution at later time.

9. Position second basin within reach but not on sterile field.

   Only inside of basin is sterile.

10. Pour hydrogen peroxide in small basin and sterile normal saline in large basin.

    Omit peroxide if metal tube (Jackson) is present.

11. Don a nonsterile glove and use gloved hand to remove soiled dressing from around tube. Discard dressing and glove.

12. Don second nonsterile glove.

13. Open second sterile drape on patient's chest.

    This drape may be used as additional work area.

14. For patients on a ventilator, disconnect oxygen source and perform ambu with inflation hold procedure. For other patients, evaluate ability to take three deep breaths to pre-oxygenate self. If patient is unable to do so, use ambu with inflation hold procedure.

    Refer to Ambu and Inflation Hold Procedure.

15. Stabilize neck plate with one hand and turn inner cannula connector to unlock cannula.

Do not touch inner cannula except at connector. Submerge cannula in solution. For patients using disposable tube, remove inner cannula and discard. Insert new sterile cannula and lock in place.

16. Remove inner cannula following natural curve of trachea, and place it in peroxide solution.

17. Insert spare inner cannula (optional).

Spare cannula must be inserted with patients on ventilator.

18. Reconnect oxygen source if on continuous O_2.

19. Remove contaminated gloves.

20. Put on sterile gloves.

21. When bubbling ceases in peroxide solution, pick up sterile brush and clean inner surface of inner cannula.

If brush does not fit, sterile pipe cleaners can be used. For pediatric tubes use sterile pipe cleaners.

22. Place inner cannula in saline solution to rinse off hydrogen peroxide. Do not dry cannula.

Peroxide solution is irritating to tissue and must always be rinsed off thoroughly before reinserting cannula. Moisture from saline rinse will provide lubricant to assist with insertion.

23. Disconnect oxygen source, and preoxygenate patient if on continuous O_2.

24. Unlock spare inner cannula, and remove it.

25. With sterile gloved hand, remove inner cannula from saline, and reinsert it in outer cannula.

26. Lock inner cannula in place by turning connector to "lock" position.

Discard used equipment in plastic bag according to infection control procedures.

27. Reconnect oxygen source if on continuous O_2. Remove sterile gloves, and put on nonsterile gloves (optional).

28. Pick up cotton-tip applicator, and dip it in peroxide or saline solution.

A sterile gauze may be used instead of cotton-tip applicator.

29. Clean stoma, posterior tracheostomy plate, and anterior tracheostomy plate with applicator. Discard applicator.

30. Pick up second cotton-tip applicator, and pour small amount of saline on applicator. Repeat step 29.

31. With third applicator, dry stoma.

If there are profuse secretions, use sterile gauze to dry area. Do not touch portion of dressing that will be in contact with stoma.

32. Apply dressing under tracheostomy plate on stoma.

33. Check Velcro straps.

They should be dry and should adequately secure tube. If they are soiled or frayed, they should be changed.

34. When changing tracheostomy ties, leave original ties in place until new ones are secure.

35. Put all used equipment in plastic bag and discard.

Discard according to infection control procedures.

DOCUMENTATION

1. Document the frequency of care and routine hygiene care.

2. Document in the medical record as needed:
   - Progression of stoma healing
   - Observations of the stoma indicative of infection (redness, odor, or increased secretions) and the treatment plan
   - Observations of the stoma indicative of infection resolution
   - Any unusual occurrences

3. Document patient and family education in progress notes or appropriate chart form.

PATIENT AND FAMILY EDUCATION

1. Explain procedures and complications to the patient and family.

2. Teach the procedures as appropriate.

Types of Tracheostomy Tubes

PURPOSE

Identify commonly seen tubes and pertinent safety concerns (Table 5-2)

STAFF RESPONSIBLE

REFERENCES

Mathews, P.J., Mathews, L.M., and Mitchell, R.R. (1992) "Artificial Airways Resuscitation Guidelines You Can Follow" *Nursing92* 12(1):53–58.

Shapiro, B.A., Harrison, R.A., and Trout, C.A. (1979) *Clinical Applications of Respiratory Care* Chicago: YearBook Medical Publications; pp. 255–280, 293–395.

Table 5-2 Types of Tracheostomy Tubes									
Name	**Material**	**Cuffed**	**Noncuffed**	**Fenestrated**	**Nonfenestrated**	**Inner Cannula**	**Obturator**	**Other**	
Jackson	Stainless steel		X	X	X	X	X	1. Notify respiratory therapy to provide adaptor for ambuing. For most effective ventilation change trach to Shiley. 2. Adaptor screws on inner cannula. 3. Can be resterilized. 4. Will be cold to touch in cold temperatures. 5. Do not clean with hydrogen peroxide.	
Shiley	Plastic	X, Low-pressure cuff	X Peds sizes available	X	X	X, Shiley SCT does not have inner cannula	X	1. Adaptor for suctioning is attached to inner cannula. 2. Spare (colored top) inner cannula available for short-term use. 3. Fenestrated trach has a plastic cork. 4. Disposable inner cannula is also available. 5. Suction patient before deflating cuff and corking patient.	
Portex	Siliconized plastic	X, Low-pressure cuff	X	X	X	X	X	1. May or may not have cannula, depending on model. 2. Has one-way valve to prevent leak. 3. Some styles may be used as talking tube.	
Kamen-Wilkinson (Bivona)	Silicone	Self-inflate cuff or Low-pressure cuff	X	O	X	O	X	1. When adaptor is open the cuff is up. Never push air into cuff unless an emergency seal is needed for a short period of time. When air is inserted the cuff becomes a	

Name	Material	Cuffed	Noncuffed	Fenestrated	Nonfenestrated	Inner Cannula	Obturator	Other
								high-pressure cuff. When adaptor is closed the cuff is down.
Montgomery T-tube	Plastic	O	X	O	O	O	O	1. Requires no external security as tube is surgically inserted and held in place by "T" structure. 2. In an arrest, plug stoma and ventilate from above.
Kistner Button	Plastic	O	O	O	O	O	O	1. Is minimally held in place by phalanged edges. 2. Suction through tube only in emergency situation. 3. In an arrest remove button and insert cuffed tracheostomy tube. 4. Document number of rings exposed in progress note and verify every shift.
Olympic Button	Plastic	O	O	O	O	O	O	1. Phalanged inner edge is open when inner cannula or cork is in place. 2. Inner cannula has universal trach adaptor. 3. Suctioning is not recommended except in emergency. 4. In an arrest remove button and insert cuffed reach tube.
Talking trach tubes (Portex, Communitrach)	Plastic	X	O	O (cannot be corked)	X	O (Communitrach has inner cannula but Portex does not)	O	1. Special design allows air to pass through vocal cords to produce voice. 2. Airflow is provided by attaching side port to oxygen or air with flow rate of at least 5 L/min. 3. When not in use shut off oxygen to prevent drying.

Minimal Leak Technique

PURPOSE

To prevent overinflation of the cuff; to prevent complications associated with pressure to the tracheal wall

STAFF RESPONSIBLE

EQUIPMENT

1. 10-cc syringe
2. Manual resuscitation bag (ambu)

3. Tracheostomy tube
4. Stethoscope
5. Suction machine

 ## GENERAL CONSIDERATIONS

1. "The objective of minimal leak technique is to place the minimal volume of air in the cuff to allow optimal sealing of the airway." (Shapiro, 1979) Minimal leak should be verified at least once per day with continuously inflated cuffs and with each cuff inflation.

2. This technique cannot be used on self-inflating cuffs such as the Kamen-Wilkinson or Bivona tubes.

3. Technique is based on principle that during positive-pressure ventilation the tracheal diameter is maximal on inspiration.

4. Minimal leak cannot be measured by air volumes as it can change slightly with postural changes and position changes of the tracheostomy tube.

5. Periodic cuff deflation is not necessary when minimal leak technique is used. NEVER INFLATE A CUFF WHEN THE DECANNULATION CANNULA (red cork or plug) IS IN PLACE AS THIS WILL NOT ALLOW ADEQUATE AMOUNTS OF AIR TO PASS THROUGH THE UPPER AIRWAY. *IT WILL TOTALLY OCCLUDE THE AIRWAY.*

6. Physician to write orders for cuff inflation/deflation frequency and parameters. Always check physician orders and seek clarification if orders deviate from procedure.

Procedure

 Steps

 Additional Information

1. Explain procedure to patient. Gather equipment. Wash hands.

2. Suction trachea and oral pharynx.

   To clear oral secretions which could enter lower airway when cuff is deflated.

3. Attach syringe to Luer-Lok valve of cuff inflation port.

   This is a one-way valve which allows air to enter but not exit.

4. Connect ambu bag to tracheostomy tube and give deep breath.

5. At the start of expiration of this breath, deflate cuff by aspirating with syringe.

   Expiratory flow can prevent particles above cuff from entering lower airway.

6. Position stethoscope on lateral aspect of the trachea superior to thyroid cartilage.

7. Inflate cuff until you can no longer auscultate air with stethoscope on inspiration.

   If unable to hear with stethoscope, place hand over nose and mouth and listen. Cuff is maximally inflated when you can no longer feel or hear an air leak. Using an ambu bag to provide positive pressure can facilitate auscultation of an air leak.

8. Aspirate by 0.5-cc increments until air leak is again heard with stethoscope on inspiration.

   If unable to hear with stethoscope place hand over nose and mouth and feel for air leak. When air leak is felt you have a minimal leak. For patients on positive-pressure ventilation: listen for air leak on inspiration. There should be no decreased exhaled volume or P_{max}.

9. Disconnect syringe, label, and store in clean area at bedside.

   If no minimal leak is detected or if cuff leak is present, notify the physician.

 DOCUMENTATION

1. Document:
   - Frequency of minimal leak checks
   - Scheduled times

2. Implementation of procedure.

3. Documented as they arise:
   - Any unusual occurrences.

4. Patient/family education and practice.

REFERENCES

Shapiro, B.A., Harrison, R.A., Trout, C.A. (1979) *Clinical Applications of Respiratory Care* Chicago: YearBook Medical Publishers; p. 273.

Tracheostomy Tube Changes

PURPOSE

To safely replace well-established tracheostomy tubes

EQUIPMENT

1. Appropriate type and size tracheostomy tube and spare
2. Ambu bag with oxygen source
3. Suction equipment
4. Sterile gloves
5. Water-soluble lubricant
6. Drain sponge
7. Sterile disposable cup
8. Sterile water

 ## GENERAL CONSIDERATIONS

1. Auscultation for bilateral breath sounds should be performed following insertion.
2. Minimal leak should be performed if cuff is to be inflated (see Minimal Leak Procedure).

3. If tracheostomy tube of the same size is difficult to replace and the patient is dependent on the airway, insert a tracheostomy tube one size smaller and immediately notify the appropriate physician service and respiratory therapy for further instructions.

4. Patients with long-term tracheostomy tubes have a high incidence of obstructive airway lesions. Be sure to assess the patency of the upper airway before a tracheostomy tube is permanently removed.

5. Patient hazards and safety precautions:
   - Bleeding: use obturator when inserting trach tube.
   - Pneumothorax.
   - Air embolism.
   - Subcutaneous or mediastinal emphysema.
   - Airway contamination and infection: use clean technique.
   - Airway obstruction may occur. Auscultate immediately after cannulation or decannulation to verify breath sounds.
   - Tracheostomy tube malposition.
   - Sterile technique should be followed when handling all artificial airways and during suctioning.

Procedure

Recannulation Following Unplanned Decannulation:

 ### Steps

 ### Additional Information

1. Instruct and comfort the patient
2. Ensure that the patient is adequately ventilating or being ventilated before proceeding with the following steps.
3. Take appropriate size and type tracheostomy tube and remove inner cannula.
4. To insure cuff integrity, inflate the cuff while maintaining sterile technique and observe for leakage while immersing in sterile water or saline.
5. Deflate cuff slowly while tapering cuff by pulling toward flange with sterile gloves.
6. Insert obturator, then lubricate distal tip of obturator and outer cannula with water-soluble lubricant.
7. Insert tracheostomy tube through stoma, and following its contour, slide the tube into the trachea.
8. Inflate cuff, if indicated, using minimal leak technique.
9. Auscultate for bilateral breath sounds.
10. Tie trach ties so that one finger only can slide under the ties.

If the situation is urgent, a quick leak check may be performed by inflating the cuff and checking for gross leaks by squeezing cuff and observing for volume loss.

Procedure

Elective Trach Tube Insertion/Removal

 Steps

 Additional Information

1. Suction patient via tracheostomy tube and oropharyngeally.

2. Deflate cuff completely and remove tracheostomy tube after new tube has been checked for leaks and prepared for insertion.

3. Proceed as in Steps 6–10. See Recannulation Procedure.

4. If tracheostomy tube is to be permanently removed, the patient's airway must be assessed for patency before stoma is allowed to close. To do this, remove old trach tube and cover stoma completely to prevent air from entering stoma. With stoma covered, assess patient's breathing through his or her upper airway by listening for stridor and observing for increased work or breathing. If any signs of difficulty breathing through upper airway are observed, replace trach tube and notify physician about observations. If no signs of upper airway problems are seen, cover stoma with a sterile 4 × 4 gauze and tape.

5. Encourage patient to deep breathe and cough.

 DOCUMENTATION

Document:
1. Procedure performed
2. Reason procedure performed

3. Size of trach removed and replaced
4. Drainage
5. Condition of stoma
6. Patient's tolerance of the procedure
7. Patient and family education

Corking a Tracheostomy Tube

PURPOSE

To assess patient's ability to breathe via upper airway, mobilize secretions, or to protect airway in preparation for decannulation

STAFF RESPONSIBLE

EQUIPMENT

1. Syringe: 10 cc
2. Inner cannula

3. Decannulation cannula (red) plug
4. Stethoscope
5. Gloves
6. Suction catheters/suction machine
7. Storage container for inner cannula

 GENERAL CONSIDERATIONS

1. In order to cork a cuffed tracheostomy tube the tube must be fenestrated and cuff deflated. ALWAYS VERIFY ORDER WITH RESPIRATORY BEFORE CORKING A NONFENESTRATED TUBE. *NEVER CORK A CUFFED NONFENESTRATED TUBE.*

2. Fenestrated tube is a tracheostomy tube in which a "window" has been cut in posterior wall of the outer cannula.

3. Customized fenestration tubes are available.

4. With long-term use periodically check for granulation tissue which can occlude fenestration and restrict airflow.

This can be done by removing inner cannula and shining flashlight at fenestration. If tissue is seen at the fenestration, notify the physician.

5. For resuscitation purposes insert inner cannula and inflate cuff.

Procedure

 Steps

 Additional Information

1. Obtain physician order.

2. Explain procedure to patient.

3. Gather equipment. Check trach face plate to verify fenestration. Check with respiratory therapy if trach is not fenestrated before initial corking.

4. Observe patient's current respiratory rate, effort, and subjective feelings.

5. Wash hands. Don gloves.

6. Suction trachea then suction oropharynx or have patient clear throat with a cough.

7. Check balloon inflation line for damage. If damage is noted notify respiratory therapy and physician as a new trach may be needed.

8. Insert Luer-Lok tip of syringe into Luer-Lok valve on pilot line.

9. Withdraw all the air into syringe until resistance is met. Note how much is removed.

10. Disconnect syringe, expel all air out.

11. Reconnect to balloon and attempt to withdraw additional air with syringe. If resistance is felt disconnect syringe.

12. Remove inner cannula.

13. Check fenestration for granulation tissue.

14. Insert decannulation cannula (red plug) and twist to lock into place.

15. Observe patient closely for respiratory distress when red decannulation cannula is in place.

16. Remove decannulation cannula and insert inner cannula if distress occurs.

To specify duration and frequency of corking procedure.

A nonfenestrated trach may be used when a custom trach is made. At times a noncuffed nonfenestrated trach may be corked. NEVER CORK A CUFFED NONFENESTRATED TRACH.
Used as baseline parameters.

Prevents secretions which have collected on cuff from falling into trachea.
When balloon inflation line is damaged it may be difficult to adequately deflate cuff to allow for corking.

All air must be removed from balloon as airflow through fenestration is not adequate. With balloon down, air will flow around tube.

Place in closed container.
Use flashlight.
Hold only the outer portion. Avoid touching the inner lumen.
Distress can occur if upper airway is obstructed. If this is initial corking attempt, closely monitor patient for at least 2 h. If this is not initial attempt, keep patient within sight for approximately 10 min. Notify therapist to return patient if respiratory distress occurs or patient complains of shortness of breath.
Determine duration and frequency of corking program with physician and therapist. Initially insert decannulation cannula during the day and remove it at night, replacing it with inner cannula.

17. After each use rinse with H_2O_2 and normal saline. Store inner cannula in a clean, dry container at patient bedside.

If patient requires suctioning in therapy, send container with inner cannula and other necessary equipment with the patient to the therapy.

 DOCUMENTATION

1. Document in progress note for initial corking:
   * Initial respiratory status: rate, rhythm, effort, patient response to corking, any changes in respiratory rate, effort, or signs of distress
   * Duration of corking
   * Patient's ability to mobilize secretions while corked
   * Ability to speak
2. Indicate frequency procedure to be performed.
3. Document corking schedule and routine implementation on performance of procedure on functional care plan.
4. The respiratory therapist and speech language pathologist document in progress note

* Respiratory status: rate, rhythm, effort, patient response to corking, any changes in respiratory rate, effort, or signs of distress
* Duration of corking
* Patient's ability to mobilize secretions while corked
* Ability to speak

5. Document any occurrences of respiratory distress and actions taken in progress note in medical record.
6. The registered nurse documents in the progress note or on teaching checklist patient-family education.

REFERENCES

Shapiro, B.A., Harrison, R.A., and Trout, C.A. (1979) *Clinical Applications of Respiratory Care* Chicago: YearBook Publications.

Tracheal Suctioning

PURPOSE

To provide for removal of secretions by application of negative pressure to the patient's airway; to maintain bronchial hygiene; to maintain a patent airway

STAFF RESPONSIBLE

EQUIPMENT

The equipment needed depends on the setting.
1. Suction catheter kit
2. Sterile normal saline
3. Plastic bag
4. Suction machine (portable or battery-operated) and tubing
5. Ambu bag
6. Oxygen source and tubing
7. Oxygen flowmeter

GENERAL CONSIDERATIONS

1. Tracheal suctioning is a routine procedure. The major complications associated with suctioning include:

* Hypoxemia
* Cardiac dysrhythmia
* Hypotension
* Lung collapse

These can be avoided by carefully selecting the appropriate size suction catheter, preoxygenating the patient, and limiting the duration of suctioning. If these complications occur, terminate the procedure, administer oxygen, and notify the physician.

2. Patients with a tracheostomy and known preexisting cardiac arrhythmias are at high risk for complications during suctioning. These patients should be suctioned initially by persons (nurses or respiratory therapists) best able to respond to potential complications. No off-unit therapy or tests should be provided for high-risk patients without a nurse accompanying the patient and/or a physician order.

3. Catheter size is based on the size of the internal lumen of the inner cannula. The suction catheter should occupy no more than half the lumen of the inner cannula. The appropriate size suction catheters must accompany the patient at all times.

4. A new sterile catheter kit is used for each suctioning session.

5. Surface suctioning of a tracheostomy tube is done with a sterile catheter.

6. Patients on oxygen therapy or mechanical ventilation must be preoxygenated by using a manual resuscitator (ambu bag) at a flow rate of 10 L/min before and after suctioning.

7. The vacuum generator on the suction machine should be set between 80 and 120 mmHg negative pressure for adults and between 80 and 90 mmHg negative pressure for children and infants.

8. Suction bottles are emptied and rinsed at least once per shift in accordance with infection control guidelines. Never allow fluid to reach the "full" level.

9. Deflation and inflation of the cuff in accord with procedure on minimal leak may only be performed by those professional trained and competent in the procedure according to protocols of your institution.

10. If a professional is unfamiliar with the type of tube in place then they should seek input from the nurse or respiratory therapist prior to attempting the suctioning procedure.

11. Special considerations with different tracheostomy tubes are as follows:
    - *Tracheostomy button (Olympic)*: suction only in case of respiratory distress and per written physician's order because damage may occur to the tracheal wall. In case of emergency, you may suction and then notify the physician.

- *Montgomery tube*: push up on the tube to guide the catheter into the lower airway. To suction the upper airway, push down on the tube and direct the catheter upward.
- *Fenestrated tracheostomy tube*: insert the inner cannula and inflate the cuff. After suctioning, *deflate the cuff*, remove the inner cannula, and cork the tube as ordered. Rinse the inner cannula with sterile water or saline, and dry it with sterile 4×4 gauze. Store the cannula in a clean, dry, capped container. Send the cannula with the patient at all times.

12. Suctioning procedures must be performed in accordance with infection control policies:
    - Sterile technique must be used at all times except in emergency situations.
    - Sterile solutions must be properly labeled and discarded 24 h after opening.
    - Goggles or eye shields are strongly recommended.

14. Respiratory equipment for home care should be ordered based on a physician prescription. Practice with the unit to be used at home should be encouraged prior to pass/ discharge.

Procedure

 Steps

 Additional Information

1. Gather equipment. Wash hands.

2. Explain procedure to patient.

3. Take baseline pulse.

4. Turn on suction machine and check vacuum source by occluding tubing.

5. Verify that cuff is inflated.

    Exception: cuffless tracheostomy tubes

6. Open sterile saline.

7. Open catheter kit in aseptic manner and position it on flat surface close to patient.

8. Don sterile gloves.

    One or two gloves may be provided, depending on the manufacturer. Two gloves are recommended. One hand is kept sterile throughout the procedure.

9. Pop open basin and, with nonsterile hand, pour saline into basin.

10. With sterile gloved hand, pick up catheter, exposing only connector end.

11. With nonsterile hand, pick up connecting tube attached to suction machine and attach it to connector end of catheter.

12. Preoxygenate patient:
    - Method 1: hand ventilate patient three to five times with ambu bag, giving inflation hold on last breath.
    - Method 2: instruct patient to take three to five quick deep breaths and to hold last breath for a few additional seconds.

For patients on oxygen therapy or mechanical ventilation, Method 1 must be used and ambu bag connected to 10 L/min flow rate.

13. Disconnect ambu bag. Lubricate catheter in saline.

14. Insert catheter with sterile hand into airway without applying suction until resistance is felt.

Catheter should reach level of carina.

15. Withdraw catheter ½ to 1 in. before applying suction.

This is done to avoid carinal irritation.
Do not apply suction for more than 10 s at a time.

16. Apply suction with nonsterile hand as you withdraw catheter with your sterile hand. Twirl catheter with fingers of sterile gloved hand as you withdraw it.

17. Oxygenate patient, and rinse catheter by suctioning small amount of saline through catheter.

18. Repeat procedure as needed. Always oxygenate before and after each pass of catheter.

Do not suction more than three times consecutively without allowing a few minutes for patient to rest and reoxygenate by deep breathing or ambu.

Only those persons qualified to perform cuff deflation/inflation may perform minimal leak.

19. Inflate cuff according to physician orders.

20. Shut off machine.

21. Pull glove back over catheter, and discard all materials in plastic bag.

22. Empty suction container.

23. Check patient's pulse.

24. Obtain new catheter kit and replenish saline if necessary. Place equipment with suction machine. Return manual resuscitation bag to proper storage at bedside.

DOCUMENTATION

1. Document the time and frequency of suctioning required.

2. Document with the initial suction procedure and when unusual situations occur during the procedure or periodically thereafter:
   - Baseline pulse and any rate change
   - Color, amount, and consistency of secretions
   - Patient's response to the procedure, and any actions taken

3. Report any unusual circumstances to the physician or respiratory therapist.

PATIENT AND FAMILY EDUCATION

Teaching for patient and/or family suctioning procedures must be completed and their competencies must be documented prior to pass/discharge. Patient/family teaching should include:
- Anatomy and physiology of respiratory system
- Effects of injury on respiratory status
- Measures to maintain airway
- Measures to improve vital capacity
- Tracheostomy care

REFERENCES

AARC Clinical Practice Guideline (1993) "Endotracheal Suctioning of Mechanically Ventilated Adults and Children with Artifical Airways" *Respiratory Care* 38:500–504.

Shapiro, B., Harrison, R., and Trout, CA. (1979) *Clinical Application of Respiratory Care*, 2d ed. Chicago: YearBook Medical Publishers.

Tracheal Suctioning with Red Rubber Catheters

PURPOSE

To decrease trauma to the tracheobronchial structure when suctioning or when recent tracheal trauma has occurred; to provide for removal of secretions by application of negative pressure to patient's airway; to maintain bronchial hygiene and maintain patent airway

STAFF RESPONSIBLE

EQUIPMENT

1. Sterile normal saline
2. 6 in 1 adaptor
   (or)
3. Y connector
4. Sterile gloves
5. Eye shields
6. Plastic bag
7. Suction machine
8. Red rubber catheters (May be straight or coudé tip of appropriate size for trach.)
9. Sterile specimen container

 ## GENERAL CONSIDERATIONS

1. Tracheal suctioning is a routine procedure. The major complications associated with suctioning include:
   • Hypoxemia
   • Cardiac dysrhythmia
   • Hypotension
   • Lung collapse
   These can be avoided by carefully selecting appropriate size suction catheter, preoxygenating patient, and limiting the duration of suctioning. If these complications occur terminate procedure, administer oxygen, and notify physician.
2. Catheter size is based on size of the internal lumen of the inner cannula. The suction catheter should occupy no more than one half the lumen of the inner cannula. See chart for recommended sizes.

Tracheostomy Tube-Catheter Size Chart	
Recommended Trach Size	Suction Catheter Size
0	4
1	5
2	6
4	10
6	12 or 14
8	12 or 14
10	14

3. A new sterile catheter kit is used for each suctioning session.
4. Surface suctioning of tracheostomy tube is done with a sterile catheter.
5. Patients on oxygen therapy or on mechanical ventilation should be preoxygenated using a manual resuscitator (ambu bag) with oxygen at flow rate of 10 L/min before and after suctioning.
6. The vacuum generator on the suction machine should be set in range of 80 to 120 mmHg negative pressure for adults and between 80 to 90 mmHg negative pressure for children and infants.
7. Suction containers are emptied and rinsed at least once per shift in accordance with infection control guidelines. Never allow fluid to reach "full" level.
8. *Fenestrated Trach Tube*: To suction insert inner cannula and inflate cuff. After suctioning *deflate cuff*, remove inner cannula, and cork trach as ordered. Rinse inner cannula with sterile water or saline and dry with sterile 4 × 4 gauze. Store inner cannula in clean, dry, container at bedside. Send cannula with patient if frequent suctioning is required.
9. Suctioning procedures must be performed in accordance with infection control policies:
   • Sterile technique must be used at all times except in emergency situations.
   • Sterile solutions must be properly labeled and are discarded 24 h after opening.
   • Goggles or eye shields are recommended.
10. The nurse is responsible for teaching patient/family suctioning procedures and documenting their competence.
11. Respiratory equipment for home care is ordered by nursing based on physician prescription. See equipment manual. Practice these skills on the unit; this can be arranged and should be encouraged.

Procedure

 Steps

Additional Information

1. Gather equipment, wash hands.
2. Explain procedure to the patient.
3. Take a baseline pulse.
4. Turn on suction machine and check vacuum source by occluding the tubing.
5. Verify cuff is inflated.

   Exception: cuffless tracheostomy tubes.
6. Open sterile saline and pour into sterile cup.

   If using small single-dose saline, then skip this step.
7. Open red rubber catheter kit in aseptic manner and position on flat surface in close proximity to patient.
8. Don sterile glove.

   One or two gloves may be provided, depending on manufacturer. Two gloves are recommended. One hand is kept sterile throughout procedure.
9. With sterile gloved hand, pick up catheter, exposing only connector end.
10. With nonsterile hand, pick up suction tubing with Y connector or 6 in 1 adaptor attached.
11. Preoxygenate the patient.
    - Method 1: hand ventilate three to five times with ambu bag giving inflation hold on last breath.
    - Method 2: have patient take three deep breaths in quick succession.

    For patients on oxygen therapy or mechanical ventilation, Method 1 must be used and ambu bag connected to oxygen at 10 L/min flow rate.
12. Disconnect ambu bag. Lubricate catheter in saline.
13. Insert catheter with sterile gloved hand into airway without applying suction until resistance is felt.

    Catheter should reach level of carina.
14. Withdraw catheter ½ to 1 in. before applying suction.

    This is done to avoid carinal irritation.
15. Intermittently apply suction as catheter is withdrawn using sterile gloved hand. Twirl catheter with fingers as it is withdrawn.

    Do not apply suction for more than 10 s at a time.
16. Oxygenate patient, and rinse catheter by suctioning a small amount of saline through catheter.
17. Repeat procedure as needed. Oxygenate patient before and after each pass of the catheter.
18. Shut off suction machine.
19. Pull glove back over catheter, and discard all materials in plastic bag.

    Dispose of all materials according to infection control procedures.
20. Empty suction container at least once per shift and as needed when filled.
21. Check patient's pulse.

    Notify physician of significant rate and/or rhythm changes, especially bradycardia or dysrhythmias.

DOCUMENTATION

1. Document the time and frequency of suctioning performed or therapists reported frequency.

2. Document in a progress note when unusual situations occur during procedure including:
   - Baseline pulse and any rate changes,
   - Color, amount, and consistency of secretions
   - Patient response to procedure
   - Actions taken.

3. Document patient/family education on teaching checklist or progress note.

PATIENT AND FAMILY EDUCATION

Patient/family teaching prior to weekend pass/discharge should include:
- Anatomy and physiology of respiratory system
- Effects of injury on respiratory status
- Measures to maintain patent airway
- Measures to improve vital capacity
- Tracheostomy care

REFERENCES

Shapiro, B.A., Harrison, R.A., and Trout, C.A. (1979) *Clinical Applications of Respiratory Care* Chicago: YearBook Publications.

Suctioning (Oral, Nasal, or Pharyngeal) in Patients Without an Artificial Airway

PURPOSE

To maintain a patent airway; to provide for removal of secretions by application of negative pressure in patients without an artificial airway

STAFF RESPONSIBLE

EQUIPMENT

1. Suction catheter kit
2. Sterile normal saline/water
3. Plastic bag
4. Water-soluble lubricant
5. Suction machine and tubing
6. Ambu bag
7. Oxygen source and tubing
8. Oxygen flow meter
9. Nasal airway (if appropriate)
10. Eye shields
11. Gloves

GENERAL CONSIDERATIONS

1. Do not unnecessarily suction a patient. Attempt a cough first and, if ineffective, then suction. Suctioning is a common procedure but not without its risks. The major complications include:

- Hypoxemia
- Cardiac dysrhythmias
- Hypotension
- Lung collapse
- Tracheal edema

These can be avoided by selecting the appropriate size catheters, preoxygenating the patient, and limiting the duration of suctioning. If complications occur, terminate the procedure, administer oxygen, and notify the physician (Shapiro, Harrison, and Trout, 1979).

2. Frequent suctioning via the nasal, oral, or pharyngeal routes can be uncomfortable and irritating. Complications related to suctioning of the upper airway include tissue trauma, bleeding, and gagging. To minimize trauma to the nasal mucosa, consider the use of a nasal airway. A nasal airway may be readily obtained and inserted.

3. Catheter size is based on the size of the lumen of the catheter. The common catheter size for an adult is 12 to 14 French, for a child is 6 to 8 French, and for an infant is 4 to 8 French.

4. A new catheter kit is used for each suctioning session. The same catheter may be used for an upper airway only after lower airway suctioning is completed.

5. If the patient is on oxygen therapy, preoxygenate him or her by placing on oxygen delivery device for 30 s before and after suctioning attempts.

6. The vacuum generator on the suction machine should be set between 80 and 120 mmHg negative pressure for adults and between 80 and 90 mmHg negative pressure for children and infants.

7. Suction bottles should be rinsed at least once per shift and emptied as needed. Replace the connecting tubing daily and the collecting bottles as needed.

8. Suctioning procedures are performed in accordance with infection control policies. All patients should be considered on Body Substance Precautions, gloves must be worn and eye shields as appropriate.

9. Patients requiring frequent nasopharyngeal suctioning should be assessed for placement of an artificial airway.

Procedure

 Steps

 Additional Information

1. Assemble all equipment. Explain procedure to patient.

2. Turn machine on, and test vacuum source by occluding tubing and observing manometer.

3. Wash hands.

4. Take baseline pulse.

   Assess rate and rhythm of pulse.

5. Open bottle of sterile solution.

6. Open suction catheter kit in aseptic manner, and position it on flat surface close to patient.

7. Don sterile gloves.

   One or two gloves may be provided, depending on the manufacturer.

8. Open basin and, with nonsterile hand, pour solution into basin.

9. With sterile hand pick up catheter, expose connector end, and attach to connecting tubing on suction machine.

   Only sterile hand should come in contact with catheter.

10. Preoxygenate patient. Ask patient to take three to five deep breaths.
    • Nasal route
      • Lubricate catheter with water-soluble lubricant.
      • Check nasal passage for patency.
      • Insert catheter gently into airway following anatomic floor of nare.
      • If unable to pass catheter, pull it back, and try again in other nasal passage.
      • Insert to just above epiglottis and apply intermittent suction as you slowly withdraw catheter.

      • Release suction; do not remove catheter from nose.

      • Repeat procedure until secretions are cleared.

    • Oral route
      • Insert catheter along side of patient's tongue along oral floor.
      • Insert catheter to level of the epiglottis and apply intermittent suction as you withdraw catheter.
      • Replace oxygen device.
      • Repeat procedure until secretions are cleared.

    If on oxygen make certain patient breathes the supplemented environment.
    • *Nasal route*

    • *Prior to inserting catheter, estimate length of tubing from nose to epiglottis. Do not apply suction for more than 10 s.*
    • *This minimizes trauma and helps to reduce contamination from upper airway.*
    • *Listen to breath sounds to determine when secretions are cleared. Preoxygenate before and after each attempt.*
    • *Oral route*

    • *Do not suction for period in excess of 10 s.*

    • *Preoxygenate before and after each attempt.*

11. Shut off machine.

12. Pull glove back over catheter, and discard all materials in plastic bag.

    Discard according to appropriate infection control procedures.

13. Empty suction bottle if needed.

14. Check patient's pulse and listen to breath sounds.

Notify physician of significant rate and/or rhythm changes, especially bradycardia or dysrhythmias.

15. Wash hands.

DOCUMENTATION

1. Document the time, route, and frequency.

2. Document in a progress note the initial procedure and any unusual situations on periodic basis:
   - Pulse rate changes with the procedure
   - Color, amount, and consistency of secretions
   - Patient response to the procedure
   - Effectiveness of the procedure

3. Report any unusual circumstances to the physician.

4. Document patient and family teaching and response.

PATIENT AND FAMILY EDUCATION

Teach procedures and precautions to the patient and family, documenting competence.

REFERENCES

AARC Clinical Practice Guideline (1992) "Nasotracheal Suctioning" *Respiratory Care* 37:898–901.

Shapiro, B., Harrison, R.A., and Trout, C.A. (1979) *Clinical Application of Respiratory Care*, 2d ed. Chicago: YearBook Medical Publishers.

Obtaining Sputum Specimen in Patient with Tracheostomy

PURPOSE

To obtain a sterile sputum specimen by way of a tracheostomy for laboratory examination

STAFF RESPONSIBLE

EQUIPMENT

1. Sterile normal saline

2. Suctioning machine and tubing

3. Oxygen source and tubing

4. Ambu bag

5. Plastic bag

6. Leuken's tubes/sterile sputum trap

7. Oxygen flowmeter

8. Suction catheter kit

9. Face mask or goggles/eye shields (may be necessary)

GENERAL CONSIDERATIONS

1. Sputum specimens are ordered by physician.

2. There are multiple methods that may be used to induce a productive cough for a specimen.

3. Obtaining sterile specimens may require sterile suctioning.

4. If culture is needed and can not be obtained, notify respiratory therapy staff and request physician order for sputum to be induced.

5. Adhere to infection control practices when obtaining a sputum culture. Gloves are to be worn at all times and eye shields as needed.

6. Suctioning a tracheostomy with the use of the Leukens tube/sputum trap provides for a sterile sputum specimen.

7. For specific suctioning directions see appropriate procedures.

Procedure

 Steps

 Additional Information

1. Gather equipment. Explain procedure to patient.

2. Wash hands and don protective gear necessary according to patient status. NOTE: Gloves must be worn.

   Gown, mask, and eye shields may be necessary if patient has a forceful cough, secretions, or airborne microbes which would contaminate clothing.

3. Set up suctioning equipment according to the Suctioning Procedure with the following exceptions:
   - Attach the male port of the sputum trap to the female port of the suction machine tubing.
   - Attach male adaptor of suction catheter to female adaptor of sputum trap.

4. Suction the patient as directed. Amount of sputum obtained should be at least 2 to 3 cc. Small amounts of sterile saline are suctioned as needed to move secretions into specimen container.

   Large amounts of normal saline may interfere with proper processing of the specimen.

5. Disassemble equipment and attach the female adaptor of the sputum trap to its male adaptor.

6. Dispose of supplies and wash hands.

7. After specimen is obtained, close lid tightly.

8. Label container with patient's name, physician's name, room number, specimen number, date, and time of collection. Place in plastic bag and seal bag tightly.

9. Ensure sample gets to lab.

   Do not refrigerate.

10. Dispose of supplies.

11. Wash hands.

 DOCUMENTATION

Document that the specimen has been collected.

REFERENCES

Demus, R.R. (1982) "Complications of Endotracheal Suctioning Procedures" *Respiratory Care* 27:453–457.

Fuchs, P. L. (1984) "Streamlining Your Suctioning Techniques: Part 1. Nasotracheal Suctioning" *Nursing* 84:14.

Fuchs, P. L. (1984) "Streamlining Your Suctioning Techniques: Part III. Tracheostomy Suctioning" *Nursing* 84:14.

Shapiro, B., Harrison, R. and Trout, C.A. (1979) *Clinical Application of Respiratory Care*, 2d ed. Chicago: Year Book Medical Publishers.

Stevens, K. (1987) "Autonomic Regulation and Respiratory Function: Section 2. Respiratory Function: Alterations in Airway Clearance" In P. Matthews and C.E. Carlson (Eds.) *Spinal Cord Injury: A Guide to Rehabilitation Nursing* Rockville, MD: Aspen.

Assistive Ventilation

Bi-PAP Ventilatory Support

PURPOSE

To improve alveolar ventilation, treatment of sleep apnea, prevent ventilatory fatigue

STAFF RESPONSIBLE

EQUIPMENT

1. Bi-PAP machine
2. Tubing

CONTRAINDICATIONS

1. Patients incapable of maintaining life-sustaining ventilation in the event of malposition of face mask.
2. Patients with or susceptible to pneumothorax or pneumomediastinum require very close monitoring. Persons with preexisting bullous lung disease may represent a relative contraindication to any positive-pressure ventilation.
3. Allergy to the material of which the mask is made.

 ### GENERAL CONSIDERATIONS

1. Hypotension may be induced by positive-pressure ventilation.

2. Patient status may require the placement of suitable alarms (i.e., low pressure, oxygen saturation).
3. Caution should be exercised in applying a snug or tight-fitting full-face mask to patients because of the increased possibility of aspirating gastric contents. This is particularly true in patients who are at risk for, or who have been, vomiting.
4. Mask ventilation does not guarantee either a patent or protected airway.
5. If not tolerated and patient continually fails use of machine or wearing mask, another mode of ventilatory support should be considered.
6. If using a full-face mask (nasal/oral), advise the patient not to eat or drink 2 to 3 h prior to bedtime.
7. If skin irritation or breakdown develops due to the mask:
   - Consider changing the mask from nasal to full-face or vice versa as appropriate.
   - Place a patch of wound care dressing on the bridge of the nose to provide a cushion between the bridge and the mask.
   - Skin irritation may be due to an allergy to the mask material. Consider using a skin barrier such as Duoderm or Micropore tape to prevent mask contact with the skin.
   - Verify the mask spacer is being used. Check spacer size. If skin irritation develops under spacer, it may be due to excessive pressure or a skin reaction. Consider using a skin barrier as described above.
   - Observe patient for development of ear discomfort or conjunctivitis.
   - Consider adding humidification.

Procedures

 ### Steps

1. Check physician order.

 ### Additional Information

Physician order should include:
- *Settings*
- *Oxygen concentration (F_{IO_2})*
- *Mode*

2. Explain indication for and procedure to patient and family.

Patient understanding and acceptance is important for the success of the modality.

3. Fit mask to face.

Proper mask sizing and application are crucial to the success of noninvasive ventilation. Mask discomfort is often the limiting factor to continued use. Mask should be the smallest size to fit the patient.

If mask rests on or too close to lips it may increase the likelihood for leaks, be uncomfortable, and cause gum irritation.

4. Mask should fit from proximal end of nasal bone to just below the nares. *Hint:* To prevent abrasion, place a patch of wound care dressing on the bridge of the nose.

5. Place the mask over the patient's nose and select proper spacer size.

6. Attach spacer to mask.

7. Attach headstrap to mask.

8. Apply mask and headstrap to patient.

9. Adjust straps until all significant leaks are eliminated.

Avoid overtightening as this will cause patient discomfort and may cause leaks due to the distortion of the mask cushion. If possible, have the patient vary head position to confirm mask seal during normal range of motion. Be careful not to overstress an anxious patient with attempts to place the mask.

 ## DOCUMENTATION

Document:

1. Patient condition before and during treatment, include:
   - Pulse and respiratory rate
   - Skin color, temperature, and perfusion
   - Use of accessory muscles of ventilation
   - Lung sounds

2. Report patient's tolerance to wearing face mask.

3. Patient and family education.

REFERENCES

Suggested Protocol for Initiation of the BiPAP S/T-D Ventilatory Support System. Respironics, Inc. (1993).

Care of the Patient Requiring Mechanical Ventilation

PURPOSE

To care for a patient requiring mechanical ventilation; to describe safety measures required for the apneic individual on mechanical ventilation

STAFF RESPONSIBLE

EMERGENCY PROCEDURE

All staff involved in direct care of patient on mechanical ventilation are responsible for instituting manual ventilation and calling for assistance as proper response to ventilator alarms.

 ## GENERAL CONSIDERATIONS

1. All patients admitted on mechanical ventilation will be prescreened prior to admission. If possible meet the patient while the individual is in the acute care hospital.

2. Prepare the necessary equipment and initiate therapy according to the physician order and maintain routine checking of its function. Ensure operation of ventilator and availability of extra equipment. All ventilator setting changes are made by the appropriate staff member(s) as ordered by the physician.

3. It is necessary to have a procedure in place to insure individuals working with the patient on mechanical ventilation are knowledgeable and able to respond to alarm situations.

4. If mechanical failure or clinical emergency occurs, initiate manual ventilation with ambu bag and oxygen immediately.

5. A back-up alarm is used at the bedside in addition to alarms on the ventilator if nursing personnel are not with the patient. VENTILATOR ALARMS MUST NEVER BE TURNED OFF AT ANY TIME. A test lung may be used to silence the alarms during suctioning.

6. Contact the vendor if problems with equipment occur.

7. Ventilatory support may be provided by:
   • Phrenic nerve stimulators
   • Volume-cycled portable ventilators (LP-10, LP-20)

8. All staff working with patients on mechanical ventilation should be aware of complications which can occur, basic operation of the ventilator, how to respond to alarms, and how to MANUALLY VENTILATE AND CALL FOR HELP. Initially all patients will receive therapy on the nursing unit. A physician order will be required to start off-unit therapy. In order to attend off-unit therapy, the therapist treating the patient must demonstrate ambu, suctioning, and emergency procedures to the nurse. The nurse must then document therapist proficiency. If therapist is unable to perform these procedures a nurse must accompany the patient off the unit. When the patient leaves the unit they must have the following equipment:
   • Ambu bag
   • Oxygen (if not available in therapy)
   • Battery-operated suction machine with full charge
   • Appropriate size suction catheter kit
   • Sterile saline
   • Spare trach of same size and type

9. A nurse will accompany the patient to appointments outside of the facility.

10. All procedures must be performed in accordance with infection control policies and procedures.

11. An emergency tension pneumothorax kit (thoracentesis kit) is available at all times.

Procedure

✓ Steps

1. Ensure that the necessary equipment is at the bedside:
   • Portable ventilator and circuits
   • Ambu bag and emergency trach equipment
   • Suction machine and catheter kits

2. Check that the following are as ordered. Notify respiratory therapy of any discrepancies:

   • Parameters: rate/volume/F_{IO_2}/PEEP pressure settings

   • Alarms are in ON position
   • Extra equipment is available with the patient

3. Assess current status of the patient; auscultate breath sounds every 4 to 8 h:
   • Perfusion status
   • Pulse rate

   • Blood pressure

4. Notify physician of any findings which deviate from the patient's norm.

5. Observe patient for signs and symptoms of tension pneumothorax:
   • Sudden absence or decrease of breath sounds
   • Inability to ventilate

Additional Information

Respiratory therapy is responsible for setting up the ventilator and its alarm systems.

The nurse checks the alarms and settings at the start of each shift. Only the respiratory therapist may adjust ventilator settings.
   • *Parameters are routinely documented by the RT on flow sheet at bedside.*

   • *See General Consideration # 9.*

   • *A change in pulse rate may indicate a decrease in cardiac output.*
   • *A decreased blood pressure may also indicate a decrease in cardiac output.*

- Rapid drop in blood pressure
- Rapid increase in pulse rate
- Deviation of trachea to opposite side

NOTE: If these occur notify the physician immediately as this is a life-threatening event.

6. Monitor function of the ventilator and respond to alarms:

- LOW PRESSURE

- HIGH PRESSURE

- ALTERNATE POWER

- *Low pressure indicates a leak or disconnect in the system. Manually ventilate the patient and check circuitry for leak.*
- *High-pressure alarm indicates an increase in airway resistance or decrease in compliance. Check need for suctioning, repositioning, or manual ventilation to decrease anxiety. Check tubing for excess fluid and drain.*
- *When the ventilator changes from one power source to another, an alarm will sound. Investigate the cause. Internal battery carries charge for 1 h of operation.*

 ## DOCUMENTATION

1. The registered nurse documents parameters as ordered by the physician and pertinent nursing orders.
2. Document:
   - Alarm checks every shift
   - Breath sounds checked during shift
3. Document:
   - Patient/family education and competency in responding to alarm situations and performing manual ventilation with ambu bag.
   - Unusual occurrences (mechanical failure, change in patient status) include:
     - Time
     - Action taken
     - Personnel notified
     - Patient response

PATIENT AND FAMILY EDUCATION

REFERENCES

Johnson, D., Giovannoni, R., and Driscoll, S. (1986) *Ventilator-Assisted Patient Care*, Rockville, MD: Aspen Publishing Inc.

Shapiro, B.A., Harrison, R.A., and Trout, C.A. (1979) *Clinical Applications of Respiratory Care* Chicago: YearBook Publications.

CHAPTER 6

Procedures to Provide Safety

Introduction

Safety considerations are a common concern in the care of patients with neuromusculoskeletal conditions due to cognitive, sensory, and mobility changes. This chapter addresses several types of patient safety issues (hazards of immobility, medical complications, behavior issues, falls, and environmental issues) that have implications for safety of the individual. Each individual should be assessed for risk, and a specific plan developed to provide safety for the patient and others. These guidelines can be used to direct this process.

Many nursing interventions involve designing or altering the environment to enhance patient goal achievement. For example, the guidelines for care of the agitated patient and fall prevention are included in this chapter because they are used to create a safe environment for the individual. Throughout rehabilitation, every effort is made to respect patient dignity and rights, promote function, and insure safety within a therapeutic milieu.

Preventing Hazards of Immobility

Prevention of Thromboembolism

PURPOSE

To institute prevention measures to minimize risk of thromboembolism; to monitor patient for signs and symptoms of thromboembolism and pulmonary embolus

STAFF RESPONSIBLE

EQUIPMENT

No equipment necessary.

GENERAL CONSIDERATIONS

1. Thromboemboli, or clots in the extremities or pulmonary vasculature, are associated with immobility and are a major cause of death for immobilized patients. Contributing factors to clot formation include venous stasis, intimal trauma, and hypercoagulability.

2. Patients at risk for thromboemboli include those with:
   - Spinal cord injury
   - Multiple fractures
   - Post–total hip or knee replacements
   - Immobility
   - Post–hip fracture
   - Hormonal therapy
   - Post–stroke
   - History of thrombus
   - Cancer or malignancy
   - Increasing age (over 40)

3. Deep vein thrombosis, if not treated, can result in embolization, whereby all or part of the clot is dislodged and gives rise to pulmonary emboli which are often life-threatening.

4. Prophylactic treatment is controversial so always check with physician regarding preferred prevention measures.

5. Signs and symptoms associated with thrombophlebitis are:
   - Unilateral swelling of an extremity
   - Warmth and/or redness at site of inflammation
   - Low-grade temperature
   - Pain or tenderness
   - Increased spasticity

6. Diagnosis of thromboemboli is difficult. The definitive study for diagnosis is contrast venographic studies.

7. Signs and symptoms of pulmonary emboli include: tachypnea, dyspnea, pleuritic chest pain, crackles, syncope, hypoxia, cough, and tachycardia.

8. Heparin-induced thrombocytopenia usually occurs after 5 days of parenteral heparin therapy. Closely monitor platelet count. Heparin is usually discontinued when present.

Procedure

 Steps

1. Assess patient risk status on admission. Assessment should include:
   - Concurrent medical conditions
     - Peripheral vascular disease
     - Dehydration
     - Intimal trauma
     - Cholesterol levels
     - Recent surgery
     - Fractures
     - Cancer/Malignancy
   - Diagnostic exams
     - Date and findings from last Doppler ultrasound exam

 Additional Information

316

- Current management
  - Antiemboli stockings
  - Pneumatic compression boots
  - Range of motion
  - Activity
- Medications
  - Birth control pills
  - Anticoagulants

Anticoagulants should be started as soon as possible and continued for a period of 8 to 12 weeks. Medications which enhance anticoagulation such as aspirin, dextran, non-steroidal anti-inflammatory agents should be used with care while on anticoagulant therapy.

  - Hormonal replacement medication
- Physical examination
  - Baseline leg measurements—thigh and calf

Measure at standard point (i.e., 10 cm above/below patella) or mark area measured to insure consistency of measurement.

  - Peripheral pulses
  - Temperature (body and extremities)
  - Breath sounds

2. Apply compression hose at all times or pneumatic compression boots when in bed.

3. Every shift inspect compression devices for proper fit and underlying skin for signs of pressure.

4. Instruct patient on preventive measures
   - Adequate hydration
   - Early mobilization
   - Range of motion two times per day

Start early mobilization and passive exercise as soon as patient is medically stable.

   - Proper fit and use of compression devices

5. Administer anticoagulant therapy per physician order.

Based on risk factors and/or physician preference.

6. Initiate serial leg measurements on weekly basis.

7. If symptoms are detected, do not move patient, notify nurse.

Inspect lower extremities daily for signs and symptoms of thromboemboli.

DOCUMENTATION

1. Document baseline leg measurements in the medical record.

2. Document prevention interventions (leg measurements, use of compression boots, application of antiemboli hose) in the medical record.

3. Document in the medical record signs and symptoms of complications, action taken, and patient response.

PATIENT AND FAMILY EDUCATION

1. Instruct patient and family in signs and symptoms and actions to take.

2. Instruct patient and family re: prevention measures and care of antiemboli devices.

3. Instruct patient and family on purpose, food–drug interactions, and administration and monitoring of anticoagulant medications.

REFERENCES

Babcock, R.B., Dumper, C.W., and Scharfman, W.B. (1976) "Heparin-Induced Immune Thrombocytopenia" *NEJM* 295(5):237–241.

Consortium for Spinal Cord Medicine (1997) *Prevention of Thromboembolism in Spinal Injury* Washington, D.C., Paralyzed Veterans of America.

Launis, B., and Graham, B.D. (1998) "Understanding and Preventing Deep Vein Thrombosis and Pulmonary Embolism" *AACN Clinical Issues* 9(1):91–99.

Matthews, P.J., and Carlson, C. (1987) *Spinal Cord Injury: A Guide to Rehabilitation Nursing* Rockville, MD: Aspen Publishers.

Swarczinski, C., and Dijkers, M. (1991) "The Value of Serial Leg Measurements for Monitoring Deep Vein Thrombosis in Spinal Cord Injury" *Journal of Neuroscience Nursing* 23(5):306–314.

Cardiac Precautions

PURPOSE

To establish a plan for monitoring patients at risk for cardiac complications

STAFF RESPONSIBLE

EQUIPMENT

1. Watch/clock with sweep second hand
2. Sphygmomanometer
3. Stethoscope
4. Nitroglycerine tablets, if ordered

GENERAL CONSIDERATIONS

1. Cardiac precautions are recommended for patients who have had:
   - A myocardial infarction within 6 months of admission to rehabilitation service
   - Cardiac surgery within 6 months of admission
   - A history of angina pectoris
   - A history of congestive heart failure
   - Any recent cardiac dysrhythmia or pacemaker implant
   - Other cardiac conditions requiring more frequent monitoring with activity/therapy
2. Cardiac precautions with parameters require therapists (PT/OT) to perform monitoring of vital signs before, during, and after activity. Patients on cardiac precautions with parameters are generally not allowed to participate in activities such as pool therapy or group exercise classes which preclude close individual monitoring of vital signs.
3. Physician order for precautions is sent to all clinical departments.
4. Activities/therapy should be planned to include:
   - Warm-up period: 10 min of light activity (passive, ROM, stretching, etc.)
   - Short rest period: 5 min
   - Exercise period: initially 10 to 20 min of activities that are closely monitored to reach target heart rate without producing any signs of decompensation (shortness of breath, chest/abdominal pain, decreased heart rate, decreased blood pressure, increased heart rate, increased blood pressure that exceeds parameters) of up to 2 to 3 min
   - Short rest period: 5 min
   - Cool down period: 10 min of light activity (ROM, stretching, etc.)
   - Rest period
5. Rest periods should be sitting, with legs down in well-supported chair, or if lying is more comfortable, with head slightly elevated. Avoid raising leg, which may increase venous return and further stress the heart.
6. If nitroglycerine tablets have been ordered, administer according to physician order.
7. When working with patients with a pacemaker and/or implanted cardiac defibrillator, the healthcare practitioner should be completely aware of the programmed values in each device. For patients with automatic implanted cardiac defibrillators (AICDs), exercise is terminated when an intrinsic heart rate or rapid response atrial fibrillation develops, 15 to 20 beats below the heart rate programmed in the cardioverter.
8. When signs and/or symptoms of cardiac distress occur, the patient should rest, stop all activities, and be monitored (vital signs, time the pain interval, etc.).

Procedure

 Steps

1. The physician evaluates the need for precautions with parameters and enters order in the medical record.

2. Document cardiac history and assessment on admission form including apical pulse rate (1 min) and rhythm.

3. Establish plan for monitoring on the care plan. Orders may include:
   - Scheduled rest periods between activities or therapy
   - Apical pulse (1 min) monitoring with new activity
   - Monitoring vital signs before, during, and after activity
   - Monitoring patient during activity for signs of fatigue, diaphoresis, pain, shortness of breath, dizziness, syncope, and/or alteration in heart rate or rhythm
   - Avoidance of activities that may result in a Valsalva maneuver: straining with urination or defecation, pushing or pulling against resistance, bending, lifting more than 5 to 10 lb, gagging, vomiting, or spasmodic coughing
   - A fluid/weight schedule for patients with congestive heart failure that includes:
     - Amount of fluids allowed
     - Intake/output
     - Weights at a minimum of three times per week
   - A plan of management of angina for patients with a known history; this includes:
     - Measures to take when pain occurs
     - Parameters for use of nitroglycerine
     - Amount of activity that triggers angina

4. PT/OT therapists monitor vital signs before, during, and after activity and notify the physician/nurse when findings are outside of parameters.

 ## DOCUMENTATION

1. Document in the medical record:
   - Patient tolerance of new activities
   - Any signs of fatigue, diaphoresis, pain, shortness of breath, dizziness, syncope, or alteration in heart rhythm, rate, or blood pressure
   - Any episode of cardiac origin
   - Any deviation from parameters listed in physician order
   - Patient/family education re: precautions
   - Intervention implemented and patient reaction

PATIENT AND FAMILY EDUCATION

1. Signs and symptoms of angina and appropriate actions to take.

2. Safe medication use.

3. Safe performance of activities and activities to be avoided.

REFERENCES

American Heart Association (1985) *Target Heart Rate* Dallas, TX: AHA

Berkhuysen, M.A., Nieuwland, W., Buunk, B.P., et al. (1999) "Effects of High- versus Low-Frequency Exercise Training in Multidisciplinary Cardiac Rehabilitation on Health-Related Quality of Life" *Journal of Cardiopulmonary Rehabilitation* 19:22–28.

Cundey, P.E., and Frank, M.J. (1995) "Cardiac Rehabilitation and Secondary Prevention after a Myocardial Event" *Clinical Cardiology* 18:547–553.

Rehabilitation Nursing Foundation (1987) *Rehabilitation Nursing Concepts and Practice—A Core Curriculum* Skokie, IL.

Sharp, C.T., Busse, E.F., Burgess, J.J., and Haennel, R.G. (1998) "Exercise Prescription for Patients with Pacemakers" *Journal of Cardiopulmonary Rehabilitation* 18:421–431.

U.S. Department of Health and Human Services (1994) "Clinical Practice Guidelines Heart Failure: Management of Patients with Left-Ventricular Systolic Dysfunction" Agency for Health Care Policy and Research.

Aspiration Precautions: Initiation and Implementation

PURPOSE

To establish a plan of management for patients at risk for aspiration

STAFF RESPONSIBLE

EQUIPMENT

1. Latex gloves
2. Suction machine as appropriate
3. Dysphagia evaluation tray
4. Flashlight
5. Dysphagia bag
6. Dysphagia folder
7. Laryngeal mirror
8. Flashlight

 ## GENERAL CONSIDERATIONS

1. Patients at risk for aspiration pneumonia or aspiration of fluid/food include those with:
   - History of aspiration pneumonia or respiratory compromise
   - Presence of dysphagia (see Chap. 1)
   - Impaired cough reflex and/or reduced cough strength
   - Cough associated with feeding/drinking
   - Reduced level of awareness and responsiveness
   - History of gastroesophageal reflux
   - Presence of a tracheostomy
   - History of chronic pulmonary disease
   - Parenteral feeding (nasogastric/gastric)
   - Children under 6 years of age

2. Aspiration syndromes include:
   - Bilateral infectious pneumonia from aspiration of oral-pharyngeal secretions containing bacteria
   - Chemical pneumonitis from aspiration of acidic gastric contents
   - Aspiration of inert nontoxic substances (e.g., water, blood, food particles) may lead to mechanical obstruction of the airway

3. Symptoms of aspiration include gradual onset of fever, fatigue, productive cough, respiratory distress, obstructive symptoms of cough, wheezing, and inability to speak or aphonia.

4. Strategies to prevent aspiration of gastric material include:
   - Sitting upright during meals/drinking and remaining upright at 60 to 90 degrees for 30 to 60 min after meals or tube feedings
   - Positioning bed in reverse Trendelenburg (bed flat with head section higher than foot) when patient is fed in bed
   - Administering antacids and/or other medications to stimulate esophageal motility and gastric emptying
   - Monitoring gastric residuals prior to tube feedings

5. Other strategies to reduce colonization of oral-pharyngeal flora with bacteria include:
   - Maintain good oral hygiene
   - Decrease presence of tooth decay and periodontal disease
   - Provide good denture care
   - Decrease risk for airway infections through routine coughing and/or bronchial hygiene

6. For patients assessed to be at high risk, the nurse enters orders on the patient care plan for monitoring and specific frequency that may include temperature and checking breath sounds.

7. A dysphagia bag contains specialized equipment for feeding and individualized instructions. Anyone can access the bag and see what fluid or food restrictions/modifications and feeding techniques to use with a particular patient (not always a bag).

Procedure

 Steps

1. Assess swallowing on admission.

2. If an in-depth dysphagia evaluation is needed, contact the speech-language pathologist for clinical evaluation and recommendations.
   - Clinical Dysphagia Evaluation by speech-language pathologist
   - Videofluoroscopic Swallowing Evaluation
   - Respiratory Therapy Evaluation and Treatment
   - Chest x-ray if needed

3. As part of Clinical Dysphagia Evaluation the speech-language pathologist makes recommendations for:
   - Diet modification (including NPO)
   - Optimal positioning for feeding
   - Use of compensatory techniques during feeding
   - Degree of supervision needed during feeding
   - Modification of meal-time environment
   - Participation in group feeding program
   - Oral feeding by speech-language pathologist only
   - Appropriate equipment for feeding

4. Identify patient risk status and communicate to all team members.

5. Indicate on care plan daily recommended fluid volumes, specific positioning instructions based on speech recommendations, functional levels and orders for calorie counts, frequent (at least bid) oral care, and any special monitoring needed.

6. Follow recommendations when providing food/fluids and document patient response to interventions.

7. Ensure that dysphagia bag is in place prior to patient leaving unit.

8. Check dysphagia instructions in bag before providing food/fluids and indicate amount given, calories, and responses on daily record sheet within the bag.

9. If nonclinical staff are requested by the patient or family to provide food/fluid, refer the patient to appropriate clinical staff.

 DOCUMENTATION

1. Physician enters necessary orders in the medical record.

2. The speech-language pathologist documents
   - Initial findings and recommendations in the medical record
   - Results and recommendations in the Communicative Disorders Initial Evaluation Report
   - Results and recommendations in the Videofluoroscopic Swallowing Evaluation
   - Progress and current status in progress note in chart as needed

3. Document assessment of nutritional/hydration assessment in a progress note in the chart weekly.

4. All staff documents care performed, intake/output, calorie counts, and weights as ordered in the medical record.

5. Document in the progress notes as needed
   - Patient response to interventions and functional changes
   - Signs/symptoms of aspiration and actions taken
   - Patient/family instruction

PATIENT AND FAMILY EDUCATION

Patient/family education on diet texture modifications, swallowing techniques, and signs/symptoms of aspiration are provided by the speech-language pathologist and the registered nurse. The dietitian is consulted when information is needed regarding special diets and food preparation.

REFERENCES

Cherney, L.R., and Souder, T.S. (1996) "Evaluating Swallowing Disorders: The Speech-Language Pathologist's Perspective" *Topics in Stroke Rehabilitation* 3(2):14–26.

Langmore, S.E., Terpenning, M.S., Schork, A., et al. (1998) "Predictors of Aspiration Pneumonia: How Important Is Dysphagia?" *Dysphagia* 13:69–81.

Orthopedic Precautions

Hip Precautions: Post–Total Hip Arthroplasty

PURPOSE

To describe common orthopedic precautions required after hip arthroplasty surgery

STAFF RESPONSIBLE

EQUIPMENT

1. Abductor splint or two to three pillows
2. Raised toilet seat
3. Assistive device: walker or crutches as prescribed by physical therapist
4. Reacher

GENERAL CONSIDERATIONS

1. Because of the nature of hip joint replacement surgery, all patients who have had a hip arthroplasty (joint replacement) are required to follow the general principles of hip precautions (Fig. 6-1). Specific precautions may vary by surgeon so always verify with the surgeon preferences for their patients.

2. The nurse is responsible for:
   - Initiating hip precautions on admission
   - Communicating the need for hip precautions to all caregivers
   - Ordering the necessary equipment
   - Assessing wound condition and monitoring for signs and symptoms of complications
   - Evaluating pain and providing analgesics and other measures to minimize pain and promote function
   - Ensuring patient and family education

Procedure

 Steps

1. Initiate hip precautions on admission and issue and review reminder sign (see Fig. 6-1) with patient. Note hip precautions on care plan.

2. Use abductor splint or two to three pillows between legs to abduct legs when lying in bed.

3. Turn to back and unaffected side only, always making certain abduction is maintained.

4. Keep leg in neutral position during bed activities. Avoid elevating head of the bed higher than 70 to 90 degrees.

5. Depending on surgeon preference, do not flex hip past 70 to 90 degrees for at least 6 weeks postoperatively. This includes during transfers and while reaching for objects when sitting. Teach patient to use dressing aids or to call for assistance to reach objects at the foot of the bed.

 Additional Information

Do not adduct or internally rotate affected leg because this movement can precipitate a hip dislocation. Simultaneous adduction with internal rotation presents a particularly high risk for dislocation.

Figure 6-1. Hip Precautions

WHEN? For a minimum of *6 weeks* after hip replacement surgery. All newly admitted hip surgery patients are placed on hip precautions until physician orders indicate otherwise.

DO	DON'T

DO

1. Keep legs abducted. Use abductor splint between your legs at all times. Use splint or at least two pillows between your legs when turning. Always use Velcro knee straps to keep hips abducted when you are in a wheelchair.

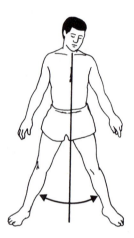

Leg Abduction

2. Turn to back and unaffected hip only.
3. Keep operated leg in neutral position when you are in bed and during activities.
4. Use elevated toilet seat. In community, you should use handicapped toilets, which are generally raised seats.
5. Report the following to physician:
   - Swelling of operated leg
   - Redness or discoloration of hip
   - Pain at hip
   - Drainage from incision line
   - Chest pain
6. Tell your physicians and dentists about your hip surgery.
7. Report any infections to your physician for immediate treatment.

DON'T

1. Adduct legs (cross operated leg over midline).

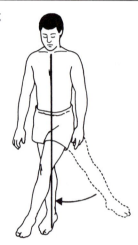

Leg Adduction

2. Flex legs past 90 degrees for first 6 weeks after your operation.
3. Flex hip when in side-lying position.
4. Bend forward at hip during transfers or when sitting in wheelchair, pulling pants on, or reaching for object on the floor.

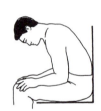

Hip Flexion

5. Elevate footrests on wheelchair.
6. Sit for long periods. (You should raise up or stand for 1 to 2 min to relieve pressure. Every 30 min to 1 h).
7. Turn onto operated side.
8. Internally rotate operated leg.

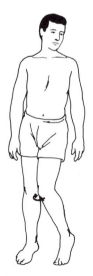

Internal Rotation

6. When in the wheelchair use pillows, Velcro straps, or abductor splint to maintain abduction. Remind patients to avoid crossing legs while sitting.

7. Check incision line daily, noting healing, signs/symptoms of inflammation or infection. Report delayed healing to the physician. Consult surgeon regarding showering while staples are in place.

Generally, showering is allowed once staples have been removed.

8. Provide analgesics prior to therapy to minimize pain and promote function. After therapy ice packs to joints may further reduce pain and swelling.

9. Order and use raised toilet seat to facilitate maintaining precautions during toilet transfers.

If raised toilet seat is not available, use raised commode chair.

10. Monitor for signs and symptoms of hip dislocation:
    - Swelling of operated leg
    - Redness or discoloration of hip
    - Pain at operated hip (sudden or severe)
    - Unusual positioning of extremity

 ## DOCUMENTATION

1. Document all nursing orders and interventions in the medical record.

2. Document any unusual situations, signs, symptoms of complications, and actions taken in the medical record.

3. Document the patient and family teaching of hip precautions and the patient's ability to comply.

PATIENT AND FAMILY EDUCATION

1. Teach the patient and family proper positioning and the use of the equipment.

2. Teach precautions, correct movements, movements to be avoided, signs and symptoms of complications, and long-term considerations for the reconstructed joint.

3. Remind patients to avoid driving and sexual activity for a period of 6 to 8 weeks postoperatively.

4. Instruct patients to notify the physician whenever they develop an infection, such as a sore throat, urinary tract infection, or whenever dental work is needed. Prophylactic antibiotic coverage may be indicated to reduce risk for infection spread to the joint.

REFERENCES

Maker, A.B., Salmond, S.W., and Pellino, T.A. (1994) *Orthopaedic Nursing*, Philadelphia: W.B. Saunders.

Care of the Patient with a Seizure Disorder

PURPOSE

To identify high-risk patients; to describe preventive interventions; to describe treatment interventions that promote patient safety and accurate assessment of the diagnosis of a seizure disorder

STAFF RESPONSIBLE

EQUIPMENT

1. Cotton blankets and tape
2. Padded side rail protectors
3. Pillows
4. Oral airway
5. Emergency drug
6. Seizure precaution signs

 GENERAL CONSIDERATIONS

1. Seizures are sudden episodes precipitated by abnormal, excessive neuronal discharges within the brain. They are characterized by convulsive movements or other motor activity, sensory phenomena, or behavioral abnormalities. Seizures are the result of excessive release of electrical impulses by a group of neurons in different parts of the brain. Seizures are a symptom, not a disease.

2. Common etiologic categories in which seizure activity is a symptom include:
   - Cerebral injuries
   - Birth injuries
   - Infectious diseases
   - Cerebral circulatory disturbances
   - Neoplasms of the brain
   - Biochemical imbalances
   - Drug or alcohol overdose
   - Medication-induced electrolyte imbalance
   - Posttraumatic causes
   Seizures may also be idiopathic.

3. Seizures are classified as given in Fig. 6-2.

4. Status epilepticus is a medical emergency in which a series of seizures occurs in rapid succession and in which the patient is unable to regain consciousness between the seizures, thus increasing the risk of cerebral anoxia or pulmonary aspiration. When status epilepticus occurs, interventions are directed to:
   - Establish and maintain a patent airway
   - Provide oxygenation
     - Apply oxygen
     - Contact respiratory therapist
   - Prevent cardiovascular collapse
   - Prevent injury to the patient
   - Control seizure activity with IV medications
     - Prepare patient for IV insertion (IV medications commonly used include diazepam, phenytoin, and Ativan and should be available; normal saline IV fluid is required when phenytoin is given)
     - Monitor and maintain ventilation, hydration, electrolyte balance, and urine output after the medication is given because medications may precipitate respiratory depression, hypotension, or cardiac dysrhythmias.

5. The nurse is responsible for:
   - Obtaining a seizure history and documenting it on the admission form
   - Administering anticonvulsant medications per physician's order and notifying the physician when problems with administration or schedule disruption occur
   - Recognizing patients at risk for seizures and instituting safety measures

326

Figure 6-2 International Classification of Seizure Types

1. Partial seizures (seizures that involve or begin in one area of the brain):
   - Partial seizures with elementary symptomatology (seizures that have relatively uncomplicated symptoms; usually the person remains conscious):
     - With motor symptoms (symptoms affecting the muscles)
     - With sensory or somatosensory symptoms (symptoms affecting the senses)
     - With autonomic symptoms (symptoms affecting the internal organs)
     - Compounded forms (symptoms of more than one of the above types)
   - Partial seizures with complex symptomatology (partial seizures with more complicated symptoms, usually with some loss of consciousness):
     - With impairment of consciousness only
     - With cognitive symptomatology (symptoms affecting thought)
     - With affective symptomatology (symptoms affecting mood or emotion)
     - With psychosensory symptomatology (symptoms affecting sense perception, such as illusions or hallucinations)
     - With psychomotor symptomatology (symptoms such as movement and behavior inappropriate to the situation)
     - Compound forms (symptoms of more than one of the above types)

   - Partial seizures secondarily generalized (seizures that begin as partial seizures and then become generalized)

2. Generalized seizures (seizures that involve both sides of the brain):
   - Absences (brief lapses of consciousness occurring without warning and unaccompanied by prominent movements, as in petit mal)
   - Bilateral massive epileptic myoclonus (an involuntary jerking contraction of the major muscles)
   - Infantile spasms (brief muscle spasms in young children)
   - Clonic seizures (seizures consisting of jerking movements of the muscles)
   - Tonic seizures (seizures in which the muscles are rigid)
   - Tonic-clonic seizures (seizures that begin with muscle rigidity and progress to jerking muscular movement; commonly known as grand mal seizures)
   - Atonic seizures (seizures in which there is a loss of muscle tone and the person falls to the ground)
   - Akinetic seizures (seizures in which there is a loss of muscle movement)

3. Unilateral seizures (seizures involving one hemisphere, or half, of the brain and consequently affecting one side of the body)

4. Unclassified epileptic seizures (seizures that, because of incomplete information, cannot be put in a category)

SOURCE: From "Clinical and electrocephalographical classification of epileptic seizures" by H. Gestaut, 1970, *Epilepsia*, *11*, p. 102. Copyright © 1970 by Raven Press. Reprinted by permission.

Procedure

Identification and Preventive Safety Measures for Patients on Seizure Precautions

 Steps

 Additional Information

1. Gather seizure history if possible from patient and family or from referral material.
   Information to be included:
   - Length of known seizure history
   - Date of last seizure (type and duration)
   - Common symptoms experienced
   - Presence of aura and type
   - Known precipitating factors
   - Current medications
   - Patient and family knowledge

2. Initiate seizure precautions.

3. Initiate safety measures.

4. Pad side rails of bed with cotton blankets or pads as judged necessary.

5. Obtain a protective helmet for patients with skull defect.

Physician's order is necessary. Once surgical plate is inserted, helmet may be discontinued.

6. Inform caregivers that electronic thermometer is necessary to take patient's temperature.

If glass thermometer must be used, then temperature must be taken through rectal or axillary route only.

7. Obtain suction machine for bedside as judged necessary.

Consider this for patients with difficulty with airway protection or at risk for status epilepticus.

 DOCUMENTATION

1. Document assessment and seizure history on appropriate medical record(s).

2. Document preventive safety measures to be implemented as seizure precautions.

3. Document patient and family education on appropriate medical record.

PATIENT AND FAMILY EDUCATION

Instruct the patient and family about:
1. The nature of the seizure disorder

2. Signs and symptoms of seizure activity, precautions, actions to take
   - Treatment, medication regimen including common side effects of medications

3. Common precipitating factors (alcohol, caffeine, fever, anxiety, fatigue, and stress)

4. Activity limitations (safety needs, use of machinery, and driving restrictions)

5. Medical follow-up after discharge

6. Need for oral care when taking phenytoin.

7. Generally, no driving, operating machinery, or swimming until seizure-free for 1 year.

Identification and Treatment of Seizures

 Steps

 Additional Information

1. At onset of symptoms, stay with patient, time seizure, and call for help. Provide for patient's safety.

See General Consideration 1 under Care of the Patient with a Seizure Disorder.

2. Turn patient's head to side, if possible, and flex it slightly to facilitate drainage of oral secretions.

Major actions: protect patient from injury and maintain patent airway.

3. Place pillow or blanket under patient's head.

In absence of pillow, place patient's head on your lap.

4. If possible, turn patient on his or her side.

If patient is in wheelchair, tilt chair back, remove belt, and slide chair from underneath patient, thus lowering patient to floor without lifting. If patient has skull defect, turn him or her to opposite side.

5. Loosen restrictive clothing.

6. Allow freedom of movement of extremities.

Remove harmful objects from reach or pad surfaces that might injure patient. If patient falls, logroll him or her if possible.

7. Suction patient as needed.

This helps reduce risk of aspiration.

8. If patient is receiving tube feeding, *stop feeding*.

9. Observe and note pattern of seizure, progression, changes in pupils or gaze, presence of incontinence, duration of seizure activity, and respiratory involvement.

10. Once seizure has subsided, carefully move patient, take vital signs, and monitor every 30 min.

If fall occurred, institute spinal precautions until directed otherwise by physician.

11. Allow patient time to sleep.

12. Observe for presence and duration of postictal symptoms
    - Paralysis
    - Somnolence
    - Aphasia
    - Headache
    - Incontinence

13. Monitor for recurrence of seizure activity.

14. When patient wakes, provide orientation and reassurance.   *Amnesia and disorientation are common.*

 DOCUMENTATION

In the appropriate medical record, note
- Onset of symptoms (time, pattern, and duration)
- Patient's activity at the time of onset
- General description
- Pupil or gaze changes
- Any injuries

- Postictal symptoms
- Notification of physician

REFERENCES

Gestaut, H. (1970) "Clinical and Electrocephalographical Classification of Epileptic Seizures" *Epilepsia* (11), 102.

U.S. Department of Health and Human Services (1995) *Clinical Practice Guidelines Post-Stroke Rehabilation* Agency for Health Care Policy and Research.

Autonomic Dysreflexia

Protocol for Identification and Treatment of Autonomic Dysreflexia

PURPOSE

To prevent acute episodes of autonomic dysreflexia in patients at risk; to describe methods to treat safely occurrences of dysreflexia

STAFF RESPONSIBLE

EQUIPMENT

1. Sphygmomanometer
2. Stethoscope
3. Nonsterile gloves
4. Irrigation kit
5. Normal saline irrigation solution
6. Straight or indwelling catheterization kit
7. Water-soluble lubricant
8. Protective underpads
9. Urinal
10. Nupercainal ointment and applicator
11. 2% lidocaine jelly

GENERAL CONSIDERATIONS

1. Autonomic dysreflexia is a life-threatening condition that can occur in patients who have spinal cord lesions at or above the T6 level. The onset of dysreflexia or hyperreflexia requires prompt recognition and treatment of the etiologic factors to prevent significant and potentially dangerous elevations in blood pressure (Consortium for Spinal Cord Medicine, 1997).

2. A noxious stimulus, most often visceral stretching, below the level of the lesion, triggers a generalized sympathetic response below the level of the injury. Vasoconstriction occurs below the level of the injury as a result of a loss of intact inhibitory fibers; vasodilation occurs above the level of the lesion (Erickson, 1980). The patient will experience sudden hypertension that will intensify until the noxious stimulus is removed. Failure to alleviate the cause may lead to neurologic or cardiac complications as a result of prolonged sympathetic excitation.

3. Signs and symptoms of autonomic dysreflexia most often include:
   - Sudden increase in systolic and diastolic blood pressure
   - Pounding headache ranging from mild to severe and often focused over the occipital area
   - Profuse sweating above the level of the injury
   - Piloerection above the level of the injury
   - Flushing of skin above the level of injury
   - Appearance of spots in patient's visual fields
   - Nasal congestion, altered level of consciousness, blurred vision, hiccups, penile erection
   - Feelings of apprehension or anxiety over impending physical problem
   - Cardiac arrhythmias, atrial fibrillation, ventricular contractions, and atrioventricular conduction abnormalities (Consortium for Spinal Cord Medicine, 1997)

4. Etiologic factors include the following:
   - *Urinary:* distention, stones, infection, bladder spasticity, micturition, catheterization, and cystoscopy, urodynamics, or detrusor-sphincter dyssynergy
   - *Bowel:* impaction, distention, digital stimulation, suppository insertion, enema administration, evacuation, and sigmoidoscopy testing
   - *Integumentary:* pressure ulcers, ingrown toenail, burns, and blisters
   - *Vascular:* venous thrombosis and external constriction (too tight clothing or shoes, and the like)
   - *Reproductive:* sexual intercourse, manual examination, menstruation, and uterine contractions
   - *Acute medical problems:* abdominal trauma, gallstones, appendicitis, or other pathology
   - *Fractures*
   - *Dental procedures:* extraction or abscess

5. If symptoms persist after nursing interventions, immediately contact physician for further treatment. Routinely, occurrences of autonomic dysreflexia and the treatment administered are reported to the physician according to policy.

Procedure

Prevention of Autonomic Dysreflexia Episodes

 Steps

 Additional Information

1. Assess patient for risk of dysreflexia.

   See General Consideration 3.

2. Teach patient and family to follow urinary management program to prevent distention, infection, and stones. If patient experiences symptoms with routine catheterizations, notify physician, and obtain order for 2% lidocaine or Xylocaine jelly to use with catheterization.

3. Teach patient and family to follow bowel management program. If patient experiences symptoms routinely with bowel procedures, request physician order for use of Nupercainal ointment with program.

   Patients at risk should have bowel program that results in bowel movement at least every other day.

4. Teach patient and family to follow skin care programs to prevent pressure sores; to check skin twice each day, including toenails; and to check for vascular changes in lower extremities.

5. Teach patient and family about acute medical conditions and procedures that may precipitate acute episodes and to seek medical intervention should they occur.

   Patients should inform community physicians that invasive bladder and bowel procedures may induce acute episode and that premedication may be warranted. Issue wallet card or medic alert bracelet that contains information about dysreflexia causes and treatment. Such a card is particularly useful for emergency episodes that occur while patient is in community.

6. Counsel patients regarding sexual responses after spinal cord injury and preventive measures to minimize risks of dysreflexia. Female patients should be advised that dysreflexia can occur during delivery and that premedication may be necessary.

7. Evaluate patient and family understanding of dysreflexia and of programs to prevent occurrence.

DOCUMENTATION

Document the patient and family teaching in the appropriate record.

Procedure

Identification and Treatment of an Acute Episode of Dysreflexia

 Steps

1. Assess patient for signs and symptoms.
2. Check patient's blood pressure.

3. If blood pressure is elevated, sit patient up and position his or her legs in dependent position.
4. Loosen any constrictive clothing.
5. Monitor blood pressure and pulse frequently.
6. If indwelling catheter is present, check for full leg bag. If it is full, empty it. Check blood pressure and patient for relief of symptoms. If bag is empty, check for kinks in catheter tubing, and reposition tubing to allow free flow of urine. Check patient and blood pressure for relief of symptoms. If bag is upside down, reposition it correctly, check for urine drainage, and check patient and blood pressure for relief of symptoms.

7. If indwelling catheter is not in place, instill 2% lidocaine jelly into urethra, wait a few minutes, then catheterize individual.

8. If it appears to be blocked, irrigate catheter with 30 mL of sterile saline to check patency. Check patient and blood pressure for relief of symptoms.

9. Change indwelling catheter if plugged.
10. If urinary distention is not present, suspect fecal impaction. Palpate patient's abdomen for distention, insert 2% lidocaine ointment into rectum, and wait 3 to 5 min. Insert lubricated, gloved finger into rectum, gently check for stool, and gently disimpact if able to do so.

11. If rectal check is negative and if symptoms are not relieved, notify physician. Monitor patient's blood pressure every 5 min. Inspect for other etiologic factors (skin, clothing, and so forth).

12. If unable to reduce blood pressure, consider pharmacologic therapy. Use an antihypertensive with rapid onset and of short duration.

Additional Information

See General Considerations 3 and 4.

Monitor blood pressure every 5 min during and after treatment for 15 min and then every 15 min up to 2 h after occurrence.

This facilitates venous pooling and lowers venous return to heart, thus lowering blood pressure.

Abdominal binder should be loosened.

An overfilled leg bag may result in bladder distention. An empty leg bag suggests that catheter is plugged, that tubing is kinked, or that leg bag is improperly positioned.

If indwelling catheter is in urethra, urine outflow will be blocked and can result in bladder distention.

If catheter is plugged, irrigation will be impossible or may dislodge obstructing clot, resulting in urine emptying. Never drain more than 500 mL at one time because rebound hypotension can occur. Clamp catheter for 10 to 15 min before draining more urine. Repeat.

Check for relief of symptoms.

See General Consideration 4.

Medications used include Nitropaste, atropine, Hyperstat, and other antihypertensive agents. Monitor for hypotension.

 DOCUMENTATION

1. Document in the appropriate medical record:
   • Signs and symptoms noted
   • Vital signs and treatment measures employed

   • Etiologic factor precipitating the episode
   • Plan to prevent further occurrence
   • Physician notification

2. Document the patient and family teaching in the medical record.

PATIENT AND FAMILY EDUCATION

1. The nurse is responsible for teaching the patient and family about the following:
   - What is autonomic dysreflexia
   - The consequences of dysreflexia
   - Signs and symptoms
   - Common etiologic factors
   - Treatment measures for acute and chronic episodes
   - Preventive measures to be followed

2. This teaching should be completed before the patient's first pass or out-trip and should be documented on the teaching checklist or in the progress notes of the medical record.

3. The patient should be taught the common signs early in his or her hospital stay so that he or she can request assistance early if they occur.

REFERENCES

Consortium for Spinal Cord Medicine (1997) *Acute Management of Autonomic Dysreflexia: Adults with Spinal Cord Injury Presenting to Health-Care Facilities* Washington, D.C.: Paralyzed Veterans of America.

Erickson, R.P. (1980) Autonomic Hyperreflexia: Pathophysiolgoy and medical management. *Archives of Physical Medicine and Rehabilitation* 61:431–440.

Chemotherapy Precautions

PURPOSE

To describe procedure for preparing, administering, and disposing of cytotoxic medications; to identify and define chemotherapy precautions and procedures required to implement them; to describe procedures for safe management of spills, contamination, and actions to take when situation occurs; to describe measures designed to protect workers from exposure to cytotoxic drugs

STAFF RESPONSIBLE

EQUIPMENT

1. Latex gloves (sterile or nonsterile depending on procedure)
2. Disposable nonpermeable gown (as needed)
3. Plastic face shield or eye goggles (as needed)
4. Disposable plastic back absorbent liner (Chux)
5. Large yellow plastic containers with toxic waste label
6. Hamper with yellow toxic waste linen bags

 ### GENERAL CONSIDERATIONS

1. Preparation, storage, administration, and disposal of cytotoxic medications can expose hospital staff to high envi-

ronmental levels of these agents and the risks associated with long-term exposure. This procedure defines chemotherapy precautions that are the reasonable course of action required to protect workers from these occupational hazards (OSHA, 1986).

2. The risk to workers is the combined result of the drug's inherent toxicity and the extent to which workers are exposed to cytotoxic drugs on the job. The main routes of exposure are:
   - inhalation of drug dusts or droplets
   - absorption through the skin
   - ingestion through contact with contaminated food or cigarettes (OSHA, 1986)

3. Smoking, drinking, applying cosmetics, and eating should never take place in areas where cytotoxic drugs are being prepared.

4. Excreta from patients who have received cytotoxic drugs may contain high concentrations of the drug or hazardous metabolites and should be handled with caution. Any patient currently receiving cytotoxic drugs or who has received a cytotoxic drug within a period of 48 h must be on chemotherapy precautions (OSHA, 1986). All staff are to carry out the steps described in this procedure.

5. Chemotherapy precautions are required whenever the patient is receiving any of the medications listed in Table 6-1 of this procedure.

6. Cytotoxic drugs may be used in the treatment of arthritis or other non-cancer-related diseases. Examples of cytotoxic drugs that may be used in arthritis management include methotrexate. Patients receiving these meds must be treated in accordance with chemotherapy precautions according to current OSHA guidelines.

Procedure

Identifying Patients Requiring Chemotherapy Precautions

1. On admission review medications and obtain order from physician for chemotherapy precautions as appropriate.

2. Orders for chemotherapy precautions are listed on patient care plan and medication instructions and communicated to pharmacy and all allied health areas.

3. Review medication instructions for chemotherapy precautions before preparing medications.

334

Table 6-1   Antineoplastic Drugs

Generic Name	Trade Name	Generic Name	Trade Name
Altretamine		Ifosfamide	Isophosphamide
Aminoglutethimide		Interferon-A	
Azathioprine		Isotretinoin	
L-Asparaginase	Elspar	Leuprolide	
Bleomycin	Blenoxane	Levamisole	
Busulfan		Lomustine	
Carboplatin		Mechlorethamine	
Carmustine	BICNU	Medroxyprogesterone	
Chloramphenicol		Megestrol	
Chlorotrianisene		Melphalan	
Chlorozotocin		Mercaptopurine	
Cyclosporin		Methotrexate	Mexate, Folex
Cisplatin		Mitomycin	Mutamycin
Cyclophosphamide	Cytoxan, Neoscar	Mitotane	
Cytarabine		Mitoxantrone	
Dacarbazine	DTIC	Nafarelin	
Dactinomycin	Cosmegen	Pipobroman	
Daunorubicin		Plicamycin	
Diethylstilbestrol		Procarbazine	Matulane
Doxorubicin	Adriamycin	Ribavirin	
Estradiol		Streptozocin	Zanosar
Estramustine		Tamoxifen	
Ethinyl estradiol		Testolactone	
Etoposide	VePesid	Thioguanine	6-TG Thioguanine
Floxuridine		Thiotepa	Triethylene thiophosphoramide
Fluorouracil	5FU, Adrucil	Uracil mustard	Uramustine
Flutamide		Vidarabine	
Ganciclovir		Vinblastine	Velban
Hydroxyurea		Vincristine	Oncovin
Idarubicin		Zidovudine	

Preparation, Administration, and Storage of Cytotoxic Drugs

4. Oral medications
   - Wash hands
   - Apply latex gloves
   - Pour medication into the medicine cup without touching the pill
   - Dispense medication per facility policy
   - Any unusable oral medication must be disposed of in accordance with procedure on disposal
   - Place closed medication bottle in plastic bag and seal
   - Remove latex gloves. Discard in plastic toxic waste container

5. Intramuscular drugs
   - Wash hands
   - Place disposable chux on work area at nurses station
   - Gather supplies: needle, syringe, 4 × 4 gauze
   - Apply latex gloves
   - Add diluent slowly
   - Wrap 4 × 4 gauze around the vial to prevent spraying while slowly removing medication.
   - Clear drug from the needle before removing it from the vial.
   - Place used needle in plastic toxic waste container.

- Dispose of unused medication according to procedure on disposal.
- Position patient and place chux below injection site.
- Locate injection site, don gloves, swab with alcohol, and administer injection.
- Place needle and syringe in plastic toxic waste container. Dispose of gloves, gauze, and chux in accordance with procedure on disposal.
- Wash hands

6. Topical medications
   - Wash hands
   - Double glove with latex gloves.
   - Place chux below area of application.
   - Apply medication to the prescribed area until med is absorbed.
   - For meds not absorbed cover the area with gauze and secure with tape.
   - Remove gloves and dispose of gloves and gauze in accordance with procedure on disposal.

7. Caring for patient receiving cytotoxic drugs
   Drugs and/or their metabolites may be excreted in the urine, feces, or other body fluids. Personnel dealing with these fluids should follow these guidelines.
   - Wash hands
   - Wear latex gloves when in contact with urine, stool, gastric secretions. In cases where exposure may be extensive (i.e., diarrhea, urinary incontinence, emesis), gowns, double gloves, masks, and eye protection may be necessary.

8. Disposal of contaminated materials
   - Place disposable products (paper, gauze, unused medication in a plastic bag/wrapper) in plastic toxic waste container.
   - Place contaminated linen in plastic toxic waste bag in patient room or therapy area.
   - Contaminated patient clothing must be washed in soap/water separate from other clothing. Run an empty cycle of detergent/water before washing other laundry in machine.

9. Managing spills
   - Spills should be cleaned immediately.
   - Identify and mark spill area.
   - **For overt contamination of the person:** remove gloves and gown, wash area three times with non-germicidal soap (approximately 5-min wash).
     For eye exposure: flood the eye with water for at least 5 min. Notify employee health nurse for further treatment.
   - Apply latex gloves and place absorbent gauze on spill and absorb liquid. Wash area three times with detergent and water.
   - Apply latex gloves and with wet 4×4 gauze absorb solid spill waste. Wash area three times with soap/water solution and rinse well with water.
   - Large spills: Identify and mark spill area to alert other staff of the spill. NOTIFY APPROPRIATE DEPARTMENT TO REMOVE SPILL AS SPECIAL PROTECTIVE EQUIPMENT MAY BE NEEDED.

 DOCUMENTATION

1. Document medication administered in the medical record.
2. Chart implementation of chemotherapy precautions in the medical record.
3. Spills and/or exposure to cytotoxic drugs should be noted on employee unusual occurrence report.

REFERENCES

ASHP Technical Assistance Bulletin on Handling Cytotoxic and Hazardous Drugs (1990) *American Journal of Hospital Pharmacy* 47:1033–1049.

Gullo, S. (1988) "Safe Handling of Antineoplastic Drugs: Translating the Recommendations into Practice" *Oncology Nursing Forum* 15(5):595–601.

OSHA Chemotherapy Guidelines 8-1.1, January 29, 1986.

OSHA Instruction TED 1.15, September 15, 1995.

Power, L.A., Anderson, R.W., Cortopassi, R., et al. (1990) "Update on Safe Handling of Hazardous Drugs: The Advice of Experts" *American Journal of Hospital Pharmacy* 47.

Latex Allergy Precautions

PURPOSE

To identify individuals at risk for latex allergy; to describe actions to take to provide safe, therapeutic environment; to describe staff responsibilities for education of patient and family

STAFF RESPONSIBLE

EQUIPMENT

No equipment necessary.

 GENERAL CONSIDERATIONS

1. Latex allergy is an allergic or hypersensitivity reaction that occurs in response to contact with latex. The nature of the response may be:
   • Cutaneous: hives, swelling
   • Ocular: tearing, redness, swelling
   • Nasal: sneezing, discharge, congestion, itching
   • Asthmatic: wheezing, chest tightness, shortness of breath, or respiratory arrest
2. Latex products are made from the sap of the rubber tree. It is commonly used for its elasticity, strength, tear resistance, and degree of protection.
3. Individuals at risk for latex allergy include:
   • Individuals with history of food allergy to banana, kiwi, papaya, melon, pear, potato, tomato, fig, avocado, cherry, celery, peach
   • Individuals with prolonged contact with latex products such as healthcare workers and individuals with spina bifida or spinal cord damage
4. Signs and symptoms of a latex allergy include:
   • Generalized hives or rash
   • Flushing
   • Swelling
   • Vomiting, cramps, diarrhea
   • Hypotension
   • Acute asthma
   • Cardiovascular collapse

Procedure

 Steps

1. Identify patients at risk and monitor for signs and symptoms of latex allergy.
2. Look at environment and remove latex to provide a safe environment.
   • Place patient in private room or room with another patient on latex precautions.
   • Clean and remove all latex 24 h prior to admission.
   • Close door after cleaning until patient arrives.
3. Alert staff to allergy and need for non-latex product alternatives.
   • Physician documents latex allergy in medical record
   • Latex allergy precautions are communicated to staff treating patient.
   • Review treatment plan to insure patient is not exposed to latex during treatment or in treatment environments (Table 6-2).

4. Before using any product during patient care check for latex content. If latex is present check for latex-free alternative option (Table 6-3). Instruct patient and family re: latex allergy safety, signs and symptoms of allergy, and actions to take.

 DOCUMENTATION

1. Document latex allergy in medical record.
2. Place latex allergy notification in medical record and room.
3. Document patient care interventions in medical record.
4. Document patient and family teaching.

PATIENT AND FAMILY EDUCATION

Instruct patient and family re: latex allergy safety, signs and symptoms of allergy, and actions to take.

LEVELS OF CONSIDERATIONS

REFERENCES

Barton, E.C. (1993) "Latex Allergy Recognition and Management of a Modern Problem" *Nurse Practitioner* 18(11):54–58.

Charous, L. (1995) "Perspectives in Latex Allergy for Healthcare Workers, A Slide Education Program" Beckton-Dickinson.

Hancock, D.L. (1994) "Latex Allergy Prevention and Treatment" *Anesthesiology Review* 21(5):153–163.

Tomazic, V.J., Shampaine, E.L., Lamanna, A., et al. (1994) "Cornstarch Powder on Latex Products Is an Allergen Carrier" *Journal of Allergy & Clinical Immunology* 53(4):751–757.

Table 6-2 Common Latex Products and Alternatives in Healthcare

Product	Latex-Free Option	Product	Latex-Free Option
Latex gloves	Vinyl gloves	Leg bag straps	Use Velcro or nylon straps
Band-Aids	Transparent occlusive dressing	Foam lining	Transparent occlusive dressings
Ace bandages	Kling, Kerlix	IV bags	Glass bottles
Blood pressure cuff	Plastic disposable cuff	Rubber stoppers—meds, IV tubing, ABG kits	Use meds in glass ampules, use Clave connector on IV tubing
Resuscitator Bag	Plastic model	Stethoscope tubing	Use plastic models
Urinary catheters	Silicone catheters	Roho cushions	Gel or foam cushions
Condom external catheters	Silicone brands	Theraband	Latex-free option
Diapers	Tranquility brand or Huggies	Wheelchair gloves	Latex-free option
Adhesive tape	Plastic or silk tape		

Table 6-3 Common Latex Products in the Home

Art supplies	Contraceptive sponge	Rubber bands
Balloons	Cosmetic applicators	Rubber toys
Balls	Elastic clothing	Socks
Bathroom throw rugs	Erasers	Swimwear
Bungee cords	Feeding nipples	Tires
Cleaning gloves	Hoses	Wheelchair cushions and tires
Condoms	Pacifiers	Zippered storage bags

Behavior Precautions

Elopement Precautions

PURPOSE

To provide a safety management plan for patients identified as elopement risk

STAFF RESPONSIBLE

EQUIPMENT

No equipment necessary.

GENERAL CONSIDERATIONS

1. Elopement risk is determined by the physician in conjunction with the treatment team. Risk status is discussed and reviewed at team conference.

2. Individuals who have attempted to leave the unit or demonstrated behaviors that staff assesses to be a safety risk may be placed on elopement precautions.

3. Identifying characteristics which may be indicative of risk include patients:
   - Who state desire for unauthorized leave
   - Unable to follow a schedule of activities without moderate to maximal cues
   - Who are easily agitated
   - Who require 1:1 supervision for safety or wandering or are highly active
   - Who frequently talk about need to return home and are unable to understand need for hospitalization
   - Who are determined to be at risk

4. All patients on elopement precautions are to be handed off to the next therapist or returned to the patient unit by the therapist.

5. Patients on elopement precautions should be considered for therapy on the patient unit whenever possible.

6. The physician order for elopement precautions is communicated to all clinical departments.

7. Elopement precautions may be necessary to maintain safety for patients with cognitive deficits in the home. Wandering is a common problem for patients with memory loss or impaired judgment. Consider a medical alert bracelet or identification card to provide cues or alert others to identity of the person and contact information. Evaluate home environment and neighborhood for possible hazards (i.e., pools, uneven walkways, busy street intersections). A call bell system or use of baby monitors may help a caregiver monitor family member during the night.

Procedure

Steps

1. Physician, nurse, or therapist identifies patient as "elopement risk."

2. Physician enters precaution order for "elopement precautions."

3. The nurse enters a nursing order on patient care plan indicating "elopement precautions" and communicates precaution order to all clinical departments and security.

4. Therapist meets patient on the nursing unit and escorts patient to the therapy location.

5. The therapist will escort the patient to next therapist or return the patient to the nursing unit unless patient is accompanied by a private duty sitter.

6. Nursing staff are to escort patient to any group therapy. The therapist is to escort patient to next class or return patient to the nursing unit.

DOCUMENTATION

1. The nurse documents risk status in progress note in the medical record and enters necessary orders on care plan.

2. The nurse or designee reevaluates behavior, effectiveness to the interventions, and any changes in plan and documents assessment weekly.

PATIENT AND FAMILY EDUCATION

Provide patient/family instructions on activity restrictions and need for supervision.

REFERENCES

Mace, N.L., and Rabins, P.V. (1991) *The Thirty-Six Hour Day* New York: Warner Brothers Books.

Guidelines for Behavior Management

PURPOSE

To aid staff in early identification of potentially problematic situations for the patient; to guide staff in assessing the underlying sources of patient agitation; to aid staff in prevention of further escalation of a patient's unwanted behavior; to describe preventative safety measures which minimize risk of injury to the patient and staff; to describe staff treatment responsibilities for patients with potential behavioral concerns

STAFF RESPONSIBLE

EQUIPMENT

No equipment necessary.

GENERAL CONSIDERATIONS

1. These generally accepted teaching tools should be used for all patients and are effective in promoting the patient's growth and dignity and in preventing behavioral episodes:
   • Reinforce appropriate behaviors as often as possible

Signs of Patient Behavioral Distress

1. Angry facial expressions

2. Rigid defensive posture

3. Increased motor activity of extremities (often purposeless); pacing

• Ignore inappropriate behaviors when not a safety risk and verbally acknowledge patient when appropriate behavior is demonstrated

• Ignore inappropriate behaviors while redirecting patient to task at hand, then reinforce patient's engagement in the task

• Give patients a choice of activities during each session

2. Agitation is hyperarousal or excesses of behavior in response to internal or external stimuli, and it is often characterized by restlessness, inability to focus or maintain attention, irritability, and/or combative behaviors. Agitation occurs during a particular stage of recovery for many patients and will generally improve, often with no intervention.

3. Agitated and/or combative behaviors most often occur in the rehabilitation setting when patients:
   • Are frustrated with their dependence and are only beginning to address the issues of adjustment
   • Are emerging from coma, have frontal lobe damage, and/or have cognitive deficits that limit the patient's ability to understand verbal and other environmental stimuli
   • Feel they have little choice or control over their environment, and many demands are being placed on them
   • Experience change (in routine, therapists, rooms, etc.)

4. Perseveration

5. Threatening statements

6. Refusals

7. Arguing

8. Suspicion of others

Staff Responses

During a behavioral intervention, respect for individual rights and the patient's dignity, as well as protecting the safety of the patient, other patients, staff and visitors, are the key considerations. Only the least restrictive interventions are used. The most important tools for working with pateints exhibiting discomfort, anxiety, combativeness, or other unwanted behaviors are:

1. Assessment
   - Know your patient and stay alert for signs of behavioral/emotional distress
   - Keep in mind the "meaning" of the behaviors—patients often communicate in less than optimal ways; the patient may be verbal and may appear to have better communication skills than they actually possess
   - Assess the possibility of physical discomfort that might be created by noxious stimuli (nasogastric tubes, indwelling catheters, constipation, etc.); if deemed appropriate through nursing assessment, remove noxious stimuli

2. Environmental considerations
   - Create an environment that is safe, calm
   - Reduce stimuli, including verbal and visual, for those who are distractible, confused, or otherwise cognitively impaired
   - Never argue with the patient
   - Keep a calm voice and maintain some distance from patient as appropriate
   - When a patient exhibits signs of distress, stop the activity and determine next steps to help calm the patient
   - Stop all demands and begin a problem-solving process with the patient
   - Sit quietly with patient if this is helpful—reintroduce activity *only with patient's permission* and only after patient has calmed

3. Treatment plan
   If unwanted behaviors persist or escalate, a more formalized intervention may be warranted. If a formalized intervention is needed, the plan is developed by the treatment team with input from the patient and family. The team should identify the following when developing the plan:
   - Those situations which appear to "elicit" the unwanted behavior(s)
   - The reinforcers of the person served
   - The behaviors that are important for the patient to engage in—either to achieve short-term therapy goals or to improve community/social functioning

   The following elements should be included in the plan:
   - Identification of the "target behaviors"
   - Targeted behaviors that increase appropriate behaviors or skills, not merely decrease unwanted behaviors
   - Determination of the behavioral intervention that will be implemented
   - Criteria for effectiveness measurement (time limitation, measurement tools, etc.)
   - Inclusion of the behavior plan in the patient's overall treatment plan, documenting evidence of input of the person served or his/her guardian, family member, or caregiver as appropriate
   - Review of plan by a psychologist

 ## DOCUMENTATION

1. Initial assessment on admit form or progress note.
2. Interventions for behavior management program on patient care plan.
3. Indications and goals to be achieved.
4. Ongoing assessments of patient behavior and effectiveness of treatment plan.

5. Specific incidents of acute agitation and/or violent behavior in progress notes, noting antecedents, behavior, and consequences of behavior.
6. Patient/family education on teaching checklist or progress notes.
7. Implementation of prescribed behavior plan.

Guidelines for the Use of Restraints

PURPOSE

To protect patient rights and promote safety; to protect physical well-being of the patient and/or the well being of others; to guide decision making and describe proper ordering and use of restraints

STAFF RESPONSIBLE

EQUIPMENT

No equipment necessary.

GENERAL CONSIDERATIONS

1. *Restraint Philosophy:* Restraints will be used only when all identified and appropriate alternatives have been exhausted. When restraints are used, patients and families will be educated and involved regarding restraint usage. Every effort is made to continually evaluate the necessity of restraints, seek opportunities to reduce usage, and provide care to maintain patient dignity and minimize complications.

2. *Restraint Definition:* Any method of physically restricting a person's freedom of movement, physical activity, or normal access to his or her body (JCAHO TX.7, 1998).

3. *Seclusion Definition:* The involuntary confinement of a person alone in a room where the person is physically prevented from leaving (JCAHO TX.7, 1998). Seclusion does not include the therapeutic holding or comforting of children or a time-out when the person to whom it is applied is physically prevented from leaving a room for 15 min or less (JCAHO TX.7, 1998). Seclusion is not utilized at RIC.

4. Behavioral strategies should be used before use of restraints.

5. The physician/nurse assesses the need for restraints or immobilization taking into account:
   • Patient's age
   • Cognitive status
   • Underlying cause of agitation or confusion
   • Mobility
   • Skin status
   • Potential for injury to self or others

6. The interdisciplinary team discusses safety, behavior, mobility issues, and on-going need for restraints, and plans for safety and goal achievement at weekly team conference.

7. *Indications and Contraindications for Restraint Interventions*
   • These interventions are appropriate when:
     • Less restrictive measures as appropriate per the assessment have been tried and failed.
     • The patient is a potential danger to self or others.
     • The patient's behavior is not manageable within the care environment.
   • Restraint use may be contraindicated in certain conditions (i.e., burned extremities, fracture extremities, claustrophobia)
   • The benefits of restraints compared to the risks are to be evaluated on an individual basis

8. A patient when restrained or immobilized must be checked at least every 30 min for safety, circulatory status, and to insure comfort needs are attended to. The restraint is loosened and reapplied every 2 h. It is recommended that the restraint be removed at the start of each therapy session and then reapplied.

9. Knots must have appropriate quick release hitch (square knot or clove hitch) and be positioned where it can easily be reached in case of an emergency.

PROCEDURE

Restraint	Pros
Mitts/Cloth Extremity Restraints	Soft cloth extremity restraints are used to restrain extremities and prevent a patient from striking out, or pulling at tubes. This restraint is applied as follows: • One wrist • Both wrists • Both ankles and one wrist • One wrist and the opposite ankle • Both wrists and one ankle It is essential that the restraint be tied to movable part of the bed to prevent injury. Never secure to side rails or bed frame.
Jacket Restraints	Correct jacket restraint size is important for proper application so always check sizing on package to verify correct size before applying to the patient.
Vail/Optima 3000 Bed Enclosure	The Vail/Optima 3000 Bed Enclosure is considered a restrictive device. Prior to initiating use of the bed consider less restrictive measures. The Vail/Optima 3000 Bed Enclosure is a metal frame with a net covering on five sides that surrounds a standard hospital bed. The bed enclosure allows visualization of the patient at all times. The Vail/Optima Bed is appropriate for patients who are restless, agitated, and at risk due to impaired judgment as a result of primarily internal stimuli. The patient and family should be informed of the purpose and reason for the use of the bed. The appearance of the bed may be frightening to the patient and family. If use is anticipated orient family to appearance, use, and therapeutic benefits. Each bed is cleaned at regular intervals using appropriate disinfectant solution, and upon discontinuation. Notify housekeeping to clean unit. The canopy is washed in commercial-size washer with standard detergents and then hung to dry. It must never be placed in dryer as this will cause shrinkage.

Restraint	Pros
Elbow Restraints	Elbow restraints are used to prevent infants or small children from flexing their arms. The restraint consists of material with pockets into which plastic or wood tongue depressors are inserted to provide rigidity. Size of restraint may be modified by breaking tongue blade, taping the insert into pockets.

DOCUMENTATION

1. Use of restraints, criteria, behaviors, alternatives tried in medical record.

2. Any unusual occurrences in the progress notes of the medical record.

3. Patient/Family Education on teaching checklist or progress notes.

REFERENCES

Evans, L.K., and Strumpf, N.E. (1990) "Myths about Elder Restraint, IMAGE" *Journal of Nursing Scholarship* 22(2):128.

Janelli, L.M. (1995) "Physical Restraint Use in Acute Care Settings" *Journal of Nursing Care Quality* 9(3):86–92.

JCAHO (1998) *Comprehensive Accreditation Manual for Hospitals* 21–22.

Moss, R.J., and LaPuma, J. (1991) "The Ethics of Mechanical Restraints" *Hastings Center Report* 22–25.

Richmond, I., Trujillo, D., Schmelzer, J., et al. (1996) "Least Restrictive Alternatives: Do They Really Work?" *Journal of Nursing Care Quality* 11(1):29–37.

Schleenbacker, R.E., McDowell, S.M., Moore, R.W., et al. (1994) "Restraint Use in Inpatient Rehabilitation: Incidence, Predictors, and Implications" *Archives of Physical Medicine and Rehabilitation* 75(4):427–430.

Use of Bed Enclosure

PURPOSE

To decrease environmental stimuli; to provide an emotionally and physically secure environment; to prevent falls; to provide an alternative method to physical restraints

STAFF RESPONSIBLE

EQUIPMENT

1. Craig bed or Emory cubicle bed (Fig. 6-3)

2. Two to four mattresses

3. Sheet of plastic

4. Two convoluted foam mattresses

5. Two fitted sheets or one king-size fitted sheet

6. One flat sheet

7. Pillows

GENERAL CONSIDERATIONS

1. The Craig bed/Emory cubicle beds are specially designed beds. They consist of four high padded walls that sur-

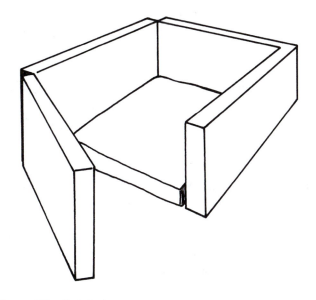

Figure 6-3 Craig bed.

round one or two mattresses placed on the floor or bed frame. The walls form a square that surrounds the mattresses. This bed works best if the patient is able to transfer himself or herself from the floor to the wheelchair with minimal assistance. Patients with tracheostomy or enteric feeding tubes may be difficult to manage in this type of bed. The bed works well with patients who have the potential for agitation or violent behavior because a wheelchair can be positioned in the center if mattresses are removed. This allows the patient a small, confined area with decreased stimulation as a time-out period. It works best for patients who can use a flat bed and who can pull themselves up to a standing position when they are restless. The inner vertical surface of the bed can be used to display orientation aids or familiar objects.

2. Check with your facility to clarify if a bed enclosure is classified as restraint or restraint alternative.

3. The decision to use a Craig bed should be made by the physician and the nurse on the basis of the amount of stimulation that the patient can tolerate, the current functional level, and the current nursing care needs. Mobile, agitated patients generally are not candidates for using the Craig bed because of safety concerns. The goals and outcomes during the use of the bed should be frequently reevaluated. A physician's order should be written for the appropriate bed.

4. Safety issues necessitating the use of the particular bed should be documented in the medical record.

5. A private room may be needed when using the large bed.

6. Each bed should be cleaned at regular intervals with antiseptic solution and on discontinuation of use. Notify housekeeping of the need to clean the unit. When using the bed with incontinent patients, it is imperative that a large plastic sheet be placed on the floor beneath the mattress.

9. The bed is discontinued when the goals and outcomes are achieved, when the goals and outcomes are not realized and further use is deemed unnecessary, or when adverse effects occur (e.g., agitation increases).

Procedure

Steps

1. Obtain physician's order.
2. Describe bed and desired outcomes to patient and family.
3. Evaluate amount of stimulation that patient should receive.
4. Notify appropriate staff of need to set up bed and determine whether additional mattresses will be needed.
5. Lock entrance walls when patient is unattended.

Additional Information

Bed surface may be raised with additional mattresses stacked on top of each other.

DOCUMENTATION

1. Note in a progress note when the bed is ordered, the reason for its use, and the goals and outcomes to be achieved.
2. Enter the order for the bed in the patient's care plan and chart its daily use.
3. Document in a progress note on periodic basis the achievement of goals and any limitations.

PATIENT AND FAMILY EDUCATION

1. The patient and family should be informed about the purpose and reasons for using the bed. The appearance of the bed may be frightening to the patient and family.

2. Orient the family to the appearance, use, and therapeutic benefits of the bed.

3. Teach the family interaction skills and when and how to secure the locks on the bed.

REFERENCES

Williams, L.M., Morton, G.A., and Patrick, C.H. (1990) "The Emory Cubicle Bed: An Alternative to Restraints for Traumatically Brain Injured Clients" *Rehabilitation Nursing* 15(1):30–33.

Vail/Optima 3000 Bed Enclosure

PURPOSE

To provide minimally restrictive environment for patients at risk of injury to self; to describe appropriate use of the Vail/Optima 3000 Bed Enclosure; to describe proper maintenance of the Vail/Optima 3000

STAFF RESPONSIBLE

EQUIPMENT

1. Vail/Optima 3000 Bed Enclosure

GENERAL CONSIDERATIONS

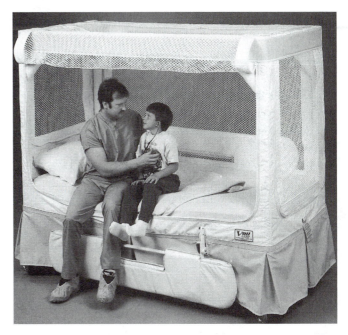

Figure 6-4 Vail/Optima enclosed bed. (Reprinted with permission, Vail Products, Inc. Toledo, Ohio.)

1. The Vail/Optima 3000 Bed Enclosure may be considered a restrictive device. Prior to initiating use of the Vail/Optima bed, consider less restrictive measures. Vail/Optima 3000 Bed Enclosure is a metal frame with a net covering on five sides that surrounds a standard hospital bed. The Vail/Optima enclosure allows visualization of the patient at all times. The Vail/Optima bed is appropriate for patients who are restless, agitated, and at risk due to impaired judgment as a result of primarily internal stimuli.

2. The decision to use a particular bed should be made by the physician and the nurse based on patient medical status, amount of stimuli the patient can tolerate, current functional level, and current nursing care needs.

3. Safety issues or documentation necessitating use of a particular bed should be documented in the medical record.

4. The patient and family should be informed of the purpose and reason for the use of the bed. The appearance of the bed may be frightening to the patient and family; if use is anticipated, orient family to appearance, use, and therapeutic benefits.

5. Current behavior, patient response to this treatment, and safety issues necessitating use of a particular bed should be documented in the progress notes in the medical record at least daily.

6. Families should be taught how to interact with the patient in the bed and when/how to close the bed.

7. Each bed is cleaned at regular intervals using appropriate disinfectant solution and upon discontinuation. Notify housekeeping to clean unit. The canopy is washed in commercial-size washer with standard detergents and then hung to dry. It must never be placed in dryer as this will cause shrinkage.

8. Staff should monitor and interact with patients in the Vail/Optima bed consistent with any other restraint device. Observations should include:
   - General safety of patient
   - All zippers are closed and secure
   - The safety ring is in place at foot of the bed
   - All tubing and lines are unobstructed

9. Do not cut or stretch the mesh as this will weaken the fabric. Do not place indwelling tubes (IVs, urinary drainage, etc.) through the mesh.

10. The bed is discontinued when:
    - Goals/outcomes are achieved
    - Goals/outcomes are not realized and further use is deemed not necessary
    - Adverse effects occur

11. See specific equipment instructions for additional product information.

Procedure

 Steps

 Additional Information

1. Obtain physician order.
2. Evaluate the amount and type of stimuli the patient should receive.
3. Remove headboard, footboard, and wall bumpers from hospital bed.
4. Position Vail/Optima 3000 bed around patient bed.
5. Pad siderails to minimize sliding and protect patient from injury.
6. Once bed is in position remove wheels on Vail/Optima bed.
7. Orient patient to the bed.
8. Close all zippers on the bed.
9. Insure the locking safety ring is in place to prevent the patient from unzipping the base and leaving enclosure.

Someone should stay with the patient initially to assess adjustment and safety needs.

 DOCUMENTATION

The registered nurse documents:
1. In progress notes on initiation of the bed:
   • When use of bed is initiated
   • Reason for use
   • Goals/outcomes to be achieved
   • Initial patient response

2. Order for bed on patient care plan.
3. In progress note, on periodic basis, achievement of goals and/or limitations, and patient response to the bed.

All Staff document on chart daily use of bed and routine monitoring.

PATIENT AND FAMILY EDUCATION

Describe the bed and desired outcomes to the patient and family.

Assisting a Patient to Prevent Falls

PURPOSE

To protect patient from injury; to minimize risk for staff injury

STAFF RESPONSIBLE

EQUIPMENT

No equipment necessary.

 GENERAL CONSIDERATIONS

1. Every effort is made to promote patient independence and function; however, in the process it is essential to be alert to potential risks to patient and staff.
2. When assisting a patient with a transfer or ambulation and the patient becomes weak or unable to continue, the safest option for the patient and staff member is for the staff member to gently lower the patient to the floor.
3. When a patient is lowered to the floor, document occurrence according to facility policy.

Procedure

 Steps

 Additional Information

1. Assess patient ability to continue activity.

2. If risk exists that the transfer cannot be completed or the patient is unable to safely ambulate to rest spot, the patient should be assisted to the floor and help summoned.

3. Staff member stops activity and positions legs with a wide base of support with one leg slightly in front of the other.

4. Staff member gently shifts patient weight to themselves, bends at knees, and lowers patient to the floor. If the patient is ambulatory, shift patient weight to anterior thigh and slide patient down thigh to the floor.

5. Position patient so as to avoid injury.

6. Stay with patient and provide comfort.

7. Call for assistance before moving the patient.

8. Report to the nurse/therapist:
   - Precipitating events
   - How lowering to the floor occurred
   - Any patient complaints or symptoms incurred prior to or during event

9. The nurse/therapist evaluates potential contributing factors and revises treatment plan accordingly.

 DOCUMENTATION

1. Document event according to facility policy.

2. Nurse/therapist documents evaluation and actions taken in the medical record.

PATIENT AND FAMILY EDUCATION

Teach patient/caregiver how to recognize problems with transfers/ambulation and provide assistance in a manner that reduces injury to individual and caregiver.

REFERENCES

Baker, L. (1992) "Developing a Safety Plan that Works for Patients and Nurses" *Rehabilitation Nursing* 17:264–266.

Brains, L., Alexander, K., Grotta, P., et al. (1991) "The Development of the RISK Tool for Fall Prevention" *Rehabilitation Nursing* 16:67–69.

Rappaport, L.J., Webster, J.S., Flemming, K.L., et al. (1993) "Predictors of Falls among Right-Hemisphere Stroke Patients in the Rehabilitation Setting" *Archives of Physical Medicine and Rehabilitation* 74:621–626.

Rogers, S. (1994) "Reducing Falls in a Rehabilitation Setting: A Safer Environment through Team Effort" *Rehabilitation Nursing* 19(5):274–276.

Vlahov, D., Myers, A.H., and Al-Ibrahim, M.S. (1990) "Epidemiology of Falls among Patients in a Rehabilitation Hospital" *Archives of Physical Medicine and Rehabilitation* 71:8–12.

Equipment Safety

Electric Wheelchair Safety

PURPOSE

To promote safe usage and care of electric wheelchairs; to reinforce patient and family teaching about care and usage of electric wheelchairs.

STAFF RESPONSIBLE

EQUIPMENT

Electric wheelchair and battery charger (as issued by physical therapist or owned by patient)

 GENERAL CONSIDERATIONS

1. Electric wheelchair batteries should be recharged in the hallways outside the patient's room.

2. Safety precautions to take when recharging electric wheelchair batteries are:
   - Chargers should be set on the ground or on shelf in hallways that are built for this purpose.
   - Wires should not be stretched, exposed, or come in contact with anything other than battery post and connector.
   - Chargers and the battery of the electric wheelchair must be dry and placed on a dry surface.
   - Only recharge battery if the electric wheelchair has been used. Recharging takes about 8 hours, depending on usage (i.e., when plugging in electric wheelchair to battery charger if charger registers 0 amps, it is fully charged—Do not overcharge.)
   - Turn electric wheelchair off before charging (except for LEVO Standup Wheelchair).
   - Colored plug on electric wheelchair battery must match colored plug on battery charger in respect to color and fit of plugs (exceptions: Amigo and LEVO Standup).

   - Amount of amperes on charger can be used to estimate amount of time battery is charged for use (i.e., 0 amps indicate electric wheelchair has 8 h of time usage).
   - Most battery rechargers are automatic. However, some older battery rechargers require setting the timer to activate recharging.

3. Safety precautions to take when using electric wheelchairs include:
   - Protective cover and straps must be over battery (protective covers are made of vinyl or hard plastic). Ideally the battery should be in a battery box.
   - Controls for manipulating electric wheelchair must be firmly and securely attached to the wheelchair. If loose or wires are exposed, return wheelchair to physical therapy for repair. Do not allow patient to use wheelchair until repaired.
   - Transfers requiring removal of wheelchair arm which has the controls on it must be avoided.

4. Battery care and maintenance includes:
   - The battery generally lasts 1 year.
   - Recharge battery daily if electric wheelchair is used daily. If electric wheelchair has not been used and was previously charged, the battery will remain charged if not used for 3 to 4 weeks.
   - When charger does not recharge battery this means one of the fuses in the charger has been blown. There are two fuses, one is accessible from the outside and one is accessible only if the whole unit is to be taken apart.
   - In the home setting, the battery charger can be plugged into any 120V outlet.

5. Types of electric wheelchairs:
   - Microswitch: Is sensitive to small movements and moves in one speed and one direction until another command is given (i.e., sip and puff controls, chin controls, toe/finger controls, etc.).
   - Proportional: The farther the switch is moved, the faster the chair moves (i.e., Joystick hand control).
   - Motor Scooter: A motor scooter is able to get into tight places and move at variable speeds. Differs for recharging by an outlet into which the recharger is plugged (e.g., Amigo).

Procedure

 Steps

 Additional Information

1. Insure that the electric wheelchair and battery is electrically safe.

2. Place electric wheelchair in hallway outside patient's room.

3. Place charger on floor or firmly on shelf.

4. Turn electric wheelchair OFF (except LEVO Standup).

5. Connect plugs from electric wheelchair battery and battery recharger.

6. Plug chargers into outlet.

7. Look to ensure battery is low on charge and in need of recharging. A high number reading indicates a charge is necessary. Overcharging the battery will destroy it.

8. Inform patient that electric wheelchair is charging and its location.

9. Inform appropriate staff of location of wheelchair.

 DOCUMENTATION

1. Indicate on care plan routine orders for charging.

CHAPTER 7

Procedures to Facilitate Self-Care Activities

Introduction

"Self-care is integral to rehabilitation" (Orem, 1985). Self-care has two phases, an investigative/decision-making phase, where the patient has control and input about an activity; and the production phase, where the patient performs the activity. Doyle and Stern's research in 1992 supports the hypothesis that individuals with a disability can control their care even if unable to perform it themselves.

After a person experiences an illness or disability that results in an inability to perform self-care activities "normally," the rehabilitation nurse and occupational therapist are often the first healthcare professionals to introduce the idea that the patient can perform the same self-care activities, but with modifications. The modifications may include a change in how the activity is performed, use of adaptive equipment, or a change in when the activity is performed. The patient must be open to new possibilities that may differ slightly or dramatically from their "normal" self-care performance.

Cultural values impact self-care activities. It is imperative that the patient's cultural values be thoroughly assessed and anticipated before alternatives are presented. In any culture, there is a range of acceptable and unacceptable behavior and performance norms. It is essential that stereotypes be avoided.

The occupational therapist is trained to observe performance in any setting and develop a treatment plan to facilitate independence in self-care activities. Other healthcare workers must assist by sharing observations about performance appropriately with one another, structuring a therapeutic environment and attitude that will encourage patient trials in performing self-care, be familiar with and reinforce use of therapeutic self-care techniques and adaptive equipment, and give constructive and supportive feedback to the patient, family, occupational therapist, and other healthcare workers.

Regardless of disability or illness, the healthcare worker must involve the patient and family in self-care activities from the very beginning of contact. Start by explaining what you are doing and why. Thoroughly assess the patient and family and aid them in developing specific self-care outcomes that encourage progress and are measurable. A positive, committed attitude is essential.

The basic self-care techniques presented are a place to start when working with patients from most disability groups. More complex or mixed disabilities may require additional consultation with the occupational therapist. Basic adaptive equipment is presented. The occupational therapist can individualize adaptive equipment for those more challenging patients.

Some basics for working with any patient in self-care activities are:

- Present information in a manner that can be understood by the patient visually and verbally
- Know and use the patient's current abilities
- Keep verbal cues/directions to one step at a time for patients with cognitive defects
- Do not distract the patient from the activity
- Rely on your own observations to determine a patient's judgment and safety level
- Structure the environment to be "therapeutic"
- Give encouragement and constructive feedback honestly

According to Hopkins and Smith (1993), energy conservation and work simplification techniques can be used with a number of physically disabled patients. Because of a disability, tasks may take much longer and require excessive amounts of energy. To determine ways to conserve energy and simplify work, analyze the task by asking:

- What needs to be improved? What takes too long, causes fatigue, or takes too much energy?
- What are the steps of the task? Include setup and cleanup.
- Why is the task necessary? What is the purpose of the task? When and where should it be done? What is the best way for the patient to get it done?
- Can a new method be developed? Can some steps be eliminated? Can some activities be combined? Can the sequence of steps be rearranged?

Use correct work height to reduce fatigue and promote good posture (standing, the work surface should be 2 in. below the bent elbow; sitting, avoid lifting the shoulders or "winging out" the elbows). Set up equipment and supplies in the work area and clear away unnecessary items. Organize a work center, so often-used supplies and equipment are nearby. Place most frequently used items within easy reach on counters and shelves right above or below counter height. Use labor-saving devices such as electric appliances. Transport heavy equipment on wheels. Plan activities allowing for rest breaks. Alternate light and heavy tasks throughout the day and week. Use proper body mechanics—wide base of support, use both sides of the body; keep objects close to the body; face objects when reaching, lifting to avoid twisting; push rather than pull; alternate positions and motions to avoid fatigue.

Dressing

PURPOSE

To dress and undress self independently

STAFF RESPONSIBLE

EQUIPMENT

1. Clothing (Table 7-1)
2. Adaptive equipment (Table 7-2)

Table 7-1 Adaptive Clothing	
Item	**Clothing Choices** **Function/Benefit**
Loose, lightweight clothing, e.g., camisole, boxer shorts, jumpers, slacks	• Easier to put on than tight clothing • Items allowing for mistakes or errors in application; lightweight allow use of weaker extremity
Front-opening clothing, e.g., shirts, bras, skirts	• Easier to fasten, can see fasteners • Can put on/remove partially buttoned
Crewneck/V neck tops	• No need to fasten
Elastic waist pants/skirts	• Stretch to put on • No need to fasten/button/zipper
Flat shoes, slip-on loafers or Velcro closures (avoid high-tops or boots)	• Slip on/slip off • Easy to fasten
Ties, scarves	• Have loosely knotted and tighten after it's on
Suspenders	• Acts as a loop to aid in pulling on clothing, but can be confusing with cognitive/perceptual deficits present
Adaptations	
Velcro	• Use instead of other fasteners • Can approximate Velcro pieces and stay fastened • The heavier the item, or more pull on the fastener, the bigger and stronger the Velcro needed. • Comes in a variety of colors and sizes • Sticks indiscriminately to rough fabrics • Close fastener to launder
Loops	• Sew inside garments near collar • Can be grasped with dressing stick or hand or weak, stiff finger(s) • Loops need to be tucked inside clothing once dressed
Zipper pull/ring	• Easier to grasp than regular zipper • May be difficult to attach or remove
Buttons on cuffs	• Move sleeve buttons to cuff edge to provide larger opening to allow putting on and removing without unbuttoning

Table 7-2	Equipment for Dressing
Button aid hook	• Can have large handle, handle with palmar strap, weighted hook, or built-up handle
Shoe horn	• Can have long handle or adapted handle
Dressing stick and/or reacher	• Extends reach in variety of directions to aid in applying/removing clothing • Loops in clothing can aid in pulling clothes up
Sock donner	• Minimizes bending at waist and hip when donning socks
Elastic shoe laces	• Allows for shoes to be donned without tying
Heel guard	• Fits snugly over shoe heel; does not need to be held in place as shoe horn does; pull on loop to remove

GENERAL CONSIDERATIONS

1. Dressing may include a wide variety of articles. Commonly, undergarments (briefs/boxers, bra, tee shirt), outer garments (shirt, pants, or skirt or dress), and footwear (stockings and shoes) are considered the basic components. However, depending on the patient's culture and personal preferences, other articles of clothing may be worn. In colder climates, hats, coats, gloves, and boots may be worn as well. Thoroughly assess your patient's particular clothing requirements to best promote independence. Medical devices may need to be applied, such as antiembolism hose, leg bags, incontinence pants, and ostomy appliances. Teaching the patient to apply/remove these items will increase their participation with the treatment plan.

2. According to Hopkins and Smith (1993), upper extremity dressing disability can result from the inability to:
   • Reach to put arm in sleeve and lift garment over head or behind back
   • Grasp shirt to pull off and on, down in back
   • Manipulate buttons, zippers, snaps
   • Lift heavy clothing
   • Attend to tasks, perceive spatial relation between clothing and body parts, and understand and learn to use adaptive methods

3. According to Hopkins and Smith (1993), lower extremity dressing disability can result from the inability to:
   • Reach to feet
   • Stand to pull pants over hips
   • Grasp to pull clothing on and pull fabric together to fasten
   • Manipulate laces, zippers, snaps, and buttons
   • Attend to tasks, perceive spatial relation between clothing and body parts, and understand and learn to use adaptive methods

4. General guidelines for dressing: Provide privacy for dressing. Encourage the patient to choose own clothing. Avoid clothing that is too tight or constricting or tight-fitting or stiff with hard seams for any patient with impaired sensation and/or mobility. Lay out the clothes in the order in which they will be needed. Allow sufficient time for patient to dress self. If certain body parts are weak or paralyzed, dress them first. Begin dressing in bed to minimize problems with sitting balance or if weak to minimize fatigue (McCourt, 1993).

5. Stable and safe positioning is essential to promote self-care activities. Patients could dress in bed and use the electric bed controls to aid in moving in bed. Patients could dress in a chair, preferably with arms, and that allows the patient to have his or her feet solidly on the floor. Patients who can stand to adjust clothing should hold onto a firm object while standing and/or lean against the wall. (Hopkins and Smith, 1993).

6. Regardless of the patient's disability, it is important for the clinician to identify the patient's specific physical deficits.

Procedure

Upper Extremity Dressing/Undressing

DONNING SHIRT: PATIENTS WITH LIMITED UPPER EXTREMITY RANGE OF MOTION OR DECREASED STRENGTH

 Steps

 Additional Information

1. Place shirt facedown on lap, with sleeves and collar near knees.

2. Slide arms through shirt into sleeves and push sleeves over elbows.

Either pull-over or button-down/front-fastening shirt may be used.

If long-sleeve shirt with button cuff is used, moving the buttons down on the edge of the cuffs will allow for donning the shirt without refastening the cuffs each time.

3. Gather shirt back and lift over head.

May rest elbows on knees or table and bend head down to push through shirt collar.

4. Protract and retract, elevate, and depress shoulders to get shirt over shoulders.

Or push shirt over one shoulder, then the other with opposite arm/hand.

5. Lean forward slightly with shoulders back, to pull shirt down in back.

6. Pull shirt front (of front-opening shirt) near the bottom to straighten and bring down fully.

Place hands inside shirt front and pull slightly away from the body, down and toward sides to bring pull-over shirt down fully.

7. Fasten shirt fastenings.

See adaptive equipment in Table 7-2.

DOFFING SHIRT: PATIENTS WITH LIMITED UPPER EXTREMITY RANGE OF MOTION OR DECREASED STRENGTH

 Steps

 Additional Information

1. Place hand inside pull-over shirt toward opposite sleeve and pull sleeve opening down over elbow. Repeat for other sleeve. Remove over head.

2. Unbutton front-fasten shirt by stabilizing shirt against body and use thumb or knuckle to push button through hole while opposite thumb pushes fabric up over the bottom.

Other adaptive equipment may be used.

3. Push collar area back over shoulders, extend arm, and retract shoulders to help sleeve drop below elbow, so arm can be freely removed from sleeve.

Alternatively, push one sleeve off shoulder, reach opposite arm/hand to sleeve hole to hold it while elevating shoulder, extending arm, and flexing elbow to remove arm from sleeve. Then pull shirt around back to other side with arm still in sleeve and slide arm out.

DONNING SHIRT: PATIENTS WITH WEAKNESS/PARALYSIS ON ONE SIDE

 Steps for front-fastening shirt

 Additional Information

1. Place front-fastening shirt on lap with front up, collar toward knees, and affected side sleeve opening exposed between legs.

2. Place affected arm into sleeve.

Lean forward to drop arm into sleeve as far as possible.

3. Pull sleeve up arm beyond elbow.

4. With stronger hand, grasp collar and sleeve that goes around to that side.

5. Lift stronger arm over head, pulling shirt around back.

6. Slip unaffected arm into sleeve, letting shirt fall onto arm, and pushing arm into sleeve as shirt is pulled around.

7. Fasten shirt.

Other adaptive equipment may be used.

 Steps for pull-over shirt

 Additional Information

1. Place shirt collar down on lap, front up, collar near thighs, and sleeve opening of affected side exposed between legs.

2. Place weak/affected arm in sleeve opening.

Lean forward to drop it in as far as possible.

3. Pull sleeve up affected arm, at least above elbow.

4. Place stronger arm in its sleeve.

5. Grasp collar with stronger hand, gather up back material, and lift over head.

The higher the sleeve is pulled up, the better.

DOFFING SHIRT: PATIENTS WITH WEAKNESS/PARALYSIS ON ONE SIDE

 Steps for front-fastening shirt

 Additional Information

1. Unfasten fastening.

2. Pull fabric toward stronger side.

3. Grasp stronger side of shirt, reach back and to the side to get it off the shoulder, then pull it down and wriggle elbow out of shirt.

4. Pull fabric to affected side, and remove affected arm.

Adaptive equipment may be used.

This will make it as loose as possible.

Alternatively, grasp sleeve of stronger side with that hand, and work it down until elbow can be worked out of the sleeve.

 Steps for pull-over shirt

 Additional Information

1. Pull fabric toward unaffected side to loosen it.

2. Pull bottom of shirt on unaffected side down, squeeze elbow through sleeve hole, and remove stronger arm from sleeve.

3. Gather fabric and grasp collar to lift garment over head.

4. Remove stronger arm from sleeve.

5. Remove sleeve from weaker arm.

Alternatively, grasp collar near nape of neck, gather back fabric with hand, and pull back over head.

Procedure

Lower Extremity Dressing/Undressing

DONNING AND DOFFING PANTS: PATIENTS WITH LIMITED UPPER AND LOWER EXTREMITY RANGE OF MOTION

 Steps

 Additional Information

1. Sit with legs extended in bed, with or without back support, with clothing nearby on bed or chair.

2. Use weak grasp or drape garment over hand to hold it in preparation for putting it over foot.

3. Pull leg with forearm, lift under knee to bend leg, and bring foot up to opposite knee.

4. Drape garment over foot through leg opening, and pull it up to knee.

5. Lift leg and push on knee to extend it.

6. Pull pants over the foot and up to the knee.

Either apply underwear and outer pants at the same time or repeat steps 2 through 6 with outer pants after underwear is pulled completely up.

7. Pull pants over knees and partially over thighs by pulling on crotch of pants with forearm and pulling with hand in pocket of pants.

Alternatively, use both hands together to grasp and pull.

8. Lie down and roll from side to side, pulling pants up over hip that is on top with each roll.

Pull pants up using hand in pocket, thumb in belt loop, or hand inside pants under waistband.

9. Fasten pants.

Elastic waistbands eliminate need for fasteners. Adaptive equipment may be used to fasten pants.

10. Reverse process to remove pants.

DONNING AND DOFFING PANTS: PATIENTS WITH ONE-SIDED WEAKNESS OR PARALYSIS

 Steps

 Additional Information

1. Sit in chair that allows for a stable base of support for both feet.

If unable to stand to pull up pants, sitting in bed is preferable.

2. Cross weak leg over stronger leg.

3. Place pants over foot and pull up to or over knee.

Make sure foot is through bottom of leg opening.

4. Replace foot on floor.

5. Hold pants near waist with stronger arm/hand and reach down to allow lifting of stronger leg into opening.

6. Pull pants up over thighs as far as possible while sitting.

7. Use weaker arm/hand to hold pants up while coming to standing, if possible.

If unable to stand, lie back in bed, and partially roll from side to side to pull pants up. Use upper trunk and shoulders to roll.

8. Fasten openings.

Clothing is looser when standing. Adaptive equipment may be used for fastening pants.

DONNING AND DOFFING SOCKS AND SHOES

 Steps

 Additional Information

1. Put on loose socks by putting stronger hand in sock opening and spreading fingers to start sock over toes.

Adaptive equipment may be used for patients with bilateral poor grasp/hand control or limited lower extremity range of motion.

2. Place weaker foot on a footstool or lift to opposite knee to stabilize it during sock donning.

3. Pull up using the stronger hand, once sock is over the toes.

Repeat with other foot.

4. Put shoe on by lifting the foot to the opposite knee, then using the stronger hand to place the shoe on the foot.

Some shoes may be applied by placing the shoe on the floor and lifting the foot into the shoe, then pushing on the knee to push the heel into the shoe.

5. Fasten shoe closures, if necessary.

Shoes may have elastic shoe laces or straps or Velcro closures for easy fastening.

 DOCUMENTATION

1. Techniques used successfully.

2. Any adaptive equipment or clothing to be used.

3. Special adaptations of the process for individual patients, based on their culture, personal desires, medical needs.

4. Patient and family teaching and return demonstration of skills.

REFERENCES

Doyle, D.L. and Stern, P.N. (1992) "Negotiating Self-Care in Rehabilitation Nursing" *Rehabilitation Nursing* 17:319–321, 326.

Hopkins, H.L. and Smith, H.D. (1993) *Willard and Spackman's Occupational Therapy*, 8th ed. Philadelphia: J. B. Lippincott Company.

McCourt, A.E. (1993) *The Specialty Practice of Rehabilitation Nursing: A Core Curriculum*, 3d ed. Skokie, IL: Rehabilitation Nursing Foundation.

Orem, D. (1985) "A Concept of Self-Care for the Rehabilitation Client" *Rehabilitation Nursing* 10(3):33–36.

Sine, R.D., Holcomb, J.D., Roush, R.E., et al. (1983) *Basic Rehabilitation Techniques: A Self-Instructional Guide*, 2d ed. Rockville, MD: Aspen.

Grooming

PURPOSE

To wash face and hands, comb/brush/style hair, brush teeth, glasses/contact lens care and donning, cosmetic application, shaving, deodorant application, and nail care independently

STAFF RESPONSIBLE

EQUIPMENT

1. Grooming aids (Table 7-3)
2. Liquid soap in push-button dispenser

 GENERAL CONSIDERATIONS

1. According to Hopkins and Smith (1993), grooming deficits can result from the inability to
   - Reach face, all areas of head, and faucets
   - Pick up, hold, and manipulate brushes, washcloth, razor, contact lenses, nail file, and other tools
   - Use both hands simultaneously to open containers or file nails
   - Attend to the activity, locate the items needed, and use them appropriately

2. General grooming guidelines: Provide privacy. Encourage patient to direct grooming activities, especially hair care, cosmetic application, and shaving. These areas may be very sensitive and private for patients. Allow sufficient time to perform these tasks. Provide verbal and/or visual cues and feedback. Gently encourage patients to consider changes in grooming so they could perform them independently.

3. Some grooming activities also have a social component. Many people go to the "beauty shop" and socialize with the other clients and stylists. Spas offer many services that are included in grooming, such as manicures, leg waxes (or bikini waxes). Department and specialty shops offer "make-overs" and other cosmetic applications. Some people do perform all their own grooming. It is a personal decision.

Table 7-3   Grooming Aids

• Antigravity assistive arm placement devices[a] to reach face and head	• Shaving cream dispenser adaptation
• Prostheses for reaching face, head and for grasping	• Extended-handle toothbrush, hairbrush
• Mechanical grasp-release orthoses[b] when grasp is absent	• Proximal interphalangeal (PIP) finger-joint stabilizer for holding finger stable to put in contact lens
• Orthosis with utensil slot when wrist stability and grasp are absent	• Wash mitt
• Utensil or universal cuff when grasp is absent or inadequate	• Octopus soap stabilizer
• Built-up handles on hairbrush, toothbrush	• Extended faucet levers to allow reach and operation
• Velcro D-ring closure strap on hairbrush	• Mount toothbrush and razor on gooseneck or other stable mounts and move head to accomplish task without use of upper extremities
• Toothpaste dispenser	• Electric toothbrush, razor
• Deodorant spray adaptation	• Suction cup–mounted brush for brushing dentures, cleaning nails
• Deodorant holder to stabilize can on hand	• Nail file taped to table
• Make-up basket that secures cosmetics in place while opening them	• Adapted nail clipper
• Razor holder	

[a]Swedish sling, deltoid aid, mobile arm support, overhead sling
[b]Wrist-driven flexor hinge, externally powered flexor hinge, cable-driven flexor hinge, RIC tenodesis orthosis

Procedure

Self-Grooming Activities

 Steps

1. Gather and set out equipment.

2. Use mouth to help open containers.

3. Use both hands or one hand stabilizing the other to hold glass, toothbrush, hairbrush, razor.

4. Tape nail file down to hold it, if grasp is too weak.

5. Set dentures on wet towel in sink.

6. Hold hairbrush close to bristles or on back where bristles are mounted for stability.

7. Place toothbrush on counter and squeeze toothpaste onto it.

8. Assist one arm/hand with the other.

9. Choose an easy care hairstyle.

10. Stabilize arms against the trunk, or elbows and wrists on sink or counter while performing grooming tasks.

 Additional Information

Patient may prefer to perform some of these tasks in a social setting (nail care).

Place containers between the knees to hold them or to stabilize them to open.

Use tenodesis to pick up larger items and adaptive equipment for smaller items, such as a universal cuff to hold toothbrush.

Move nails across file.

This will prevent sliding while brushing them.

This will help if coordination is a problem.

Toothpaste pumps can be helpful.

This can improve reach.

 ## DOCUMENTATION

1. Techniques used successfully.

2. Any adaptive equipment to be used.

3. Special adaptations of the process for individual patients, based on their culture, personal desires, and medical needs.

4. Patient and family education and return demonstration of skills.

PATIENT AND FAMILY EDUCATION

Teach patient and family how to set up, use adaptive techniques and adaptive equipment appropriately.

REFERENCES

Doyle, D.L., and Stern, P.N. (1992) "Negotiating Self-Care in Rehabilitation Nursing" *Rehabilitation Nursing* 17:319–321, 326.

Hopkins, H.L. and Smith, H.D. (1993) *Willard and Spackman's Occupational Therapy*, 8th ed. Philadelphia: J. B. Lippincott Company.

McCourt, A.E. (1993) *The Specialty Practice of Rehabilitation Nursing: A Core Curriculum*, 3d ed. Skokie, IL: Rehabilitation Nursing Foundation.

Orem, D. (1985) "A Concept of Self-Care for the Rehabilitation Client" *Rehabilitation Nursing* 10(3):33–36.

Sine, R.D., Holcomb, J.D., Roush, R.E., et al. (1983) *Basic Rehabilitation Techniques: A Self-Instructional Guide*, 2d ed. Rockville, MD: Aspen.

Bathing/Showering

PURPOSE

To clean the body through bathing or showering independently

STAFF RESPONSIBLE

EQUIPMENT

1. Bathing adaptive equipment and aids (Table 7-4)
2. Liquid soap/shampoo with push-button dispenser
3. Towels and faceclothes
4. Shower cap

GENERAL CONSIDERATIONS

1. According to Hopkins and Smith (1993), bathing disability can result from the inability to:
   - Get into tub or shower
   - Grasp and manipulate faucets, soap, sponge, washcloth, or towel
   - Reach all areas of body and faucets
2. General guidelines include: provide privacy while bathing; help patient use the shower or tub as soon as possible after onset of disability; arrange a routine that is consistent with patient's prior routine; place all bathing equipment within easy reach; provide a safe environment—rubber mats, grab bars, tub or shower chair/seat; arrange rest periods between self-care activities; determine if wheelchair fits into the bathroom; and consult with other team members to integrate care into the community.
3. Place rubber sheet or flannel-backed tablecloth on bed, for bed bathing, if bathroom is not accessible.
4. Use thermometer to check water temperature before entering shower to prevent burns in patients with sensory and mobility changes. Water causes a scalding burn in 6 s at 180°F. Turning down the water heater setting to 140°F allows more reaction time before a scalding burn occurs.

Table 7-4   Bathing Aids
Roll-in shower and/or commode chair
Bath bench
Long-handled bath sponges
Wash mitt or washcloth with loops if grasp is inadequate
Soap on a rope or soap bag on a rope
Loops on towels
Grab bars
Handheld showerhead
Single-lever faucet
Thermometer (cooking type)
Scald guard
Soap dispenser mounted in shower

Procedure

Bathing/Showering

 Steps

1. Use separate cloths for washing and rinsing.
2. Drape towel over back of shower chair to rub back against to cleanse.
3. Place soapy towel in tub bottom to cleanse feet.
4. Place soapy towel over knee and bend forward to wash arms against it.

 Additional Information

This will keep rinse water clean during bed baths.
Repeat with dry towel afterwards to dry back after shower.

If feet cannot be reached.
This is helpful for one-sided paralysis or weakness.

DOCUMENTATION

1. Techniques used successfully.
2. Any adaptive equipment to be used.
3. Special adaptations of the process for individual patients based on their culture, personal desires, and medical needs.
4. Patient and family education and return demonstration of skills.

REFERENCES

Doyle, D.L. and Stern, P.N. (1992) "Negotiating Self-Care in Rehabilitation Nursing" *Rehabilitation Nursing* 17:319–321, 326.

Hopkins, H.L. and Smith, H.D. (1993) *Willard and Spackman's Occupational Therapy*, 8th ed. Philadelphia: J. B. Lippincott Company.

McCourt, A.E. (1993) *The Specialty Practice of Rehabilitation Nursing: A Core Curriculum*, 3d ed. Skokie, IL: Rehabilitation Nursing Foundation.

Orem, D. (1985) "A Concept of Self-Care for the Rehabilitation Client" *Rehabilitation Nursing* 10(3):33–36.

Sine, R.D., Holcomb, J.D., Roush, R.E., et al. (1983) *Basic Rehabilitation Techniques: A Self-Instructional Guide*, 2d ed. Rockville, MD: Aspen.

Toileting

PURPOSE

To safely eliminate on the toilet or commode chair independently; safe use of urinal and/or bedpan; sanitary emptying of urinal, bedpan, or commode chair

STAFF RESPONSIBLE

EQUIPMENT

1. Toilet or commode chair
2. Adaptive equipment (Table 7-5)

GENERAL CONSIDERATIONS

1. According to Hopkins and Smith (1993), toileting disability can result from the inability to
   - Access and get onto the toilet
   - Move quickly enough to get to toilet
   - Reach perineum
   - Grasp and use toilet paper
   - Manage clothing
   - Insert suppository
   - Empty colostomy, perform colostomy care
2. General guidelines for toileting (McCourt, 1993) include: maintain bowel and bladder record to determine evacua-

Table 7-5 Toileting Aids
Extended-reach toilet paper holder or tongs
Bidet for cleansing
Grab bars for transfer to toilet and stabilizing while reaching to cleanse
Raised toilet seat
Urinal (male or female)
Bedside commode
Bedpan (regular or fracture)
Incontinent pads
Bowel program items and catheters for patients with loss of bowel/bladder continence: • Mechanical grasp-release orthosis or other catheter insertion device   • Adapted urinary drainage bag valve   • Labia spreader   • Adapted urinal or other collection device   • Adapted posey sheath strap for male external catheter   • Leg abductor   • Suppository inserter   • Digital stimulator

tion pattern; maintain regular, consistent schedule; allow sufficient time for toileting; provide privacy; provide assistance and caring; provide a safe, clear access to toilet area with a night light, if possible; ensure the availability of a call system on the nursing unit and in the community setting, if indicated.

3. Some patients may need to learn to use the urinal, bedpan, or bedside commode at night only. It may be safer and quicker.

Procedure

Toileting

 Steps

1. Practice toilet transfers without rearranging clothing.

2. Use lower extremity dressing/undressing techniques for clothing management.

3. Wrap toilet paper around hand if grasp is weak.

 Additional Information

When actual toileting is needed, the patient will already have done the transfer at least once before.

Adaptive equipment may also be used.

DOCUMENTATION

1. Record of toileting/elimination.

2. Intake and output record, if needed.

3. Improvement in self-care skills, level of independence.

4. Techniques used successfully.

5. Any equipment to be used.

6. Special adaptations of the process for individual patients based on their culture, personal desire, and medical needs.

7. Patient and family education and return demonstration of skills.

REFERENCES

Doyle, D.L. and Stern, P.N. (1992) "Negotiating Self-Care in Rehabilitation Nursing" *Rehabilitation Nursing* 17:319–321, 326.

Hopkins, H.L. and Smith, H.D. (1993) *Willard and Spackman's Occupational Therapy*, 8th ed. Philadelphia: J. B. Lippincott Company.

McCourt, A.E. (1993) *The Specialty Practice of Rehabilitation Nursing: A Core Curriculum*, 3d ed. Skokie, IL: Rehabilitation Nursing Foundation.

Orem, D. (1985) "A Concept of Self-Care for the Rehabilitation Client" *Rehabilitation Nursing* 10(3):33–36.

Sine, R.D., Holcomb, J.D., Roush, R.E., et al. (1983) *Basic Rehabilitation Techniques: A Self-Instructional Guide*, 2d ed. Rockville, MD: Aspen.

Feeding

PURPOSE

To feed self independently

STAFF RESPONSIBLE

EQUIPMENT

1. Adaptive equipment (Table 7-6)

GENERAL CONSIDERATIONS

1. According to Hopkins and Smith (1993), feeding disabilities can result from the inability to
   - Swallow food and drink safely
   - Reach the hand to the mouth
   - Pick up and hold utensils, finger foods, and beverage containers
   - Use both hands simultaneously to cut food
   - Attend to the activity, see the various items on the plate, locate them with the utensil, and then locate the mouth with the utensil

2. General guidelines for feeding: provide safety for the patient with swallowing problems; provide comfortable and pleasant eating environment; allow sufficient time for

Table 7-6   Feeding Equipment
Antigravity assistive arm placement devices[a] for reach to mouth
Prostheses for reach to mouth and grasp
Mechanical grasp-release orthoses when grasp is absent
Orthosis with utensil slot when wrist stability and grasp are absent
Utensil or universal cuff when grasp is absent or inadequate
Built-up handles on utensils when grasp is weak
Knife adapted to utensil cuff to secure to hand when grasp is absent or weak
Extended utensils
Swivel utensils if food slips off utensil during reach to mouth
Long straw and straw holder if cup cannot be lifted to mouth
Drinking equipment set up on wheelchair/bedside (cup holder and extended long straw)
Nonskid placemat
Plate guard or scoop dish to prevent food from being pushed off the plate
Rocker knife or regular knife used with rocking motion for one-handed cutting

[a]Swedish sling, deltoid aid, mobile arm support, overhead sling

eating; provide supervision and assistance as needed for relearning or adaptation; provide instructions for rationale and appropriate use of adaptive devices.

3. Meals are often a social time. When beginning with adaptive techniques, however, privacy can build confidence and skill with equipment and techniques. Encourage transition to social or group setting as quickly as possible.

Procedure

Self-Feeding

 Steps

1. Position patient sitting up at 90 degrees, with trunk upright and in midline, extremities symmetric, head in neutral or slightly flexed forward.

2. Set up food items.

3. Cue patient to use one hand/arm to assist the other, or both hands to pick up an item.

Additional Information

If seated in chair, position in an anterior pelvic tilt with feet flat on floor. Position chair in close to table.

Open containers, cut meat, season food, prepare drinks (coffee with cream, tea with lemon, etc.)

Rest one elbow on a high surface to facilitate reaching the mouth.

4. Weave utensil between weak fingers or teach tenodesis grasp.

5. Stabilize one hand/arm against the other or the trunk, if coordination is a problem.

6. Use a rocking motion with the knife to cut items for one-handed techniques.

Other adaptive equipment may be used.

Other techniques may be recommended by the occupational therapist, such as weighing the extremity.

Other adaptive equipment may be used, such as a rocker knife.

 ## DOCUMENTATION

1. Techniques used successfully.

2. Any adaptive equipment to be used.

3. Special adaptations of the process for individual patients, based on their culture, personal desires, medical needs.

4. Patient and family teaching and return demonstration of skills.

REFERENCES

Doyle, D.L. and Stern, P.N. (1992) "Negotiating Self-Care in Rehabilitation Nursing" *Rehabilitation Nursing* 17:319–321, 326.

Hopkins, H.L. and Smith, H.D. (1993) *Willard and Spackman's Occupational Therapy*, 8th ed. Philadelphia: J. B. Lippincott Company.

McCourt, A.E. (1993) *The Specialty Practice of Rehabilitation Nursing: A Core Curriculum*, 3d ed. Skokie, IL: Rehabilitation Nursing Foundation.

Orem, D. (1985) "A Concept of Self-Care for the Rehabilitation Client" *Rehabilitation Nursing* 10(3):33–36.

Sine, R.D., Holcomb, J.D., Roush, R.E., et al. (1983) *Basic Rehabilitation Techniques: A Self-Instructional Guide*, 2d ed. Rockville, MD: Aspen.

Self-Administration of Medications

PURPOSE

To safely prepare and self-administer medications

STAFF RESPONSIBLE

EQUIPMENT

1. Insulin syringe scale magnifier and needle guide
2. Exacta-Med Dispenser and liquid medication bottle caps (Baxa Corporation, Denver, CO 80112)
3. Medication chart (individualized for each patient; Figs. 7-1, 7-2)
4. Pill box (7-day with one compartment per day or four compartments per day or timer)

 GENERAL CONSIDERATIONS

1. Safe medication administration is essential to ensure optimal medical treatment effects.

2. The patient/family/caregivers should have an individualized, specific list of medications. This list should include:
   - Name of drug (generic and brand)
   - Dose of drug (if dose varies during the day, this should be thoroughly explained and written)
   - Times of administration (include before, with, or after meals)
   - Desired actions of the drug
   - Side effects to watch for and what to do if they occur.

3. Prior to preparing this specific list, a discussion with the physician to analyze what drugs are really necessary and consideration of the financial cost is important.

4. Smooth integration of medication administration occurs when only essential medications are used in an organized routine that complements the patient/family/caregiver's routine in the community.

5. Refer to current nursing drug books or consult with the pharmacist for drug administration instructions.

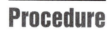 # Procedure

 Steps

 Additional Information

1. Assess:
   - Patient's current medication needs

   - Patient's postdischarge needs
   - Patient's medicaiton route (PO, tube, ocular, inhalers, optic, parenteral)
   - Patient's physical self-medication abilities
   - Patient's cognitive self-medication abilities.

2. Collaborate with physician to minimize drug administration.

3. Devise medication schedule/program list.

4. Have patient use medication schedule/program list to pour medications at least one time.

Consider over-the-counter and nonprescription supplements, as well as prn medications.

Minimize cost and number of medications if possible.

The first draft of medication list.
Closely observe for difficulty understanding which medication to administer, amount, or time.

368

5. Revise medication schedule/program list to make medication easier.

6. Have patient use medication schedule/program list to pour medications at least one more time.

7. Provide detailed description of medication schedule/program list (including duplicate) to family member(s) and home health nurse.

Consider color-coding of bottles, having someone prepour medications for a week using pill boxes.

DOCUMENTATION

1. Techniques used successfully.

2. Any adaptive equipment to be used.

3. Special adaptations of the process for individual patients based on their culture, personal desires, and medical needs.

PATIENT AND FAMILY EDUCATION

Give specific individualized administration instructions; observe return demonstration of skills.

REFERENCES

Doyle, D.L. and Stern, P.N. (1992) "Negotiating Self-Care in Rehabilitation Nursing" *Rehabilitation Nursing* 17:319–321, 326.

Hopkins, H.L. and Smith, H.D. (1993) *Willard and Spackman's Occupational Therapy*, 8th ed. Philadelphia: J. B. Lippincott Company.

McCourt, A.E. (1993) *The Specialty Practice of Rehabilitation Nursing: A Core Curriculum*, 3d ed. Skokie, IL: Rehabilitation Nursing Foundation.

Orem, D. (1985) "A Concept of Self-Care for the Rehabilitation Client" *Rehabilitation Nursing* 10(3):33–36.

Sine, R.D., Holcomb, J.D., Roush, R.E., et al. (1983) *Basic Rehabilitation Techniques: A Self-Instructional Guide*, 2d ed. Rockville, MD: Aspen.

Figure 7-1. Medication Chart.

Medication List for: _____ (Patient Name)

Doctor: _____   **Primary Nurse Instructor** _____
(Attending or Prescribing Physician)

Time to Take Drug

Name of Drug	7–8 AM	12 NOON	4–5 PM	8–9 PM
Med: mg:				
Med: mg:				
Med: mg:				
Med: mg:				
Med: mg:				
Med: mg:				
Med: mg:				

Figure 7-1.   Medication Chart (*continued*).

Name of Drug	7–8 AM	12 NOON	4–5 PM	8–9 PM
Med: mg:				
Med: mg:				
Med: mg:				
Med: mg:				
Med: mg:				
Med: mg:				
Med: mg:				

Figure 7-2.

Some Important Medication Tips

1. Do not stop taking ordered medication just because you feel better without talking to your doctor.
2. Do not share medication with anyone.
3. Keep out of reach of children.
4. Throw away unused or old medication (contact your pharmacist for proper disposal procedures for your community).
5. Tell your nurse or doctor of any new symptoms.
6. Do NOT double-dose if you forget to take medication.
7. Keep drugs away from heat and moisture.
8. Keep your pharmacy name and number next to your phone(s).

CHAPTER 8

Considerations for Reintegration into the Community

Adrienne J. Sarnecki

Reintegration into the Community

PURPOSE

To assist patients and families to adapt to life with a disability and maximize independence

GENERAL CONSIDERATIONS

1. Rehabilitation nurses begin the discharge planning process immediately on admission to the acute inpatient rehabilitation unit. Working with the interdisciplinary team, nurses provide care with the intent of maximizing functional independence and preserving quality of life. Rehabilitation is a dynamic ongoing process that does not end with discharge from the acute inpatient unit. It begins a life-long rehabilitation process.

    Rehabilitation may take place in a variety of settings: acute rehab facilities, transitional hospitals, subacute care facilities, skilled long-term nursing care institutions, assisted-living facilities, and while living in their own home with home health-care, adult day care, and outpatient rehab therapy (Table 8-1).

Table 8-1 Post–Acute Rehabilitation Care Locations

Transitional hospitals

Subacute care

Skilled long-term nursing care

Assisted-living facilities

Home health care

Adult day care

Outpatient rehabilitation therapy

2. Current trends show that inpatient rehabilitation providers are providing rehabilitation care sooner after the initial injury while lengths of stay in inpatient rehabilitation settings are decreasing. Patients are admitted from acute care hospital settings quicker and sicker. Post–acute rehabilitation services (Table 8-2) continue to grow as the shift from acute inpatient hospital settings continues. "As care has shifted to the outpatient arena, patients at home are likely to be more acutely ill and to have greater needs for ongoing care than their counterparts in years past. However, healthcare providers, accustomed to spending time on health education during inpatient admissions, are finding precious little time to prepare patients to care for themselves at home" (Kantz et al., 1998, p. 11). Therefore, rehab nurses must interact with the patient and family in all these settings to maximize independence and adaptation to life with a disability.

3. Contributing factors to unsuccessful home transitions include: "(1) family members unwilling or unprepared for their new roles as caregivers; (2) patients' inability to generalize the skills reacquired in the acute setting to the home setting; (3) physical barriers in the home that made adjustment difficult; (4) dramatic reduction of preexisting social and vocational opportunities secondary to cognitive, physical, and/or emotional challenges or other social and environmental barriers" (Evans, 1997, p. 17). The successful transition of the patient and family to the community is significant as when the needs of patients are not met at the time of discharge from the rehabilitation unit; increased rehospitalization rates and decreased favorable outcomes follow (Steinwachs, 1989). This inevitably leads to increased costs in providing care (Kantz et al., 1998). Healthcare providers need to continually attempt to limit the costs of care. Even when insurance coverage is available, it is not uncommon for individuals to have reached the maximum amount of insurance dollars available early in the life of the disability.

4. Family caregiving is an ever-increasing reality. "In the limited time between diagnosis and discharge, there is much to teach family members about caring for a disabled relative. Sensitivity to the wants and needs of prospective family caregivers is essential in helping families as they assimilate the disability into their own lives, face the uncertainty of the new caregiver role, and learn to provide assistance needed by the disabled adult" (Weeks and O'Connor, 1996, p. 16). Nurses are directly involved with the disabled and their families from initial injury to the community and are therefore in a key position to assess the needs of both the patient and family throughout the entire continuum of care (Davidhizar, 1997).

5. Patient and family educational needs may be different. Identifying needs of both patients and families ensures that the needed information is available and assists the patient and caregiver in their adaptation to life with a disability. The inclusion of family members in the entire rehabilitation process is necessary throughout each type of community setting. Family is defined as anyone who will take on the primary responsibility for care provision for the disabled individual. Traditional and nontraditional family structures are important to consider. Many patients and families are unaware of the time commitment and depletion of physical and emotional resources required to care for the disabled in the community, often at the expense of their own needs (Weeks, 1995).

6. Family caregivers experience a multitude of challenges as they take on the role of caregiver for the disabled individual.

Table 8-2 Post–Acute Rehabilitation Care

Name of Type of Facility	Key Points
Transitional Hospitals	• Provides long-term care for patients with acute, yet stable, conditions • Min. stay = 25 days • Nursing care per day = 9–12 h • Common diagnoses: ventilator dependent, low-level head injury, severe diabetes with amputation
Subacute Care	• Abides by long-term care rules and regulations • Short-term care is limited and goal oriented • Min. stay = 5–14 days • Nursing care per day = 4–6 h • Therapy per day = 2–3 h • Common diagnoses: infections, nutritional problems, circulatory impairments, respiratory diseases, skin disorders
Skilled Long-Term Nursing Care Assisted-Living Facilities	• Specialty units, especially for dementia • Regulated by each state • ALFA (Assisted Living Federation of America) is developing standards • Variety of services: special accommodations for housing, personalized support services, health-care designed to meet the needs (scheduled and unscheduled) and help with ADLs • Usually privately funded
Home Health Care	• Must have strong social support system, adaptable home, private funds, as Medicare covers skilled services ordered by the physician and administered by licensed nurse/therapist • Provides portable equipment • Home care trained nurses and therapists • Can provide telemedicine and telemetry

Adult Day Care	• Provides assisted living, subacute care, and skilled nursing
	• CARF developing accreditation criteria
	• Levels of care:
	  1: Core: unskilled assisted living
	  2: Enhanced: skilled nursing which requires little supervision or support
	  3: Intensive: max care and includes skilled nursing and therapies
	• Private and state funding

Outpatient Rehab Therapy	• Provides therapies at healthcare site, including: Physical therapy, Occupational therapy, Recreational therapy, Social work, Speech services, Vocational consulting, Drivers Ed, Psychology • Nursing services may be available • Patients may attend 1–5 times per week, ongoing or short-term basis

Weeks and O'Connor (1996) identify the following challenges of family caregivers: "fear of being alone, lack of support, fatigue, social isolation, uncertainty about treatment, feelings of anger and helplessness, guilt, problems associated with helping the disabled relative with the activities of daily living, need for help with finances and transportation, and fear of the future" (p. 16). Holicky (1996) also identifies anger, insecurity, loneliness, resentment, depression, bitterness, and role fatigue. Ongoing assessment by all nurses throughout all levels of care that responds to changing need is an important step in developing a unique and individualized plan of care that will meet the needs of the family and facilitate adjustment in the community (Table 8-3).

7. Early identification and use of community resources aids in the transition to the community. Several barriers impede the full utilization of the available community resources. The attitudes of healthcare workers toward resources in the community, costs of services, and limited accessibility can each significantly impact whether or not the patient and family will utilize available resources.

Patient barriers include the following: lack of motivation, low on priority list, previous negative experience with resource, lack of knowledge, lack of understanding of the need, poor self-image, incongruence with cultural beliefs, and limited financial resources (Clemen-Stone et al., 1995). When resource services are refused by the patient and family the rehabilitation nurse needs to identify the reasons behind the refusal. Understanding specific concerns may facilitate identification of alternate resources that are more comfortable for the patient and/or family. Often, there is initial resistance to utilize the resources. Even if refusal continues to be an issue, it is beneficial to leave the resource information with the patient and family as the passage of time or a change in the situation may precipitate utilization of available resources (Fig. 8-1 and Tables 8-4 to 8-6).

8. Rehabilitation nurses play an instrumental role as advocates for the disabled. Rehabilitation nurses have the knowledge, experience, and expertise to help educate a variety of groups in serving the needs of the disabled. The disabled often report that healthcare providers other than

Table 8-3	Emotional/Psychosocial Responses of Primary Care Givers
Emotional/Psychosocial Response	Rehabilitation Nursing Interventions
Anger Bitterness Caregiver Role Strain Depression Grief Guilt Insecurity Loneliness Powerlessness	• Ongoing data collection and assessment • Acknowledgment of responses and individualized assistance for the caregiver separate from the person with a disability • Identification of the need for and assistance with arrangements for respite care • Identification of and assistance in utilizing available resources • Enhancement of familiar strengths and minimization of weaknesses • Assistance with the development of healthy coping strategies • Education regarding increased health risks of caregivers • Support of health-promoting behaviors • Identification of specific goals and expected outcomes • Ongoing evaluation and dynamic changes in the nursing plan of care to respond to changing needs

Table 8-4   Selected Formal Community Resources

Aging
National Council of Independent Living   (703) 525-3406
1916 Wilson Blvd
Suite 209
Arlington, VA 22201

National Institute on Aging Information Center (301) 496-1752
31 Center Drive
Building 31, Room 5C27
Bethesda, MD 20892-2292

Alzheimer's Disease
Alzheimer's Association   (800) 621-0379
919 North Michigan Ave
Suite 1000
Chicago, IL 60611

Americans with Disabilities Act (ADA)
US Department of Justice   (202) 541-0301
Civil Rights Division
PO Box 66738
Washington, DC 20035-6738

Arthritis
Arthritis Foundation   (404) 872-7100
1330 West Peachtree Street
Atlanta, GA 30309

Brain Tumor
National Brain Tumor Foundation   (800) 934-2873 (CURE)
785 Market Street
Suite 1600
San Francisco, CA 94103

Table 8-4   Selected Formal Community Resources
(continued)

Caregiver
Family Caregiver Alliance   (415) 434-3388
425 Bush Street, Suite 500
San Francisco, CA 94108

Head Injury
National Head Injury Foundation   (800) 444-6443 (NHIF)
105 North Alfred Street
Alexandria, VA 22314

Heart Disease
American Heart Association, National Center   (214) 373-6300
7272 Greenville Avenue
Dallas, TX 75231

Multiple Sclerosis
National Multiple Sclerosis Society   (800) 344-4867
733 3rd Avenue, 6th Floor
New York, NY 10017

Parkinson's Disease
American Parkinson Disease Association   (800) 223-2732
1250 Hylan Blvd.
Suite B
Staten Island, NY 10305

Spinal Cord Injury
National Spinal Cord Injury Association   (800) 962-9629
8300 Colesville Road   (301) 588-6959
Suite 551
Silver Spring, MD 20910

Stroke
National Stroke Association   (800) 787-6537
96 Inverness Drive East   (800-STR-OKES)
Suite I
Englewood, CO 80112-5112

NOTE: All addresses and phone numbers are accurate as of September, 1998.
SOURCE: Adapted from: *Patient Education and Discharge Planning Manual.*

Table 8-5   Selected Informal Community Resources

Extended Family Members
Network of Friends
Church Groups
School Affiliations
Work Affiliations
Neighbors

Table 8-6   Selected Internet Resources for the Disabled

• Yahoo
• Disability-Specific Web Sites
• Organizations Serving Specific Disabilities and Conditions
• Disability Infocenter
• Disability Resources on the Internet
• National Center on Accessibility

NOTE: Please note that the information in chat rooms is not always reliable and needs to be checked for source, accuracy, and reliability.

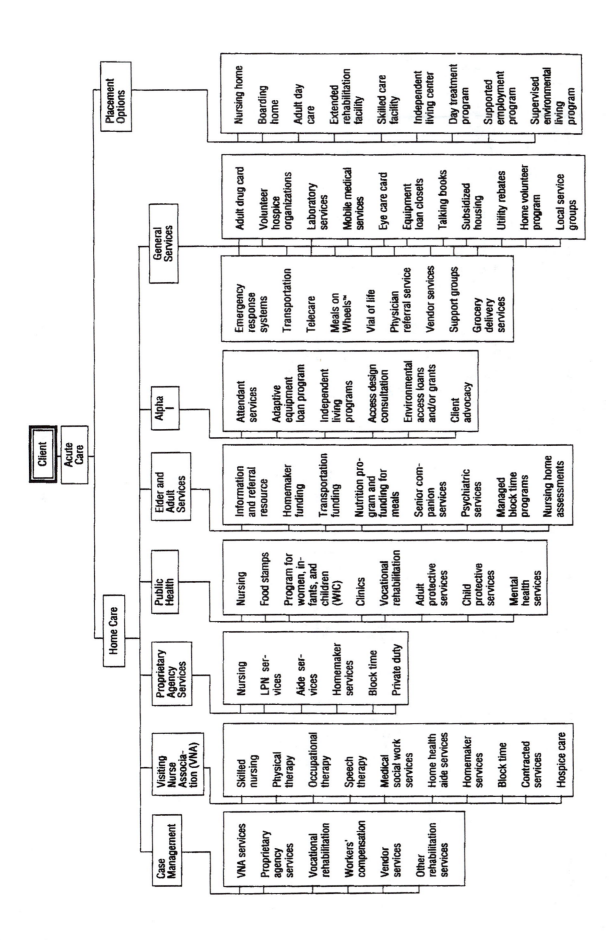

Figure 8-1 Selected formal community resources. (Reprinted from *The Specialty Practice of Rehabilitation Nursing: A Core Curriculum*, 3d ed, with permission of the Association of Rehabilitation Nurses, Skokie, IL. Copyright ©1993.)

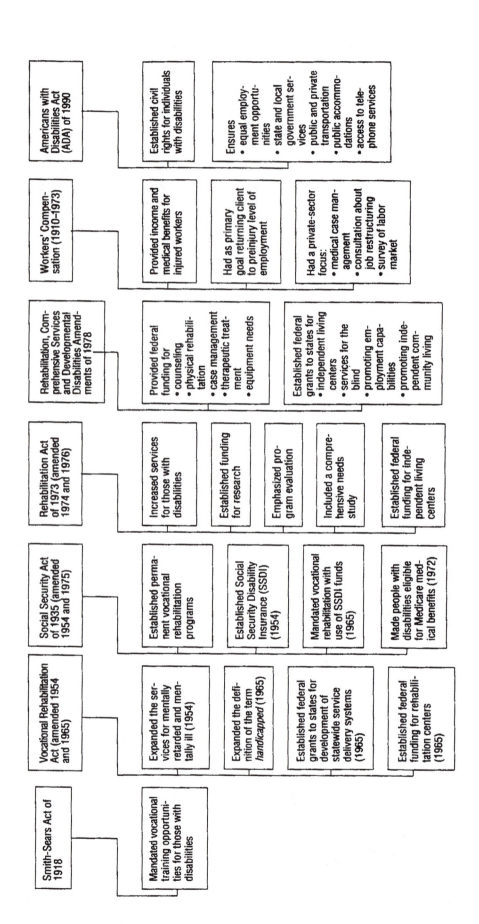

Figure 8-2 Laws governing access to rehabilitation services. (Reprinted from *The Specialty Practice of Rehabilitation Nursing: A Core Curriculum*, 3d ed, with permission of the Association of Rehabilitation Nurses, Skokie, IL. Copyright ©1993.)

those encountered within the acute rehabilitation setting are unaware of the multitude of issues for the disabled. The passage of the Americans with Disabilities Act in 1990 has allowed great strides to be made in the removal of architectural barriers, yet many attitudinal barriers remain. Figure 8-2 provides an overview of federal legislation regarding the rights of the disabled. Rehabilitation nurses need to work as patient advocates for the follow-

ing issues: housing, transportation, vocational training and employment opportunities, education, equipment/medical supplies, financial entitlements, benefits coverage, and coordination of care. Nurses need to pay attention "to the full range of human experiences and responses to health and illness without restriction to a problem-focused orientation" (American Nurses Association, 1995, p. 6).

Procedure

 Steps

 Additional Information

Clemen-Stone, Eigsti, and McGuire, 1995, p. 346

1. Gather discharge planning data:
   - Patient's desired ultimate living situation
   - Family's desired ultimate living situation
   - Financial resources available, insurance, entitlements
   - Accessibility of living arrangements (inside and outside the home)
   - Availability, willingness, and capability of family to learn and provide care (social support systems)
   - Patient's physical health
   - Functional status
   - Level of education
   - Health values and attitudes
   - Cultural, ethnic, and religious background
   - Perceptions of the situation
   - Barriers to care
   - Care preferences

2. Collaborate with interdisciplinary team to identify:
   - Realistic goals/outcomes for this admission and beyond
   - Feasibility of patient's desired living situation
   - Patient and family educational program

   Communicate results to patient and family. Begin patient and family teaching.

3. Identifying resources available to the patient and family in their community.

   Involve patient and family in this process and assist them in accessing the resources.

4. Weekly interdisciplinary conferences to determine progress toward desired outcomes, limiting factors, changes in plan of care or discharge plan.

   Patient and family need to be informed of any changes that impact the discharge plan.

5. Pass to evaluate effectiveness of discharge plan, or home evaluation with physical therapist and occupational therapist if unsure desired living situation is safe and accessible for the patient.

   Insurance coverage varies. Some insurances may not allow for passes.

6. Immediate discharge planning:
   - Durable medical equipment order
   - Medical supply list for monthly supplies prepared and supplies ordered
   - Prescriptions for medications written
   - Insurance coverage for discharge items verified
   - Home programs by therapists and nurses reviewed with patient and family

   Insurance coverage must be verified before any prescriptions or orders are placed.

- Referrals for additional/follow-up healthcare services made.
- Nursing discharge summary/plan of care
- Transportation to discharge location

7. Discharge patient.

REFERENCES

American Nurses Association (1995) *Nursing's Social Policy Statement* Washington, DC: American Nurses Publishing.

Carlson, R. and Keller, M.L. (1992) "Control over Daily Life and Caregiver Burden: Little Things Do Count" *Rehabilitation Nursing Research* 1:6–13.

Clemen-Stone, S., Eigsti, D. G. and McGuire, S.L. (1995) *Comprehensive Community Health Nursing*, 4th ed. St. Louis: Mosby-Year Book, Inc.

Davidhizar, R. (1997) "Disability Does Not Have to Be the Grief that Never Ends: Helping Patients Adjust" *Rehabilitation Nursing* 22(1):87–91.

DesRosier, M.B., Cantazaro, M. and Piller, J. (1992) "Living with Chronic Illness: Social Support and the Well Spouse Perspective" *Rehabilitation Nursing* 17:87–91.

Evans, R.W. (1997) "Postacute Neurorehabilitation: Roles and Responsibilities within a National Information System" *Archives of Physical Medicine and Rehabilitation* 78(8):S17–S25.

Holicky, R. (1996) "Caring for the Caregivers: The Hidden Victims of Illness and Disability" *Rehabilitation Nursing* 21(5):247–252.

Johnson, J., Pearson, V, and McDivitt, L. (1997) "Stroke Rehabilitation: Assessing Stroke Survivors' Long-Term Learning Needs" *Rehabilitation Nursing* 22(5):243–248.

Kantz, B., et al. (1998) "Developing Patient and Family Education Services" *Journal of Nursing Administration* 28(2):11–18.

Lindgren, C.L. (1993) "The Caregiver Career" *Image: Journal of Nursing Scholarship* 25:214–219.

McCourt, A.E. (Ed.) (1993) *The Specialty Practice of Rehabilitation Nursing: A Core Curriculum*, 3d ed. Skokie, IL: Rehabilitation Nursing Foundation.

Neal, L.J. (1995) "The Rehabilitation Nursing Team in the Home Healthcare Setting" *Rehabilitation Nursing* 20(1):32–36.

Pierce, L.L. (1994) "Fear Held by Caregivers of People with Stroke: A Concept Analysis" *Rehabilitation Nursing Research* 3:69–74.

Ruppert, R.A. (1996) "Psychological Aspects of Lay Caregiving" *Rehabilitation Nursing* 21(6):315–320.

Sayles-Cross, S. (1993) "Perceptions of Familial Caregivers of Elder Adults" *Image: Journal of Nursing Scholarship* 25:88–92.

Steinwachs, D.M. (1989) *Impact of Discharge Planning on Patient Outcome (Final Report to the Agency for Health Care Policy and Research)* Baltimore: U.S. Department of Health and Human Services.

Weeks, S. K. (1995) "What are the Educational Needs of Prospective Family Caregivers of Newly Disabled Adults?" *Rehabilitation Nursing* 20(5):256–260.

Weeks, S.K., and O'Connor, P.C. (1996) "Taking on the Family Caregiver Role" *Rehabilitation Nursing Research* 5(1):16–22.

Wood, F.G. (1991) "The Meaning of Caregiving" *Rehabilitation Nursing* 16:195–198.

CHAPTER 9

Patient/Family Centered Teaching and Learning

Introduction

Educating patients, families, and caregivers about a healthy lifestyle, adaptive behaviors, and prevention of secondary problems is an integral component of care in all rehabilitation settings. Providing individuals with chronic illness, disability, or development disorders the needed knowledge and skills to reach their optimal level of self-reliance and self-care is a major goal of the rehabilitation team. Clinicians play a central role in assessing learning needs, establishing teaching plans, and evaluating the effectiveness of the educational sessions. A defined set of principles and skills are associated with the ability of clinicians to teach others. Research shows that informed individuals are more successful at following their healthcare regimen after returning home (Newhouse, 1994).

This chapter will discuss the teaching-learning process, age-appropriate teaching-learning strategies, contrast a variety of teaching mediums, and identify evaluation methods used to measure learning outcomes. Potential learning barriers such as low literacy, differing cultural beliefs, and non-English speaking individuals will require special consideration. Evaluation and documentation of each teaching-learning experience, either planned or spontaneous, is necessary to measure progress and insure continuity of care. The last consideration is cost-effectiveness and reimbursement issues related to various programs. The format used for this chapter is designed for quick reference to plan and execute a quality teaching-learning experience.

Technology, such as cassette players, VCRs, and computers, has become widely available and affordable. Patients, family members, and caregivers are able to take home important information and review it at their own pace in the privacy of their homes. This educational medium can be used to empower patients and families to take charge of their own healthcare and make informed decisions.

JCAHO CONSIDERATIONS

The Joint Commission on Accreditation of Healthcare Organizations (JCAHO) (1997) standards for patient education underscore the need for an organization-wide plan for patient/family education activities, establishing program goals, and showing evidence of resource allocation. Patient education is a professional responsibility listed in many state nurse practice acts as well as in standards by accrediting organizations. Table 9-1 identifies some highlights of the JCAHO patient/family education standards.

Table 9-1   Highlights of JCAHO Patient/Family Education

1. The process of determining the educational needs
   - Promote patient input in determining needs
   - Identify methods that promote interactive communication
   - Increase patient decision-making ability
   - Provide plan to meet identified needs
   - Prioritize specific needs
2. The plan should include
   - An explanation of present health status
   - Treatment options, possible risks, and benefits of each
   - Financial responsibilities for treatment
   - Methods to increase amenability to care plan
   - Ways to promote a healthy lifestyle
   - Ways to incorporate coping skills
   - Sensitivity to cultural values

TEACHING-LEARNING PRINCIPLES AND PROCESS

The teaching-learning process mirrors the nursing process. The nurse uses the problem-solving approach to assess learning needs, readiness to learn, barriers to learning, and an appropriate environment for learning. The process of identifying learning needs begins with the initial admission assessment and continues through all levels of care. Table 9-2 lists the areas to be assessed and characteristics to explain each category.

Table 9-2 Teaching-Learning Assessment	
Assessment	**Characteristics**
1. Learning needs	Determined by direct observation or requested by patient, family member, or caregiver
	Physical functioning: mobility, dressing, eating, hygiene, elimination, etc.
	Psychosocial functioning: adjustment to disability, financial situation, role change, self-esteem, family relationships, etc.
	Community reentry: living arrangements, modification of home, employment, etc.
2. Readiness to learn	
Physical state	Fatigue, pain, sleepy
Mental state	Confused, overwhelmed, unable to concentrate
Emotional state	Fear, anxiety, denial
3. Motivation	
Usefulness of information	How does this apply to me?
Perception of health and situation	Does this fit into my belief system?
Seeking a solution to real problems	Will this improve my life?
4. Ability to learn	
Level of knowledge	Intellectual level, literacy
Past knowledge on subject	Build on or relate to past experiences, makes information realistic
Language barriers	Interpreter if needed, use native language teaching materials
Visual and hearing ability	Glasses, hearing aid in place, need for assistive technology
Cultural influences	Does this fit into belief system? Does trust exist?
Optimal learning style	How we process information and make it our own: visual, tactile, auditory, concrete vs. conceptual style
5. Assessing the environment	
Stress-free	Free of distractions
	Show sensitivity in your tone of voice
	Nonthreatening
	Nonjudgmental
Physical comfort	Warm
	Well lit
	Comfortable chair or bed

LEARNING DOMAINS (OBJECTIVES)

Learning is a process in which a measurable change takes place or sometimes a seed is planted for eventual change. These changes are maintained over time and can not be attributed only to growth. Learning occurs when a person makes sense out of what he or she has encountered or experienced and can integrate this new information into daily routines. The behavioral changes are the measured outcomes. Educators establish measurable, time-limited objectives within the three domains of learning based on a learning needs assessment and patient input (Bloom, 1956; Moss, 1994). Table 9-3 lists the domains, skill levels within each domain, and expected outcomes.

Learners remember 10 percent of what is read, 20 percent of what is heard, 30 percent of what is seen, 50 percent of what is heard and seen, and 80 percent of what the learner says and does (Humphrey and Milone-Nuzzo, 1996). Learner participation in the learning process has been shown to make learning more meaningful and increase retention (Moss, 1994).

"Health education is evaluated on the basis of patient outcomes rather than provider inputs" (Cravener, 1996, p. 140). Learning objectives identify the expected outcome of the learning experience. Objectives can be short-term or long-term and are mutually agreed on. Each learning objective indicates the specific behavior and content the learner should master, under what conditions, and under what criteria. The behavior is described using an active verb and should be measurable and observable, for example; state, select, or demonstrate. The objective always describes what the learner should be able to do after the learning experience, not the action of the teacher. The conditions under which the behavior occurs should be realistic and fit the learner's need; for example, walk using crutches from the bedroom to the bathroom. The desired level of accuracy is described in the criteria, which makes the objective more specific; for example, walk using crutches from the bedroom to the bathroom within 2 days. Learning objectives are written in the domain in which the learning deficit exists.

Table 9-3 Learning Domains and Expected Outcomes

Learning Domain	Skill Level	Expected Outcomes
Cognitive: Intellectual ability	Acquire knowledge Comprehension Application	Recall newly learned information Grasp meaning of information Use information in a situation
Affective: Principles that guide attitudes, beliefs, and feelings	Listening Reacting Valuing	Being exposed to new ideas or information Reacts to new ideas or information Internalizing ideas or behaviors
Psychomotor: Motor skills, gross and fine	Observing skills Performing skill using trial and error Performing skill with confidence and proficiency Adapt skill to fit lifestyle	Watching someone perform a skill, touching equipment, asking questions Staff watching, giving guidance Performs skill safely Teaches others

AGE-APPROPRIATE TEACHING-LEARNING

Learning needs and abilities change throughout the life cycle. Developmental level is taken into consideration when modifying teaching plans for each individual. Keep in mind that dysfunctional homes may have anxiety and fear that is much more elevated because of the life history. See Table 9-4 for teaching strategies appropriate for children, adolescents, adults, and older adults.

Table 9-4 Developmental Level with Corresponding Teaching Strategies

Age	Teaching Strategies
Child	• Focus on external body concept. • Use sensory terms to describe the experience. • Describe the exact parts of the procedure. • Use nonthreatening words. • Assess both the parent and child's level of understanding and knowledge. • Adapt teaching according to the child's developmental level. • Involve parents in the teaching as much as possible. • Allow plenty of time for questions, discussion, and feedback.

Table 9-4   Developmental Level with Corresponding Teaching Strategies (*continued*)

Age	Teaching Strategies
Child	• Use concrete terms and visual aids. • The older child can be taught some internal organ functions and may be interested in disease cause and prevention. • Be honest about unpleasant sensations without producing unnecessary concern.
• For toddlers	• Allow them to handle equipment and use play to teach. • Limit teaching sessions to 5 to 10 min.
• For preschoolers	• Use play and verbal explanations. • Point on a child, doll, or drawing where the procedure will be performed. • Teaching sessions can be 10 to 15 min.
• For school-aged children	• Use correct medical terms. • Use simple anatomy and physiology. • Two or more children can be in a group.
Adolescent	• Simple abstract concepts may be used. • Include friends in programs since strong peer relationships are important to adolescents. • Involve the adolescent in the decision-making and planning process. • Provide privacy and discuss long-term consequences.
Adult	• Ask learners what they expect to learn and their goals at the beginning of the session. • Let learner decide the direction and pace of learning. • Build on past knowledge and experiences. • Relate new information to learner's need to know or solution to identified problem.
Older adult	• Carefully assess for physiologic (hearing or vision losses), psychological (depression), educational barriers, Alzheimer's Disease, other cognitive disorders, and social isolation. • One or two concepts should be presented at a time and reinforced with pictures or key words in large black letters on white paper. • If the person wears a hearing aid, be sure it is in the ear and switched on. • Limit use of the metric system. • Use upper and lower case letters for easier reading.

SPECIAL CONSIDERATIONS

Special learning needs can greatly impact the ability of the patient to learn. The two areas creating the greatest teaching challenges are low literacy and cultural differences.

Occasionally, healthcare professionals inaccurately assess noncompliance when the real problem is the inability to read or understand instructions. Nurses are likely to encounter illiterate families who are in need of extensive healthcare education. Suggestions to better prepare nurses for assessing and teaching patients and their families are reviewed in Table 9-5.

Table 9-5   Suggestions for Low-Literacy Teaching

Signs of low literacy	Strategies
May respond to teaching efforts with anger, embarrassment, or shame	Create a shame-free environment
	Have a family member or friend review the information
Make excuses for their inability to read by blaming their eyesight or forgetting glasses	Attempt to give learners a sense of control in a nonjudgmental environment
Escape the situation by stating that they will read the material later	Use multiple mediums, not just written
Watching others to understand	Allow plenty of time for questions and discussion
Asking staff or other patients for help or may not ask many questions	Asking a patient to spell the names of medications instead of just reciting the names of the medicines
	Ask a patient to read the patient's bill of rights and observe if eyes move from left to right. Ask questions about the form.
	Hospital staff should be discreetly informed about the problems
	Patients should also be assured that their inability to read will not be carelessly discussed

Table 9-5   Suggestions for Low-Literacy Teaching (*continued*)

Signs of low literacy	Strategies
	Use audio and visual aids and provide as many opportunities for hands-on instructional activities as possible
	Try to pattern instructions after techniques the person already has used to learn in the past
	Teach the smallest amount possible to do the job
	Make the point as vividly as possible
	Use simple language (avoiding medical jargon, polysyllabic words, and long explanations)
	Use short, precise sentences and active words
	Illustrate points simply and summarize the important content
	Have the patient restate and perform a return demonstration
	Pick out the most important information for the first session
	Use pictorial cues

CULTURAL DIFFERENCES

When a patient or family speaks a different language, or is part of another culture, effective education can become more challenging. Cultural and language barriers need to be taken into account for effective education to occur. Bear in mind that some customs may impede learning. With patients to whom English is a second language, many can read English but may not be able to read or write in their primary language. In stressful situations such as rehabilitation, some patients and their families may only be able to communicate in their native language.

Cultural differences can affect patients' attitudes about rehabilitation care. Cultural beliefs, norms, and values influence attitudes about the causes of illness and the effectiveness of medical treatment. Culturally based ideas about family roles, gender roles, communication patterns (extremes in verbal and nonverbal methods), and religious beliefs can also influence the patient and family teaching-learning process. For some cultures, needing the assistance of persons outside of the family or community will produce a stigma, shame, or loss of status. See Table 9-6 for suggestions when working with people from different cultures.

Table 9-6   Working with People from Different Cultures

Suggestions

- Use audio tapes in the native language.
- Do not assume the patient understands what is being said when he or she nods head. The patient may be attempting to please the teacher.
- Whenever informed consent is being sought, use an official interpreter.
- Use nonverbal means of communication whenever possible.
- Ask family members for assistance.
- Provide written and audiovisuals in both English and the native language.
- Present material so that it respects cultural values.
- Incorporate dietary preferences and herbal remedies into the educational process.
- Develop and maintain a respectful attitude concerning cultural differences and their importance to patients and their families.
- Develop a method to become updated on the predominant cultures treated in the institution.
- Try to incorporate appropriate indigenous practitioners and medicines that may encourage and enhance the relationship with the patient and family.
- Respectfully disagree if any practices would conflict with modern medicine—If possible incorporate safe nontraditional practices into rehabilitation.

GENERAL CONSIDERATIONS

The following suggestions can be incorporated into many teaching plans for all age groups. Teaching is most successful:

- If the patient and/or family are calm and receptive

- Following an acute attack, the patient can be highly motivated to prevent a repeat episode
- When patient autonomy is developed

- When being respectful of the patient's values, preferences, and expressed needs
- By providing emotional support and alleviating fear and anxiety
- If the family and friends are involved
- If physical comfort is provided for
- When plenty of time is allowed for questions and discussion
- If immediate feedback is given
- When given important information at the beginning— 20-min attention span
- When explaining the normal before going into the abnormal
- By telling the learner what to expect

- By using interactive games and role playing as it relates to daily life
- By using as many senses as possible
- By using a sense of humor
- By finding out what works best for the learner to perform a task
- By offering review, repetition, and reinforcement
- By speaking slowly and distinctly and looking directly at the person
- By using the pronoun YOU to engage the person
- When clearly defining any unfamiliar terms
- When free of cultural, ethnic, age, race, disability, and sexual biases

MOTIVATION

Motivation greatly influences the outcome of rehabilitation and is the result of the interaction of the person with his or her environment. Motivation is influenced by the following three variables:

- The subjective perception on the part of the patient of the likelihood of a positive outcome of the rehabilitation process
- The perceived utility or value of a successful rehabilitation process
- The perception of the cost of the outcome and the costs of the rehabilitation process itself

Changes in any one of these variables will impact the other variables. Just because a patient refuses rehabilitation does not mean he or she is not motivated. A thorough assessment should discover the underlying problem. The rehabilitation process may place the patient in an embarrassing and confusing role as he or she confronts new challenges and limitations.

Motivational problems can be expressed by:

- Expressing anger toward the team members
- Stagnation or stopping of the rehabilitation program
- An overly critical view of the rehabilitation team

Motivational techniques:

- Learn how the patient perceives his or her situation and prognosis
- Attempt to keep the patient as an active participant in the program
- Give the patient several options to choose from when designing the program
- Be alert to motivational blocks (fear of failure)

- Identify the blocks and use them as a starting point for communication
- Try to individualize information to his or her frame of reference
- Use metaphors if possible
- Keep in mind patients can selectively remember, neglect, and/or distort information
- Set small, short-term objectives
- Relabel the patient's critical attitude, behavior, and performance in a positive way
- Assess for commitment on behalf of the patient and attempt to translate that into the rehabilitation program
- Talk openly and empathetically with the patient about possible costs
- Attempt to focus the patient on realistic estimates of the costs
- Identify any hidden costs that may occur if the patient improves (less family interactions) creating feelings of ambivalence
- Find out how and if these can be worked out with the patient
- Focus the patient on the idea that rehabilitation will lead to greater self-sufficiency
- Seek ways to make the rehabilitation process less emotionally demanding
- Build pleasant distractions or focus the patient on the pleasant experiences during exercises
- Referral to a psychologist as needed

NURSES AS TEACHERS

Multiple ongoing changes in today's healthcare settings have deeply impacted the nurses' ability to engage in meaningful patient/family teaching. Decreases in staffing and increases in

patient-to-nurse ratio have created new challenges. Barriers to teaching include:

- Limited time for teaching

- Concentrating on acute care medical needs versus long-term chronic care of the medical condition
- Use of medical jargon patients and families do not understand
- The time and materials needed for patient education are not reimbursable
- Media aids are not available when needed
- Lack of storage space for educational materials
- Poor teaching skills
- Poorly prepared or uncomfortable with subject content
- Decreased length of stay
- Increased patient acuity—multiple barriers to learning

In order to provide patients and their family members with adequate education, nurses need to know how to teach effectively. This can be accomplished through:

- Standardizing patient teaching
- Finding another nurse to teach an uncomfortable topic such as sexuality

- Setting a warm and accepting tone for learning to occur
- Providing support materials for nurses, and when the materials are requested give teaching tips
- Implementing self-paced programs on how to teach patients and their families
- Having packets available that contain information on available teaching materials
- Creating a family/patient library and resource center
- Providing instructions on how staff can obtain materials on educational videos or home care instructions
- Purchasing a teaching program for staff if resources are limited versus creating one
- Drawing upon experts in the field to provide the information to patients or have the experts develop inservices for the staff
- Video recording of the teaching session and feedback with critiquing by educator
- Management support must be available (resources, time, financial)

MEDIA TYPES

A variety of media can be used from the spoken word, printed material, audiotapes, videotapes, and computer simulations. The location of teaching, availability of resources, and patient characteristics, such as sensory losses, will influence the choice of medium. When printed education material is used in combination with personalized reinforcement, better learning outcomes occur.

Printed education materials include written booklets, leaflets, pamphlets, or information sheets. Many measures are involved in developing an effective and useful printed educational tool. When selecting any educational tool, the readability of the material needs to be evaluated. There are more than 30 formulas for assessing the readability of written tools. Com-

puter software programs to calculate readability are also available. Use any of the following authors as resources to create or evaluate printed education materials (Bernier, 1993; Ethier, 1996; Harper and Van Riper, 1993; Reiley et al., 1996).

Multiple sources exist for creating health education programs. The development of educational programs is beyond the scope of this chapter. However, Becker and coworkers (1994) and Grassman (1993) provide examples of how to create programs.

Patient education occurs through the use of many types of media. See Table 9-7 for advantages and disadvantages of printed education materials, programs, videos, and computers.

Table 9-7 Advantages and Disadvantages of Education Materials

Type	Advantages	Disadvantages
Printed Educational Materials	These items are the most common form of instructional materials: • Flexibility of delivery • Easy portability • Reusability • Consistency of the message content • Permanence of information • Low cost to produce and update • Can be prepared quickly • Can be designed per institution or chosen from the many already available • Any preprinted material costs, accessibility, and usability of the product	• Difficult to develop • Requires knowledge of instructional design and learning theory needed to critique usefulness • The lack of quality control in the available materials • May not necessarily be readable • May not be an effective teaching tool with many persons

Table 9-7	Advantages and Disadvantages of Education Materials *(continued)*	
Type	**Advantages**	**Disadvantages**
Group Programs	• Allow nurses to teach more patients in a group format • This increases cost-effectiveness if many participants attend the program	• It can be a budget drain if the turnout is limited. • The educator may fear a lack of acceptance by the group • Fear discussing an individual problem • Instructor may poorly express the subject matter
Videos	• They are successful in increasing knowledge, teaching new skills, or changing target behavior when used as a supplement to one to one teaching • Encourage discussion • The tapes can be viewed at any time by any patient with access to a video player • Frees staff time • Uses tapes in the native language	• Set aside space with a VCR unit • Staff still needs to reinforce teaching • Tape recorders and VCRs may be too costly if an illiterate family also has a low income • The videotapes may be too fast paced, and the message is missed • Costly to create • Costly to purchase • English tapes used for patients for whom English is a second language can be a poor choice
Computers	• Alternates relaxing interludes with educational messages • Offers unhurried learning in a relaxed and quiet environment with one-on-one teaching • A one-time fee is charged and is covered by most insurance • Increased autonomy of participants • The computers allow for user privacy • It is self-paced • It can be easily updated • Graphics enhance sensory stimulation • It is a cost-effective use of staff time • Reduces participant passiveness • Limited input by an educator • The text can be written free of medical jargon • The results of the user are stored on the hard disk to guide future educational sessions and to assist with statistical analysis on the computer users	• The computer requires space • The available software is limited • Patients, families, and nurses fear the use of computers • The participants need to be oriented to how to use the computer program • Costly to purchase

COST-EFFECTIVENESS

Multiple studies suggest patient education is effective. However, many times individual teaching sessions, while educationally effective, are not cost-effective.

The best way to illustrate economic benefits from a program is evaluation through cost-effectiveness analysis. While many programs may generate revenue, it rarely reflects the true cost of the program. Costs to be considered include direct, indirect, and intangible. See Table 9-8 for an explanation of costs and examples.

Cost-effectiveness uses natural measurable clinical units like exacerbations. The output is the cost per case of exacerbation averted. Comparison of programs within a particular clinical domain is straightforward; however, comparison across domains is not. Therefore, cost-effectiveness ratios with unequally valued denominators must be compared.

Cost-utility analysis converts health effects into common units, most frequently converted into quality adjusted life years. Quality adjusted life expectancy includes health status improvement.

Cost-benefit analysis expresses health effects in dollars. It subtracts net costs from net benefits, deeming the program either cost-effective or not cost-effective. This method, however, fails to value exacerbations averted from the benefit of education. This is the reason that most health professionals prefer cost-utility analysis as a method to measure cost-effectiveness.

REIMBURSEMENT

Education for inpatients is not usually reimbursable. However, some fees for patient education services have been included in self-care supplies such as central line equipment. The most common method of outpatient and community health education is through a fee-for-service charge. Third-party payers are beginning to reimburse for programs that include specialized staff members such as clinical nurse specialists. The future of reimbursement of educational services will be based on documented educational program successes that show healthcare cost savings.

Table 9-8   Program Costs

Type of Cost	Definition	Examples
Direct	Those costs that actually consume resources	Program costs, inpatient care, outpatient care, physician services (for inpatients and outpatients), emergency visits, ambulance use, drugs, short- and long-term treatment complications, devices, diagnostic services, nursing services, allergy testing and treatment, comorbidity costs, research (basic and applied), community education, and unpaid volunteer work.
Indirect	Those losses in productivity due to illness-related morbidity and premature mortality. These types of costs are very difficult to measure and very often are ignored in economic evaluations.	Work loss, housekeeping and school absence for patients and their family members. Other examples include mortality, traveling, and waiting time.
Intangible	Intangible costs are the value of pain and suffering, anxiety, and pyschic distress.	Short-term and long-term effects of living with or caring for someone with a chronic illness or disability.

EVALUATION AND DOCUMENTATION

The educational process is not complete until the nurse evaluates the outcomes mutually agreed on by the patient and staff. Oral or written questioning, direct observation, and return demonstration are useful methods of evaluation. The evaluation process also helps determine adequacy of teaching. If results indicate a knowledge or skill deficit, the reason for the deficit must be explored, and the teaching plan modified.

When documenting educational sessions, the nurse should be as specific as possible describing the content of the session.

Clear communication to other staff is recommended to avoid wasted time and resources. Document objective evidence of successful/unsuccessful outcomes. Include the teaching methods (pamphlets, audiovisual) that worked best and those that did not work with the individual. Many facilities have developed checklist forms (Figs. 9-1 to 9-5) for documenting teaching methods, material, and results. The following pages include several examples of teaching checklists that were developed specifically for the different rehabilitation populations.

REFERENCES

Anonymous (1995) "Break Down Age-Related Barriers to Learning" *Patient Education Management* 2(7):98, 100.

Anonymous (1995) "Do Your Staff Know How to Teach Effectively?" *Patient Education Management* 2(9):122–124.

Anonymous (1996) "5 Tips to Teach Staff to Instruct Illiterate Patients" *Homecare Education Management* 1(6):75–76.

Becker, A., McGhan, S., Dolovich, J., et al. (1994) "Essential Ingredients for an Ideal Education Program for Children with Asthma and Their Families" *Chest* 106(4):231S–234S.

Bernier, M.J. (1993) "Developing and Evaluating Printed Education Materials: A Prescriptive Model for Quality" *Orthopaedic Nursing* 12(6):39–46.

Bloom, B.S. (Ed.) (1956) *Taxonomy of Educational Objective: The Classification of Educational Goals. Handbook I: Cognitive Domain* New York: David McKay.

Boulet, L., Chapman, K.R. and Green, L.W. (1994) "Asthma Education" *Chest* 106(4):184S–196S.

Brookfield, S.D. (1986) *Understanding and Facilitating Adult Learning* San Francisco, CA: Jossey-Bass.

Chachkes, E. and Christ, G. (1996) "Cross Cultural Issues in Patient Education" *Patient Education and Counseling* 27:13–21.

Chapman, K.R., Dales, R.E., Chan-Yeung, M. and Cote, J. (1994) "Future Research in Asthma Education" *Chest* 106(4):270S–273S.

Consoli, S.M., Said, M.B., Jean, J., et al. (1995) Benefits of a Computer-Assisted Education Program for Hypertensive Patients Compared with Standard Education Tools" *Patient Education and Counseling* 26(1-3):343–347.

Cravener, P.A. (1996) "Principles of Adult Health Education" *Gastroenterology Nursing* 19(4):140–145.

Duffy, B. (1997) "Using a Creative Teaching Process with Adult Patients" *Home Healthcare Nurse* 15(2):102–108.

Dunn, M., Buckwalter, K., Weinstein, L. and Palti, H. (1985) "Teaching the Illiterate Does Not Have to Be a Problem" *Family and Community Health* 8(3):76–80.

Ethier, A.K. (1996) "Education Essentials. Developing Education Materials for Families" *Journal of Pediatric Oncology Nursing* 13(3):146–149.

Funnell, M.M., Donnelly, M.B., Anderson, R.M., et al. (1992) "Perceived Effectiveness, Cost, and Availability of

Patient Education Methods and Materials" *Diabetes Educator* 18(2):139–145.

Geelen, R., and Soons, P. (1996) "Rehabilitation: An 'Everyday' Motivation Model" *Patient Education and Counseling* 28, 69-77.

Goldstein, N.L., Snyder, M., Edin, C., et al. (1996) "Comparison of Two Teaching Strategies" *Clinical Nursing Research* 5(2):150–166.

Grassman, D. (1993) "Development of Inpatient Oncology Educational and Support Programs" *Oncology Nursing Forum* 20(4):669–676.

Green, L.W. and Frankish, C.J. (1994) "Theories and Principles of Health Education Applied to Asthma" *Chest* 106(4):219S–230S.

Harper, P. and Van Riper, S. (1993) "Implantable Cardioverter Defibrillator: A Patient Education Model for the Illiterate Patient" *Critical Care Nurse* 55–59.

Houts, P.S., Nezu, A.M., Nezu, C.M. and Bucher, J.A. (1996) "The Prepared Family Caregiver: A Problem-Solving Approach to Family Caregiver Education" *Patient Education and Counseling* 27:63–73.

Humphrey, C. and Milone-Nuzzo, P. (1996) *Client Teaching in the Home. Manual of Home Care Nursing Orientation* Gaithersburg, MD: Aspen.

JCAHO (1997) Comprehensive Accreditation Manual for Hospitals: The Official Handbook.

Kemp, J.E. (1985) *The Instructional Design Process* New York: Harper & Row.

Knowles, M. (1980) *Modern Practice of Adult Education* Chicago, IL: Association.

Krahn, M. (1994) "Issues in the Cost-Effectiveness of Asthma Education" *Chest* 106(104):264S–269S.

Lynch, M.E. (1992) "When the Patient Is Illiterate: How Nurses Can Help" *Journal of Practical Nursing* 42(1):41–42.

Meiman, S. (1996) "Education Essentials. Development of an Evaluation Tool for Educational Material" *Journal of Pediatric Oncology Nursing* 13(1):50–52.

Mohr, W.K. (1993) "Nurse-Led Educational Program in Psychiatric Setting: Developing a Curriculum" *Journal of Psychosocial Nursing* 31(3):34–38, 46.

Moss, V.A. (1994) "Assessing Learning Abilities, Readiness for Education" *Seminars in Perioperative Nursing* 3(3):113–120.

Newhouse, M.T. (1994) "Hospital-Based Asthma Education" *Chest* 106(4):237S–241S.

Nowicki, C.R. (1996) "21 Predictions for the Future of Hospital Staff Development" *Journal of Continuing Education in Nursing* 27(6):259–266.

Parikh, N.S., Parker, R.M., Nurss, J.R., et al. (1996) "Shame and Health Literacy: The Unspoken Connection" *Patient Education and Counseling* 27:33–39.

Reiley, P., Pike, A., Phipps, M., et al. (1996) "Learning from Patients: A Discharge Planning Improvement Project" *Journal on Quality Improvement* 22(5):311–322.

Rymes-Barley, C. (1989) "A Secret Inability to Comply. The Price of Illiteracy" *Canadian Pharmaceutical Journal* 122(2):86–88, 91–94.

Schaffner, M. (1995) "Patient Teaching Methods and Materials" *Gastroenterology Nursing* 18(1):16–19.

Shinn, J.A. (1994) "A Bridge to Autonomy: Using Technology and Teaching in Patient Centered Care" *Stanford Nurse* 9–11.

van Veenendaal, H., Grinspun, D.R. and Adriaanse, H.P. (1996) "Educational Needs of Stroke Survivors and Their Family Members, as Perceived by Themselves and by Health Professionals" *Patient Education and Counseling* 265–276.

Wasson, D. and Anderson, M.A. (1994) "Hospital-Patient Education. Current Status and Future Trends" *Journal of Nursing Staff Development* 10(3):147–151.

Weiss, B.D., Reed, R.L. and Klingman, E.W. (1995) "Literacy Skills and Communication Methods of Low-Income Older Persons" *Patient Education and Counseling* 25:109–119.

Williams, R.B., Boles, M. and Johnson, R.E. (1995) "Patient Use of a Computer for Prevention in Primary Care Practice" *Patient Education and Counseling* 25:283–292.

Wilson, F.L., McLemore, R. (1997) "Patient Literacy Levels: A Consideration When Designing Patient Education Programs" *Rehabilitation Nursing* 22(6):311–317.

REHABILITATION INSTITUTE OF CHICAGO
NURSING TEACHING CHECKLIST

PRIMARY NURSE ____________________

PRIMARY CARE GIVER ____________________

WEEKEND PASS TARGET DATE ____________________

PLACEMENT PLAN ____________________

IMPRINT PATIENT NAME PLATE

NAME

RIC NO.

DR.

ACCOUNT NO.

DATE

A. SKIN CARE

*GOALS ____________________

	Information Given 1 PT.	Information Given 1 PCG	Return Demonstration 2 PT.	Return Demonstration 2 PCG	NA
(1) Positions:					
a) Side					
b) Supine					
c. Prone					
(2) Prevention of Pressure Sores:					
a) Warning Signs					
b) Skin Checks					
c) Sit/Turn Tolerances					
d) Wheelchair Pressure Relief					
e) Bridging					
f) Care of Pressure Areas					
(3) Prevention & Care of:					
a) Burns: Blisters					
b) Rashes					
c) Bruising					
d) Edema					
(4) Care of Hands & Feet					

*NOTE

GOALS: Include short- and long-term goals and date to be achieved.

B. BOWEL CARE

*GOALS ____________________

	Information Given 1 PT.	Information Given 1 PCG	Return Demonstration 2 PT.	Return Demonstration 2 PCG	NA
(1) Bowel Program					
(2) Suppository Insertions					
(3) Digital Stimulation					
(4) Manual Removal					
(5) Enema					
(6) Regulation:					
a) Medication					
b) Fluid					
c) Diet					
d) Activity					
(7) Abdominal Message					
(8) Management					
a) Hyperreflexia					
b) Constipation					
c) Diarrhea					

KEY:

NA = NOT APPLICABLE
PT. = PATIENT
PCG. = PRIMARY CARE GIVER

PT. & PCG. : DATE AND INITIAL COLUMN 1 WHEN EXPLANATION, DEMONSTRATION TAUGHT: DATE AND INITIAL COLUMN 2 WHEN ACCEPTABLE RETURN DEMONSTRATION OR EXPLANATION IS COMPLETED BY PT. OR PCG.

2-040096-10

Figure 9-1

C. BLADDER CARE:

*GOALS _____

_____
_____
_____
_____
_____
_____
_____
_____
_____
_____

	Information Given		Return Demonstration		NA
	1 PT.	1 PCG	2 PT.	2 PCG	
(1) Foley Catheter:					
a) Size					
b) Removal/Insertion					
(2) Catheter Irrigation					
(3) Taping Catheter					
(4) Application of:					
a) Leg Bag					
b) Bedside Drainage Bag					
(5) Decatheterization Program:					
a) Straight Catheter					
b) Avoid Overdistention					
c) Fluid Restriction					
d) Stimulating Void					
FREQUENCY: e) Residuals/Catheterization					
f) Apply/Make External					
(6) Symptoms & Management:					
a) UTI					
b) Calculi					
c) Automatic Hyperreflexia					
Prevention: Infection (7) Calculi: Hyperreflexia					
(8) Effect: Fluids & Medication					
(9) Cleaning of Equipment					
(10) PH Check					
Signatures:					
Signatures:					

Nurse Therapist Signature _____ Date Completed _____

D. RESPIRATORY CARE:

*GOALS _____

_____
_____
_____
_____
_____
_____

	Information Given		Return Demonstration		NA
	1 PT.	1 PCG	2 PT.	2 PCG	
(1) Congestion Management					
(2) Exercise Program					
(3) Incentive Spirometry					
(4) Postural Drainage					
(5) Effect:					
a) Humidity, Fluid, Mobility					
(6) Assistive Cough					

E. GENERAL

*GOALS _____

_____
_____
_____
_____

	Information Given		Return Demonstration		NA
	1 PT.	1 PCG	2 PT.	2 PCG	
(1) Weather Management:					
a) Hot					
b) Cold					
(2) Spasticity Management					
(3) Protein, Weight Control					
(4) Hypotension Management:					
a) Support Hose					
b) Abdominal Binder					
(5) Knows Medications:					
a) Dosage/Actions/Schedule					
b) Side Effects					
(6) Medical Follow Up					
(7) Sexuality					
(8) Thrombophlebitis					
(9) Purchasing Equipment					
(10) Taking Temperature					
(11)					

REHABILITATION INSTITUTE OF CHICAGO

THERAPIST **ARTHRITIS/ORTHOPEDIC**
NURSING TEACHING CHECKLIST

PRIMARY NURSE _____

PRIMARY CARE GIVER _____

WEEKEND PASS TARGET DATE _____

PLACEMENT PLAN _____

Patient Name

RIC Number

Physician

Date

☐ Inpatient   ☐ Outpatient

NATURE OF ARTHRITIS	INFO GIVEN		RETURN DEMONSTRATION		
	PT	PCG	PT	PCG	NA
1) Definition of Main Type					
2) Effects on Body					
a) Joints					
b) Muscles					
c) Other Body Systems					
3) Chronicity: Exacerbations/Remissions					

MAINTENANCE OF FUNCTION	INFO GIVEN		RETURN DEMONSTRATION		
	PT	PCG	PT	PCG	NA
1) Exercise Program					
a) Contractures/ROM					
b) Muscle Strength					
c) Respiratory					
2) Joint Protection					
a) Modifications in Activity					
b) Splints					
c) Assistive Devices					
3) Positioning					
a) Supine					
b) Side					
c) Prone					
4) Posture					

SAFETY	INFO GIVEN		RETURN DEMONSTRATION		
	PT	PCG	PT	PCG	NA
1) Safe Home Environment					
2) Transferring					
3) Therapy Precautions (Joint)					
4) Activity Limits/Pain					

ENERGY CONSERVATION	INFO GIVEN		RETURN DEMONSTRATION		
	PT	PCG	PT	PCG	NA
1) Daily Schedule					
a) Planned Activities					
b) Frequent Rest Periods					
c) Rest & Sleep					
2) Role of Fatigue					

PAIN MANAGEMENT	INFO GIVEN		RETURN DEMONSTRATION		
	PT	PCG	PT	PCG	NA
1) Medications					
a) Dose and Time					
b) Side Effects					
c) Special Considerations					
2) Heat/Cold Therapy					
3) Stress Management/Relaxation					

KEY: NA = Not Applicable
PT = Patient
PCG = Primary Care Giver

PT & PCG: Date & Initial Column 1 When Explanation,
Demonstration Taught.
Date & Initial Column 2 When Acceptable Return
Demonstration or Explanation is Completed by PT
or PCG.

Pilot

Figure 9-2

BOWEL & BLADDER	INFO GIVEN		RETURN DEMO			PSYCHOLOGICAL IMPLICATIONS	INFO GIVEN		RETURN DEMO	
	PT	PCG	PT	PCG	NA		PT	PCG	PT	NA
1) Toileting Program						1) Self-Concept				
2) Hygiene						2) Independence/Dependence Issues				
3) Effects of:						3) Problem Solving Ability				
a) Medications										
b) Fluid & Diet										
c) Activity										
4) Management of:										
a) Constipation										
b) Diarhea										

SKIN CARE	INFO GIVEN		RETURN DEMO			MISCELLANEOUS	INFO GIVEN		RETURN DEMO		
	PT	PCG	PT	PCG	NA		PT	PCG	PT	PCG	NA
1) Preventing Pressure Sores						1) Sexuality					
a) Warning Signs						2) Vocational Planning					
b) Skin Inspection						3) Community Resources					
c) Sit/Turn Tolerances						4) Surgical Options					
d) W/C Pressure Reliefs						5) Medical Follow-up					
2) Care of hands and feet						6) Common Complications					
3) Prevention & Care of:											
a) Bruising											
b) Rashes											
c) Edema											
d) Ulcerations											

COMMENTS _____
_____
_____
_____

SIGNATURES: _____

SIGNATURES: _____

NURSE
SIGNATURES _____
_____

DATE COMPLETED: _____

<table>
<tr><td colspan="2">

REHABILITATION INSTITUTE OF CHICAGO
NURSING TEACHING CHECKLIST

PRIMARY NURSE _____

PRIMARY CARE GIVER #1 _____ #2 _____

DAY PASS _____ W/E PASS _____

PLACEMENT PLAN _____

</td><td>

IMPRINT PATIENT NAME PLATE

NAME

RIC NO.

DR.

ACCOUNT NO.

DATE

</td></tr>
</table>

BRAIN DAMAGE/STROKE TEACHING CHECKLIST

INSTRUCTIONS:
1. DATE AND INITIAL IN 1st & 2nd COLUMNS WHEN INFORMATION IS GIVEN TO PATIENT (PT) AND OR PATIENT CARE GIVER (PCG).
2. DATE AND INITIAL IN 3rd & 4th COLUMNS WHEN ACCEPTABLE RETURN DEMONSTRATION OR EXPLANATION IS COMPLETED BY PATIENT OR PRIMARY CARE GIVER.
3. PLACE ✓ IN 5th COLUMN WHEN NOT APPLICABLE.

	Info Given PT	Info Given PCG	Return Demo PT	Return Demo PCG	NA
I. NATURE OF BRAIN DAMAGE/STROKE					
1. Etiology					
2. Effects of Brain Damage on Body Systems					
3. Risk Factors					
4. Complications					
II. SKIN CARE					
1. Positioning/Turning					
2. Prevention of Pressure Sores					
A. Warning Signs					
B. Skin Inspection					
C. Sit/Turn Tolerances					
D. W/C Pressure Relief					
E. Splint/Orthosis Mgmt.					
F. Care of Pressure Areas					
3. Prevention & Maintenance					
A. Burns, Blisters, Rashes					
B. Edema					
1) Equipment Used					
2) Elevation					
C. Effects of Spasticity/Tone					
III. BOWEL CARE					
1. Bowel Program					
A. Toileting					

	Info Given PT	Info Given PCG	Return Demo PT	Return Demo PCG	NA
2. Suppository Insertion					
3. Effects of on Regulation					
A. Medication					
B. Diet and Fluids					
C. Activity					
D. Cognition					
E. Communication					
4. Bowel: Management of:					
A. Constipation					
B. Diarrhea					
IV. BLADDER CARE					
1. Toileting Program					
A. Frequency					
B. Fluid Schedule					
2. Hygiene					
3. Application of:					
A. External Catheter					
B. Leg Bag/Night Drainings					
C. Incontinent Pants					
4. Foley Catheter Care					
A. Size					
B. Insertion/Removal					
C. Taping Catheter					
D. Cleaning Equipment					
5. Prevention and Management of Complications					
A. Rashes					
B. Urinary Tract Infection					
C. Incontinence					

Figure 9-3

	Info Given PT	Info Given PCG	Return Demo PT	Return Demo PCG	NA
6. Effects of Fluid and Meds					
7. Clothing Management					
V. RESPIRATORY CARE					
1. Congestion Management					
A. Incentive Spirometry					
B. Assistive Cough					
2. Effects of Humidity, Fluids & Mobility					
3. Signs and Symptoms of Complications					
VI. SENSORY/PERCEPTUAL					
1. Recognition and/or Mgmt. of:					
A. Visual Field Deficits					
B. Neglect Syndrome					
C. Auditory Deficits					
VII. SAFETY MANAGEMENT					
1. Recognizes and Plans					
A. Safe Home Environment					
B. Need for Supervision					
C. Activity Limits					
2. Seizure Management					
3. Emergency Procedure — (please indicate skill & teaching on progress note)					
VIII. NUTRITION AND DYSPHAGIA MGMT.					
1. Oral Feedings					
A. Diet					
B. Positioning/Feeding Techniques					
2. Enteral Feedings					
A. Type/Amount Schedule					
B. Method:_____					
C. Positioning					
D. Care of Tube & Site					
E. Insertion of Tube					
3. Prevention and Management of Complications					
A. Food Intolerence					
B. Tube Displacement					
4. Weight Control					

	Info Given PT	Info Given PCG	Return Demo PT	Return Demo PCG	NA
IX. MEDICATIONS					
1. Dosage/Action/Schedule					
2. Side Effects					
3. Method of Administration					
X. COGNITIVE/COMMUNICATIVE					
1. Management Techniques					
A. Aphasia/Communication Tech.					
B. Arousal/Orientation Tech.					
C. Altered Affect Control					
D. Impaired Judgment					
E. Inappropriate Behavior					
F. Memory Deficit Compensation					
XI. GENERAL INFO					
1. Sexuality					
2. Related Diagnosis (please indicate skill & teaching on progress note)					
3. Vital Signs					
A. Pulse, Temp, Respirations					
B. Blood Pressure					
4. Purchasing Meds/Equipment					
5. Care and Maintenance of Equip.					
A. Support Hose					
B. Mattress/Wheel Chair Cushion					
6. Medical Follow-Up					
7. Community Services					
8. Rehab Follow-Up					

	INITIALS
Signature:	
Signature:	
Signature:	
Signature:	
Signature:	
Signature:	
Date Reviewed By	
NURSE SIGNATURE	

396

Rehabilitation Institute of Chicago
Amputee
Nursing Teaching Checklist

Primary Nurse _____

Primary Care Giver #1 _____ #2 _____

Day Pass _____ W/E Pass _____

Placement Plan _____

Issued Pre-prosthetic Care Guide? ☐ Yes ☐ No

Instructions:
1. Date and initial in 1st and 2nd columns when information is given to patient (PT) and/or patient caregiver (PCG).
2. Date and initial in 3rd and 4th columns when acceptable return demonstration or explanation is completed by patient or primary care giver.
3. Place a ✓ in 5th column when not applicable.

I. Etiology	Info Given PT	Info Given PCG	Return Demo PT	Return Demo PCG	N/A
A. Diabetes (see DM ✓list)					
B. PVD					
C. Trauma					
D. Other					
II. Skin Care					
A. Prevention of Pressure Sores					
1. Skin inspection					
2. Warning signs					
3. Sit/turn tolerances					
4. W/C pressure relief					
5. Splint/orthoses mgmt.					
B. Prevention & Care of:					
1. Burns, blisters					
2. Rashes					
3. Edema					
a. equipment used					
b. positioning					
C. Sensory/Circulation changes					
1. Color					
2. Temperature					
3. Pulses					

III. Care of Residual Limb	Info Given PT	Info Given PCG	Return Demo PT	Return Demo PCG	N/A
A. Hygiene					
B. Desensitization					
C. Shrinking & Shaping					
1. Wrapping					
2. Rigid dressing					
3. Shrinker socks					
D. Care of the Incision					
1. Dressing changes					
2. Mobilization of scar					
3. Prevention of trauma					
E. Prevention of Contractures					
1. Positioning in:					
a. bed					
b. wheelchair					
c. ambulation					
2. Exercise					
3. ROM					
F. Sensory/Pain Management					
1. Phantom pain/sensation					
2. Intermittent claudication					
3. Incisional pain					
4. Medication					
G. Diet & Weight Control					

Figure 9-4

	Info Given		Return Demo		N/A
	PT	PCG	PT	PCG	
IV. Prosthetic Care					
A. Artificial Limb					
B. Socks					
C. Shrinkers					
D. Follow-up					
V. Bowel & Bladder					
A. Signs & Symptoms					
B. Potential Complications					
1. Incontinency					
2. Clothing management					
C. Complication Management					
1. Fluids					
2. Diet					
3. Medications					
4. Mobility					
D. Other					
VI. General Information					
A. Psychological Considerations					
1. Body image					
2. Sexuality					
3. Family coping					
4. Available supports					
B. Medications					
1. Dose, frequency, action					
2. Side effects					
VII. Discharge Planning					
A. Medical Follow-up					
1. Community MD					
2. Home health care					
3. Med./supply purchase					
4. RIC follow-up					
B. Home Accessibility					
C. Community Resources					

	Info Given		Return Demo		N/A
	PT	PCG	PT	PCG	
VIII. Related Considerations					
A. Other Diagnoses					
B. Related Teaching					

	Initials
Signature:	
Signature:	
Signature:	
Signature:	
Signature:	
Signature:	
Date Reviewed By:	

Rehabilitation Institute of Chicago
Home Care Respiratory Checklist

Patient _____   Respiratory Vendor _____

Nurse _____   Contact Person _____

Caregivers   1. _____   R.T. Instructor _____

2. _____

3. _____

	Info Given		Return Demo		N/A
	PT	PCG	PT	PCG	
I. Structure & Function					
A. Normal Structure and Function of Respiratory System					
B. Changes After Injury					
II. Tracheostomy Care: Type & Size					
A. Cleaning Inner Cannula Technique					
B. Stoma Care					
C. Trach Insertion					
D. Cuff Care					
E. Trach Safety and Precautions					
F. Care of Equipment					
G. Weather Management					
H. Makes Saline					
III. Suctioning					
A. Suctioning Technique					
B. Catheter Care					
C. Using Battery Operated Machine					
D. Use of Ambu Bag					
E. Setting Up Oxygen					
IV. Prevention & Management of the Following:					
A. Atelectasis Signs/Symptoms Management					
B. Pneumonia Signs/Symptoms Management					
C. Pulmonary Emboli Signs/symptoms Management					
D. Extubation					
E. Aspiration Signs/Symptoms Management					

Figure 9-5

RIC Home Care Respiratory Checklist (continued)

	Info Given		Return Demo		N/A
	PT	PCG	PT	PCG	
V. Respiratory Program					
A. Incentive Spirometry					
B. P-Flex					
C. Assistive Cough					
D. Corking					
E. Postural Drainage					
F. Percussion/Vibration					
G. Humidity					
H. Mobility					
I. Respiratory Treatments					
VI. Ventilator Maintenance					
A. Operational Controls and Function					
B. Ventilator Circuit Changes					
C. Use of Ambu Bag					
D. Emergency Measures					
1. Power failure					
2. Tracheostomy tube coming out					
3. Emergency phone number list					
E. Trouble Shooting of Equipment when Alarm Sounds					
F. Disinfecting of Respiratory Equipment					
G. Changing of Oxygen Cylinders					
VII. Oxygen Therapy					
A. Current Program					
B. Setting Up					
C. Flow/Delivery system					
D. Care and Maintenance					
E. Safety Precautions					
F. Signs/Symptoms Decreased					
G. Signs/Symptoms Increased					
VIII. Emergency Procedures					
A. CPR Discussed					
B. States ER Plan					
C. Notifies Utility/Fire Company					
D. Vital Signs					
1. Temperature					
2. Pulse					
3. Respiratory rate					
4. Blood pressure					
E. 24-Hour Dry Run					
F. Overnight Pass					
G. Supplemental Oxygen Sources					

INDEX

NOTES

NOTES

NOTES

ISBN 0-07-048266-7

90000

9 780070 482661

OLSON/REHAB NURSING
PROCEDURES MANUAL 2/E